BODY COUNTS

Body Counts

Medical Quantification in Historical and Sociological Perspective /
La quantification medicale, perspectives historiques et sociologiques

EDITED BY
GÉRARD JORLAND, ANNICK OPINEL,
AND GEORGE WEISZ

Published for / publié pour
Fondation merieux

by / par

McGill-Queen's University Press
Montreal & Kingston • London • Ithaca

ISBN 0-7735-2829-6 (cloth)
ISBN 0-7735-2925-X (paper)

Legal deposit second quarter 2005
Bibliothèque nationale du Québec

Printed in Canada on acid-free paper that is 100% ancient forest free (100% post-consumer recycled), processed chlorine free.

McGill-Queen's University Press acknowledges the support of the Canada Council for the Arts for its publishing program. It also acknowledges the financial support of the Government of Canada through the Book Publishing Industry Development Program (BPIDP) for its publishing activities.

Library and Archives Canada Cataloguing in Publication

Body counts : medical quantification in historical and sociological perspective = la quantification médicale, perspectives historiques et sociologiques / edited by Gérard Jorland, Annick Opinel and George Weisz.

Text in English and French.
Proceedings of the symposium La quantification dans les sciences médicales et de la santé: perspective historique, held at Musée Claude-Bernard, in Saint-Julien-en-Beaujolais, France, Oct. 24–26, 2002.
Includes index.
ISBN 0-7735-2829-6 (bound).—ISBN 0-7735-2925-X (pbk.)

1. Medical statistics—History—Congresses. 2. Epidemiology—Statistical methods—History—Congresses. 3. Medical instruments and apparatus—History—Congresses. I. Jorland, Gérard II. Opinel, Annick III. Weisz, George IV. Fondation Marcel-Mérieux V. Title: Quantification médicale, perspectives historiques et sociologiques.

RA407.B62 2005 610'.9 C2004-906136-4E

Catalogage avant publication de Bibliothèque et Archives Canada

Body counts : medical quantification in historical and sociological perspective = la quantification médicale, perspectives historiques et sociologiques / edited by Gérard Jorland, Annick Opinel and George Weisz.

Textes en anglais et en français.
Compte-rendu du symposium La quantification dans les sciences médicales et de la santé: perspective historique, présentée au Musée Claude-Bernard, in Saint-Julien-en-Beaujolais, France, Oct. 24–26, 2002.
Comprend un index.
ISBN 0-7735-2829-6 (relié).—ISBN 0-7735-2925-X (br.)

1. Statistique médicale—Histoire—Congrès. 2. Épidémiologie—Méthodes statistiques—Histoire—Congrès. 3. Médicine—Appareils et instruments—Histoire—Congrès. I. Jorland, Gérard II. Opinel, Annick III. Weisz, George IV. Fondation Marcel-Mérieux V. Titre: Quantification médicale, perspectives historiques et sociologiques.

RA407.B62 2005 610'.9 C2004-906136-4F

Typeset in 10/12 Baskerville by True to Type

Contents

Contributors ix

1 Introduction: Who Counts?
Gérard Jorland and George Weisz 3

PART ONE MEDICAL ARITHMETIC

2 Quantifying Experience and Beating Biases: A New Culture in Eighteenth-Century British Clinical Medicine
Ulrich Tröhler 19

3 When the State Counts Lives: Eighteenth-Century Quarrels over Inoculation
Harry M. Marks 51

4 Quantifying Infant Mortality in England and France, 1750–1800
Andrea Rusnock 65

PART TWO QUANTIFICATION AND INSTRUMENTATION

5 Medical Statistics at the Paris School: What Was at Stake?
Ann F. La Berge 89

6 Standardizing Body Temperature: Quantification in Hospitals and Daily Life, 1850–1900
Volker Hess 109

7 Les multiples usages de la quantification en médecine : Le cas du diabète sucré
Christiane Sinding 127

8 "Measures, Instruments, Methods, and Results": Jozefa Joteyko on Social Reforms and Physiological Measures
Ilana Löwy 145

9 The Production of Biomedical Measures: Three Platforms for Quantifying Cancer Pathology
Peter Keating and Alberto Cambrosio 173

PART THREE STATISTICS AND THE UNDERDETERMINATION OF THEORIES

10 La sous-détermination des théories médicales par les statistiques: le cas Semmelweis
Gérard Jorland 205

11 Epidemiology in Transition: Tobacco and Lung Cancer in the 1950s
Mark Parascandola 226

PART FOUR REDUCING UNCERTAINTY AND THE POLITICS OF HEALTH

12 William Farr and Quantification in Nineteenth-Century English Public Health
Michael Donnelly 251

13 La santé publique et ses instruments de mesure : Des barèmes évaluatifs américains aux indices numériques de la Société des Nations, 1915–1955
Lion Murard 266

14 Statistical Theory Was Not the Reason That Randomization Was Used in the British Medical Research Council's Clinical Trial of Streptomycin for Pulmonary Tuberculosis
Iain Chalmers 309

15 Exigence scientifique et isolement institutionnel : L'essor contrarié de l'épidémiologie française dans la seconde moitié du XXe siècle
Luc Berlivet 335

16 L'infléchissement du travail politique autour des essais contrôlés : L'épidémie de sida à la fin du XXe siècle
Nicolas Dodier 359

PART FIVE AFTERTHOUGHTS

17 From Clinical Counting to Evidence-Based Medicine
George Weisz 377

18 Medical Quantification: Science, Regulation, and the State
Theodore M. Porter 394

Index 403

Contributors

LUC BERLIVET, Centre de Recherche Médecine, Sciences, Santé et Société (INSERM, CNRS, EHESS), Paris

ALBERTO CAMBROSIO, Department of Social Studies of Medicine, McGill University, Montreal

IAIN CHALMERS, Editor, *James Lind Library*, Oxford, England

NICOLAS DODIER, École des hautes études en sciences sociales (EHESS), Paris

MICHAEL DONNELLY, Division of Social Studies, Bard College, Annandale-on-Hudson, NY

VOLKER HESS, Institute for the History of Medicine, Charité-Humboldt University, Berlin

GÉRARD JORLAND, École des hautes études des sciences sociales (CNRS), Paris

PETER KEATING, Department of History, University of Quebec at Montreal

ANN LA BERGE, Program in Science and Technology, Virginia Tech University, Blacksburg, Va.

ILANA LÖWY, Centre de Recherche Médecine, Sciences, Santé et Société (INSERM, CNRS, EHESS), Paris

HARRY M. MARKS, Institute of the History of Medicine, The Johns Hopkins University, Baltimore

LION MURARD, Centre de Recherche Médecine, Sciences, Santé et Société (INSERM, CNRS, EHESS), Paris

ANNICK OPINEL, Centre de recherches historiques, Institut Pasteur, Paris

MARK PARASCANDOLA, National Cancer Institute, Bethesda, Md.

THEODORE M. PORTER, Department of History, University of California at Los Angeles

ANDREA RUSNOCK, Department of History, University of Rhode Island, Kingston, RI

CHRISTIANE SINDING, Centre de Recherche Médecine, Sciences, Santé et Société (INSERM, CNRS, EHESS), Paris

ULRICH TRÖHLER, Institut für Geschichte der Medizin der Albert-Ludwigs-Universität, Freiburg im Breisgau

GEORGE WEISZ, Department of Social Studies of Medicine, McGill University, Montreal

BODY COUNTS

1

Introduction: Who Counts?

GÉRARD JORLAND AND GEORGE WEISZ

This book has its origins in a difference of historical opinion. Several years ago, during a colloquium on therapeutics organized for the Fondation Mérieux by Olivier Faure and Annick Opinel,[1] Gérard Jorland presented a paper on the statistical medicine of the Parisian hospital physician, Dr. P.C.A Louis. In conformity with the existing historiography, GJ viewed Louis's project as a failure and interpreted it as a rejection of quantification in medicine by French doctors of the early nineteenth century. This explanation fit in nicely with our knowledge of the French cultural landscape of the time, characterized by a shift back to the primacy of the literary from that of the scientific and reversing the order that had dominated under Napoleon: the Académie Française regained its place as the pre-eminent of the academies making up the Institut de France; Siméon-Denis Poisson's research on the probability of judgments was criticized at the Academy of Sciences and sank into oblivion, much as A.A. Cournot's research on the mathematical principles of the economy was barely noticed. In this context, the criticisms of Louis's numerical school appeared clearly as an episode in this larger cultural movement.[2]

None the less, another editor of this volume, George Weisz, directed GJ's attention to the fact that academic debates had never ceased to use statistical arguments, even after the controversy of 1837, and he referred to a relevant chapter in his book on the Academy of Medicine[3] where he suggested that received historical opinion on the subject was incorrect. If the debate on quantification has been initiated by the reading of a long paper hostile to the numerical school, a review of the interventions for and against this research program did not permit any judgments about winners and losers in this contest.

GJ and GW continued their discussions in Paris when the former invited the latter to present a number of talks, notably on the subject of medical quantification, at the École des Hautes Études en Sciences Sociales. If the failure of the numerical school could be explained by the methodological problems associated with simple counting and with the inability of the anatomo-pathological method to furnish sufficient numbers of cases for aggregation, it remained to be explained why it took until the Second World War for mathematics to become an effective tool, and not just a rhetorical one, in international medical research. GJ and GW thus decided to organize, under the aegis of the Fondation Mérieux and with the indispensable collaboration of Annick Opinel, a meeting devoted to medical quantification from its beginnings in the eighteenth century to our own day. This took place at the Musée Claude Bernard in Saint-Julien-en-Beaujolais. This volume presents the results of this colloquium.

Numbers of one sort or another now play a central role in all modern societies; they have transformed the way in which we think about and resolve a vast number of issues. While the origins and impact of statistics and quantification generally have been examined by a number of outstanding historians and philosophers of science,[4] their role in medicine has until recently received far less attention. Quantification in eighteenth-century British medicine has been extensively analysed in two recent books.[5] Several major figures who advanced quantification in British public health have received book-length studies, as has, most recently, the seminal figure in late-nineteenth-century statistics, Karl Pearson.[6] There is some work on epidemiological thinking in the early twentieth century,[7] while the rise of clinical trials has been significantly advanced by Harry Marks's major book on the American case, as well as by a number of doctoral theses.[8] There exists one synthetic study of quantification in clinical medicine, which serves as a useful starting point but is seriously incomplete.[9] A recent collection of essays on medical statistics in Britain makes an important distinction between the use of counting in medicine and reliance on sophisticated statistical techniques and points to the decisive role of Karl Pearson in this shift.[10]

The essays in this volume follow on this work (much of it written by contributors to this book) and extend it to new areas. In taking the perspective of the *longue durée*, the volume seeks to bring to the surface the changing nature of quantification in medicine as well as some of the enduring difficulties and tensions inherent in its application. Sociologists of science and of medicine have added considerably to our understanding of the subject, and we have tried to include their perspectives in this volume. We have also taken some pains to invite contributions from authors who work on different countries in order to bring a much-needed comparative dimension to this subject. Finally we seek to move beyond the usual emphasis on either public health or clinical medicine (which have in recent years moved closer together because of their common reliance on the techniques of epidemiology) to include the central role of quantification in laboratory work and many kinds of medical instrumentation.

MEDICAL ARITHMETIC

In the first essay, Ulrich Tröhler shows how British doctors of the eighteenth and early nineteenth centuries created a medical arithmetic on the model of political arithmetic. This was not limited to therapeutics but extended as well to nosology. Therapeutic statistics carried with it the notion of probability of success rather than certainty, a notion that would durably shape therapeutic research. Scurvy was the subject of some of the most sophisticated studies of this sort. These led to rigorous reflection about clinical trials – how to compare things that are in fact comparable – questions which lacked a satisfactory response for a century and a half, as Iain Chalmers shows later in the volume. As for nosology, the two most important categories of the epoch – insanity and fevers – were the primary objects of statistical inquiry.

Tröhler demonstrates further how this medical arithmetic was made possible on one hand by the practice of inoculation, which required quantified follow-up as a means of responding to those who objected to the practice, and on the other hand by the development of hospital registers, which constituted a new source of reliable data. Harry Marks and Andrea Rusnock present case studies focusing on one of these conditions. Tröhler concludes with a question: if the British did so much clinical quantification, what is left of the pioneering role of the Paris school? His answer is: not much. One possible response would be that the key Parisian innovation was to apply arithmetic not just to symptomatology but also to pathological anatomy, understood as the correlation between symptoms and anatomic lesions, in order to create a new kind of statistical medicine.

Harry Marks examines inoculation. He revisits the famous controversy on this subject that pitted Daniel Bernouilli and Jean le Rond d'Alembert and concentrates on its political dimension, largely neglected by historians. While Bernouilli constructed a mathematical model on the basis of tables of mortality in order to quantify the number of lives of every age saved by this practice, and thus adding to the power of the state, d'Alembert followed a completely different strategy. He took the position of the subject who must make a decision whether or not to inoculate his or her child. And he made use of the distinction introduced by Daniel Bernouilli himself between mathematical and moral expectations to differentiate between the point of view of the state and that of the individual subject; in the latter case, he took account of interpersonal differences of attitude when facing risk. This opposition between public and private perspectives would recur throughout the history of medical quantification.

Andrea Rusnock focuses on hospital registers. She shows that quantified representations of infant mortality appeared in eighteenth-century England and France as the first serious public health measure. She describes the move from use of parish registers, necessarily inexact because of the problem of baptisms, for this purpose, to use of hospital registers as a means of establishing mortality estimates that were more rigorous and more dramatic than had been previously imagined and that precipitated sanitary reforms, most notably inoculation. She thus sheds new light on another theme that recurs throughout the history of quantification – its role in the politics of any era. Numbers, in other words, are not just mathematical entities but part of the ordinary language that seeks to understand, convince, and get people to act.

Why did reasoning with numbers become convincing in the eighteenth century and, in the case of England, possibly earlier? New sources of data, we saw are one part of the answer. Another has to do with broad social changes and needs. Both Andrea Rusnock and Phillip Kreager,[11] for instance, have in recent essays discussed a new form of quantitative reasoning that emerged in England near the end of the seventeenth century. The former calls this "Merchant's Logick," and the latter, "mercantile bookkeeping." A new kind of commercialized society was generating new business practices and new forms of reasoning and argumentation. The early and widespread development of commerce in England may well account both for the early emergence of medical quantification in that country and for its continued strength during virtually every period covered in this collection. Both Harry Marks and Ted Porter in this volume call attention to another kind of quantified reasoning, one growing out of the practices of state bureaucracies. This raises interesting questions about the kinds of quantification that each set of social practices produces. And if widespread commercial practices may be especially congruent with certain forms of quantification, one wonders whether administrative quantification may appear, as it did for d'Alembert, as a threat to individual choice and autonomy. Can the indisputable links between state administration and numbers in France explain the exceptional vehemence of anti-quantitative rhetoric in that country in the early nineteenth century and the relatively slow acceptance of such practices as random clinical trials in more recent times?

QUANTIFICATION AND INSTRUMENTATION

Epidemiological modes of reasoning have become so pervasive that we tend to identify medical quantification almost exclusively with them. The essays in this section remind us that quantification is also embedded in a wide range of technologies and instruments and that these are related in subtle but important ways to the development of clinical and public health numbers.

Ann La Berge returns to the famous academic discussion of 1837 about medical quantification in general and to Louis's numerical school in particular. She reminds us that one aspect of this complex controversy pitted the advocates of a medical *science* favourable to quantification against supporters of a medical *art* hostile to numbers on the grounds that they homogenized individual differences. This disagreement was not dissimilar to the inoculation dispute between D'Alembert and Bernouilli, which split those for whom health was a state affair from those for whom it was the responsibility of individuals. But she reinvigorates the interpretation of this discussion by showing that the stakes surrounding quantification were much more profound, involving nothing less than the possibility of objectifying disease as a necessary condition for the introduction of medical technologies – in this case, the microscope.

The microscope, like other visualization technologies, represents one form of objectification that uses instruments to extend the power of the senses to new objects. Debates about their use have characteristically concerned the reliability of representations produced, whether or not they provided information not accessible directly to the senses, and whether they are in any way useful practically. But other instruments involve a more radical transmutation from sensory impressions to something entirely different – namely, numbers or time charts. Volker Hess, in his masterful essay, discusses one of the first instruments that embodied quantification – the thermometer. It was used to diagnose one of the essential, though declining, pathologies of the nineteenth century – fevers – which, in their innumerable forms, constituted a distinct nosological entity. He describes how the thermometer represented a new way to objectify disease. The problems posed by this technique were of the same order as the ones posed by statistics: how to standardize and calibrate categories and measurements so that results across time and space would be stable and comparable and how to integrate into medical practice a technique that involved the adaptation not of the instrument to the individual but, on the contrary, of the individual to the instrument.

Despite this latter constraint, Hess finds that, surprisingly and contrary to the fears of opponents of quantification or emulators of Foucault, the thermometer served as a vector of democratization in medicine in two ways. First, objectivity of measurement freed diagnosis to some degree from the subjectivity of the physician's judgment; second and above all, by taking his or her own temperature, the sick person became the fully responsible subject of his or her malady, an active agent rather than a passive patient. This form of quantification, in other words, rather than imposing the power of the state on the body, in fact allowed subjects to reappropriate their malady. The illness of Jacques is not that of Peter or Pauline, not because the physician had a privileged relationship with each of them based on their idiosyncrasies but because Jacques, Peter, and Pauline were in a position to look after their own state of health.

In a similar manner, Christiane Sinding shows that standardized measures for diabetes preceded the arrival of insulin on the market after the First World War. This allowed for the new drug to be adapted to every individual case. In other words, quantification made possible a new kind of individuation of medicine rather than state dominance or standardized therapy for everyone. Reciprocally, each diabetic became the agent of his or her own therapy, examining urine, calculating food intake, planning meals, and doing physical exercise. In addition to all this, insulin was an extraordinarily effective medication.

Ilana Löwy presents us with a much less successful case of innovation, that of a Polish scientist, Jozefa Joteyko, who attempted to transform pedagogy into a rigorous science, pedology, based on an instrumental and quantitative physiology. This effort, like her earlier research in fatigue studies, represented an effort to use quantified scientific methods in order to promote social reform. Joteyko was largely unsuccessful, in part because of her marginal status in the scientific world and in part because of the contradictions inherent in her scientific program.

Finally, in their discussion of cancer research, Peter Keating and Alberto Cambrosio introduce a valuable distinction between quantification of pathology and quantification in pathology. The quantification of pathology does not reduce the pathological to the normal but rather "aligns" them and puts each on the same ontological plane while giving them the same epistemological status. Quantification in pathology is identified with instrumentation, which the authors study at three levels: morphology, immuno-phenotyping, and molecular genetics. They then show that objectification reaches its culminating point in the automation of testing on cells, which eliminates all traces of subjectivity. Biological instrumentation thus represents the end or at least the transformation of classical clinical medicine. The authors highlight another aspect of this history: in becoming exact, medicine brings into being the fundamental science, which it uses to advance. Consequently, the quantification of medicine appears at the same time as the biologization of medicine.

STATISTICS AND THE UNDERDETERMINATION OF THEORIES

Medical statistics were thus part of a general movement of instrumentation in medicine. But they constituted a very particular sort of instrument. When confronted with unpleasant results, one might "shoot the messenger" (or, as the French say, break the thermometer in order to put an end to the fever), instead of dealing seriously with the problem. Both essays in this section analyse debates about disease causation – nearly a century apart – in order to understand some of the limits of statistical reasoning in medicine at different times.

Gérard Jorland examines the discussion of puerperal fever in the Paris Academy of Medicine in 1858. Even though Semmelweis's argument and statistical data were well known, other statistical data produced before and after supported his conclusions, and special Parisian statistics were compiled for the purposes of the discussion, all these data proved incapable of producing belief in the infectious origins of this malady. Jorland argues that ontological realism (the belief that there must be an observable agent of disease), together with the underdetermination of theories by statistical observation (meaning that several interpretations of the evidence seemed equally plausible), blinded the leaders of Parisian medicine to the existing evidence.

This attitude was hardly unique. Medicine has had a strong penchant towards ontological realism – the belief that there must be a causal agent for any disease, whether an anatomical lesion or a physiological inflammation, a miasma propagated through the air or a microbe carried by water. A physician must see the cause in order to believe in the pathology. At the other end of the spectrum, statistics, being mathematics, is nominalistic. The only thing that it can say is that whenever you see a set of events, most of the time you also observe another set of events. Why? It cannot say. How? It cannot say. It cannot say even that it is always the case. Therefore the realism of medicine is at odds with the nominalism of statistics. And, correlatively, medical micro-determinism is at odds with statistical macro-determinism.

Mark Parascandola shows in a similar manner that a century later the statistical correlations between smoking and cancer were open to multiple interpretations, that they notably did not exclude the possibility that there existed a common cause for both variables; consequently, quantitative evidence did not convince many epidemiologists that a causal link existed. While Parascandola emphasizes the divisions inherent in a newly emerging discipline, it is possible here too to see epidemiologists' medical realism blocking their acceptance of quantitative data. To put it another way, epistemological underdeterminism was superimposed on opposition between ontological realism and nominalism. None the less, by the mid-twentieth century statistical thinking had advanced sufficiently so that uncertainty no longer led epidemiologists and doctors to reject statistical reasoning outright; they insisted instead that causal relations between tobacco and cancer be unambiguously established. Parascandola describes in detail how the techniques of statistical research were mobilized for this purpose

REDUCING UNCERTAINTY AND THE POLITICS OF HEALTH

The uncertainty associated with statistical reasoning has been lessened over time by the development of certain conceptual tools. Some of these have been mathematically based, like standard deviation and the chi-square test introduced by Karl Pearson; but others seem to have emerged from practical medicine and public health. (We shall see that the origins are sometimes contested.) The development of such tools has created a powerful set of techniques around which epidemiology has crystallized. In recent years, epidemiological techniques have become so central to the practices of health-care systems that they have become targets for pressure groups of various sorts that seek to shape the way in which they are conducted and used by experts and governments.

The first of the innovations to be discussed is that of William Farr, in many respects the most important medical hygienist of the nineteenth century. It was he who extended medical quantification as an instrument of fundamental research beyond therapy and aetiology to the domain of public health. His definition of zymotic maladies, though borrowed from the chemist Liebig, was designed to bring together all diseases susceptible to action by public authorities. Because he used this category to provide indices of public salubrity, replacing the more traditional reliance on life-span, he introduced the concept of "avoidable disease" and in effect founded contemporary epidemiology.

Lion Murard describes the appearance in the United States during the 1920s of a new indicator of public health, the Appraisal Form for Community Health Work, which local administrations could use. He also describes how these indicators were adopted by the League of Nations, under the rubric "Life, Environment and Health Indices," to measure the efficacy of public sanitary services. Conceived by Charles V. Chapin, superintendent of health of Rhode Island, and implemented by Charles Edward Winslow, head of the Department of Public Health at Yale University, these indicators were drawn from the tables of fire insurance companies. In fact, Winslow was also president of the the Committee on Administrative Practice financed by the Metropolitan Life Insurance Company. It was one of Winslow's protégés, Isidore Falk, who introduced these indices to the League of Nations, as a means of comparing the sanitary performance of its member states vis-à-vis one another and vis-à-vis the United States.

In his illuminating essay, Iain Chalmers describes how, 150 years after the appearance of medical statistics, one of the chief problems faced by early medical quantifiers – comparing the comparable – was resolved. The clinical testing of streptomycin for the treatment of pulmonary tuberculosis by the Medical Research Council in Britain after the Second World War, provided the occasion for serious reflection about ways to eliminate bias of all sorts. The techniques that were adopted were elaborated by Austin Bradford Hill. Chalmers shows how these techniques were designed to resolve two problems. The first was how to randomly distribute patients into one of two comparison groups; the choice was between alternation or some version of rolling the dice. The second involved ways of eliminating all possibility that doctors, patients, or anyone else involved in the study might gain knowledge of this patient distribution. These clinical trials have remained paradigmatic for the way in which Bradford Hill was able not only to resolve these problems but also to conceptualize his solutions. In telling his story, Chalmers takes issue with the current interpretation of the origins of clinical trials that argues that the work of statisticians such as R.A. Fisher, who theorized the role of randomization in purely statistical terms, was determinant in the acceptance of this practice. Chalmers in contrast uncovers a long-standing tradition within medicine of distributing subjects through alternation which shifted easily into randomization. This practice, he thus argues, was not based on purely statistical considerations but rather on the practical experience of physicians who had learned that knowing who was taking what medicine inevitably affected outcomes and biased results.

The development of new techniques has led to new disciplinary communities. In the case of quantification, the most visible has been epidemiologists, who emerged from the public health domain to play a significant role in clinical testing as well. Mark Parascandola's essay discussed above introduces us to the fragmented community of American epidemiologists in the mid-twentieth century. Luc Berlivet examines the professionalization of French epidemiologists after the Second World War. He describes their integration into the various loci of medical knowledge: schools of public health, medical faculties, research institutes, and the public health administration. He shows that the major impetus for this integration in France was provided by statisticians – in this case, graduates of the elite engineering school, the Ecole Polytechnique, who exported their expertise to a medical domain that was rather doubtful about its value. One consequence was the separation between scientific research and health policy, reproducing the traditional opposition between the "fundamental" and the "applied." It required doctors' entry into this domain, under the banner of Charles Mérieux and his foundation, for French epidemiology to become a multidisciplinary science and thus an effective instrument for aiding political decision-making. Berlivet shows as well that because the mathematization of medicine in France was due to forces external to medicine, quantification did not take hold of medicine in the way that it did of physics or economics. Epidemiology has thus remained to some degree at the margins of French medicine.

The gradual reduction of uncertainty and spread of epidemiological thinking to public policy did not eliminate all old problems and has in fact created quite a few new ones. Resolving an issue with statistics has turned out to be a lengthy and very expensive process. Frequently, decisions have to be made quickly on the basis of indeterminate data. Some can be put off until sufficient data accumulate, as happened with the tobacco–cancer link. But frequently either the immediacy of risk or promise of benefits leads to early decisions. The medical literature is full of issues that have yet to be resolved but that demand immediate action and of new data that call into question practices introduced on the basis of then-available evidence. In these numerous situations of uncertainty, whether one errs on the side of caution or not, whether one chooses to act or not, depends frequently on the balance of power among the groups involved. For one of the most striking things about the growing dominance of statistical thinking in the health-care sphere is the number of actors who are now involved in the process of statistical decision-making.

Nicolas Dodier illustrates this phenomenon vividly in his examination of AIDS in France. He shows how various people sought to shape clinical trials. These actors included doctors, of course, pharmaceutical laboratories, and – a relatively new phenomenon – the patients themselves. Patients' associations acted in effect as pressure groups. Dodier describes in detail how AIDS patients, transformed into militants for a cause, came to negotiate the protocols of trials, including the number of patients enrolled, criteria of inclusion, and the length of trials. In other words, far from representing a means of controlling bodies, medical statistics in this case objectified the illness and thereby called into question medical authority; this allowed AIDS sufferers to move from the status of patient to that of agent, from objects of the medical gaze to the subjects of their own illnesses. Once again, the fears of Risueno d'Amador and others to the effect that numbers would subjugate the individual were, at least in this case, not realized.

AFTERTHOUGHTS

Two final papers take a longer and more synthetic view of the history of quantification in medicine. George Weisz compares some of the main themes of debate about medical statistics in the nineteenth century with those that have accompanied the explosive appearance during the past decade of "evidence-based medicine." To some degree, the latter reflects the same urge to objectify knowledge through numbers, protocols, and instrumentation that animated nineteenth-century reformers. Consequently many of the objections sound very similar, having to do with the ability of instruments such as random clinical trials to deliver the certainty that they promise and with the apparent contradiction involved in applying knowledge relating to populations to unique individuals. As in the nineteenth century, numbers provoke fear that skills and power are being displaced from practitioners to mechanical procedures and small groups of experts. But, unlike the statistical medicine of the nineteenth century, "evidence-based medicine" (EBM) exists in an extraordinarily complex institutional environment. It has been claimed by many different groups with wildly different agendas, so that it is coming to serve as a slogan for a wide variety of sometimes-opposing interests: defending the medical profession and limiting the power of the medical profession, spending more and better on health care and saving money by paying less. Whatever its strengths and defects as a scientific program, EBM is emerging as a powerful ideological weapon in the battle to shape health care in North America and Europe.

In the final essay, Theodore M. Porter pulls together many of the themes of this collective volume. Statistics, he suggests, were initially part of a public medicine that existed alongside private medicine. This distinction between public and private partially overlapped the oppositions between medicine as a science and medicine as an art, as the processing of information versus the interpretation of signs. In addition to two institutions that made quantification both possible and necessary – the hospital and the laboratory – Porter emphasizes the role of a third institution going back to the inoculation debates, and no less efficacious, though not always as visible – the insurance company. In other words, quantification is implicated in bridging not just the opposition between public and private spheres but also the division between private enterprise and private life, with the former exercising increasing surveillance over the latter.

In fact there is little about modern life that has not in some way been deeply touched by the ever-growing influence of numbers. In medicine, this influence has become particularly striking. What medicines we take and our health status generally are frequently determined by numbers of one sort or another. The role of quantification is so ubiquitous that we have to remind ourselves that this has not always been the case. Medical statistics as a form of objectivity has had a relatively short history. The essays in this volume are meant to help us recover that history and better understand its current status.

NOTES

1 The proceedings appeared in Olivier Faure, ed., *Les thérapeutiques: savoirs et usages* (Lyon: Collections Fondation Mérieux, 1999).

2 Gérard Jorland, "La médecine statistique du docteur Louis," in ibid., 123–34.

3 George Weisz, *The Medical Mandarins: The French Academy of Medicine in the 19th and Early 20th Centuries* (Oxford: Oxford University Press, 1995), 159–88.

4 Some of the many works on the history of statistics are *Journées d'étude sur l'histoire de la statistique* (France: Vaucresson, 1976); *Pour une histoire de la statistique* (Paris: INSEE, 1977); Stephen Stigler, *The History of Statistics. The Measurement of Uncertainty before 1900* (Cambridge, Mass.: Harvard University Press, 1986); Theodore M. Porter, *The Rise of Statistical Thinking 1820–1900* (Princeton, NJ: Princeton University Press, 1986); Ian Hacking, *The Taming of Chance* (Cambridge: Cambridge University Press, 1990); Alain Desrosières, *La politique des grands nombres: histoire de la raison statistique* (Paris: La Découverte, 1993).

5 U. Tröhler, *To Improve the Evidence of Medicine: The 18th Century British Origins of a Critical Approach* (Edinburgh: Royal College of Physicians, 2000); Andrea A. Rusnock, *Vital Accounts: Quantifying Health and Population in Eighteenth-Century England and France* (Cambridge: Cambridge University Press, 2002).

6 John M. Eyler, *Victorian Social Medicine: The Ideas and Methods of William Farr* (Baltimore, Md.: Johns Hopkins University Press, 1979; and *Sir Arthur Newsholme and State Medicine, 1885–1935* (Cambridge: Cambridge University Press, 1997); Theodore Porter, *Karl Pearson: The Scientific Life in a Statistical Age* (Princeton, NJ: Princeton University Press, 2004).

7 Steven. Kunitz, "Explanations and Ideologies of Mortality Patterns," *Population and Development Revue* 13 (1987), 379–408; J. Andrew Mendelsohn, "From Eradication to Equilibrium: How Epidemics Became Complex after World War I," in Chris Lawrence and George Weisz, eds., *Greater than the Parts: Holism in Biomedicine 1920–1950* (Oxford: Oxford University Press, 1998); Mark Parascandola, "Uncertain Science and a Failure of Trust: The NIH Radioepidemiologic Tables and Compensation for Radiation-Induced Cancer," *Isis* 93 (2002), 558–84; Harry M. Marks, "Epidemiologists Explain Pellagra: Gender, Race, and Political Economy in the Work of Edgar Sydenstricker," *Journal of the History of Medicine and Allied Sciences* 58 (2003), 34–55.

8 Harry M. Marks, *The Progress of Experiment: Science and Therapeutic Reform in the United States, 1900–1990* (Cambridge: Cambridge University Press, 1997); Marcia Lynn Meldrum, "'Departures from the Design': The Randomized Clinical Trial in Historical Context, 1946–1970," PhD thesis, State University of New York at Stony Brook, 1994; Desirée Cox-Maksimov, "The Making of the Clinical Trial in Britain, 1910–1945," PhD thesis, Cambridge University, 1997; B. Toth, "Clinical Trials in British Medicine 1858–1948, with Special Reference to the Development of the Randomised Controlled Trial," PhD thesis, University of Bristol, 1998.

9 J. Rosser Matthews, *Quantification and the Quest for Medical Certainty* (Princeton, NJ: Princeton University Press, 1995).

10 Eileen Magnello and Anne Hardy, eds., *The Road to Medical Statistics* (Amsterdam: Rodopi, 2002).

11 Philip Kreager, "Death and Method: The Rhetorical Space of Seventeenth-Century Vital Measurement," in Eileen Magnello and Anne Hardy, eds., *The Road to Medical Statistics* (Amsterdam: Rodopi, 2002), 1–36; Andrea Rusnock, "'The Merchant's Logic': Numerical Debates over Smallpox Inoculation in Eighteenth-Century England," in ibid., 37–54.

PART ONE

Medical Arithmetic

2

Quantifying Experience and Beating Biases: A New Culture in Eighteenth-Century British Clinical Medicine

ULRICH TRÖHLER

The last half of the eighteenth century transformed aspects of British medicine. Several practitioners built on the earlier clinical research methods of Francis Clifton (see part I), and the emergent empiricism of these marginal physicians challenged the traditional rationalist approach to medicine (part II). An empirical approach began to transform therapeutics and nosography (part III), culminating in the medical arithmetic of William Black (part IV). The result was a new culture of knowledge-making within British clinical medicine (conclusion).[1]

CLINICAL RESEARCH: CLIFTON AND HIS SUCCESSORS

A Program for Clinical Research from the 1730s

Some eighteenth-century British doctors openly admitted doubts and ignorance about the diagnosis and treatment of disease. Francis Clifton's book *Tabular Observations Recommended as the Plainest and Surest Way of Practicing and Improving Physicks* (1731) is especially noteworthy in this respect. Clifton (who died in 1736) emphasized the unreliability of memory as a basis for the evaluation of experience and the necessity; he therefore advocated regular and frank recording of all cases, compiling the data in tables, and emphasized periodic analysis and publication. A hospital so run would correspond to Solomon's House, the research institute envisaged by Francis Bacon (1561–1626) in his

New Atlantis (1627). Bacon had intended that compilers and abstractors (statisticians?) would condense such information into "Titles and Tables to give the better light for the drawing of Observations and Axioms out of them." Clifton concluded that he would never "write upon any subject, as a Physician, for which I have not Tabular Authority."[2]

A year later, in a historico-critical work entitled *The State of Physick, Ancient and Modern,* Clifton proposed a "*plan*" for "*improving* Physick and making it more useful in our days, than ever it was before ... by cultivating the business of *Observation* in the best manner it is capable of." This meant inquiring into the natural course of diseases in contemporary England, rather than in ancient Greece, in order to properly evaluate the effects of medicine. By distinguishing "plainly ... what is done by *Nature,* and what by *Art,*" doctors would become able to "prescribe with more honour to ourselves, and more advantage to the Patient." Indeed, anatomical and even chemical observation had "surveyed" the body "inch by inch," examined the fluids "by all ways that coud be thought of," and led to many discoveries. However, "what may be done hereafter by these discoveries is another question."[3]

So far there were still an insufficient "number of *facts* together ... to ground a good system upon." There were but "Theories in abundance ... Almost every physician has had a system of his own, ... and this seems the reason, why so many unaccountable things have been said and unsaid by physicians of every nation in Europe." In this situation the "matters really important, for the Patient, whatever it may be for the Physician" had hitherto stemmed "not from any *Theory,* or philosophical speculation, but from regular and judicious experiments, made ... by weight and measure" on the effect of medical interventions.[4]

Clifton knew that some of these ideas were not new. Besides referring to Bacon, he also quoted the papal physician, Giorgio Baglivi (1668–1707), criticizing him for not having adhered to his principles in actual practice. For implementation of his plan, regular clinical recordings in systematic order were essential. Thus Clifton proposed, as practical aids, tables containing one column each for sex, age, temperament, occupation, and cause of disease; two columns for daily entries of the symptoms; and one column each for the calendar dates on which the remedies were used and the event occurred. In this way even the busy practitioner could contribute to the observational sciences. He further suggested the use of abbreviations of Latin and Greek terms because of their conciseness and precision, "for to do a thing of this kind by halves, is much the same with not doing it at all."[5]

In his 1732 book, Clifton specified his practical recommendations in particular for hospitals, where "three or four persons of proper qualifications should be employed ... to set down the cases of the patients there from day to day, candidly and judiciously, without any regard to private opinions or publick systems, and at the year's end publish these facts just as they are, leaving every one to make the best uses of 'em he can for himself."

If such a program were put into effect, diseases would be better understood and more easily cured, even if the *materia medica* were not to improve. Clifton asserted, however, that if the latter were reformed and put on an observational footing, "everything would then be done, that the *Art* is capable of."[6]

Although Clifton did not explicitly mention quantification in the sense of numerical assessment, his principles and practical guidelines set an indispensable stage for the application of quantification in evaluating therapy, as well as for describing and distinguishing among diseases. He pointed to the necessity of a sufficient number of authentic "facts" and of regularly abstracting the complete records over a given period of time. Therapy should be based, for the good of the patients, on outcome assessment, rather than on recommendations 'rationally' derived from pathophysiological systems and/or from "laboratory" generated data. For it was the result from the patient's – rather than from the doctor's – point of view that really mattered in medicine!

Did Clifton's constructive criticism of medicine, with his prioritization of empirical experience over rationalist theories, have any direct influence on his contemporaries? His historical book containing a "plan for improving Physick" appeared in French in 1742, and Jean Colombier (1736–1789),the reformer of French military medicine under the *ancien régime,* referred to it in his own similar program of 1772.[7] And in Britain the same principles and guidelines were still being emphasized a hundred years later.[8] In 1784 a method of concise recording in Latin appeared in a London periodical, and in 1793 the London physician George Fordyce (1736–1802) again proposed tables for collecting group data and as a basis for their evaluation. Was this a sign of success or rather failure?[9]

In this chapter, I explore this question with respect to both therapeutics and nosography. Using printed sources prepared by private and hospital practitioners, in civilian as well as military and naval medicine, I argue that Fordyce's *Attempt to Improve the Evidence of Medicine* (1793) epitomizes a hitherto-largely-unacknowledged movement among British doctors.

From "Ordinary" to "Ordered" Experience

Let us first consider, in Clifton's spirit, the epistemic basis that led to the introduction of digitalis – one of these outstanding contributions to the *materia medica* to which Clifton had been looking forward – some 50 years after his book appeared.

William Withering (1741–1799) wrote *Account of the Foxglove and some of its Medical Uses with Practical Remarks on Dropsy and Other Diseases* (1785), highly valued by contemporaries and now a medico-historical "classic."[10] Born in the Midlands, Withering studied medicine in Edinburgh and then settled in Stafford in 1767. Having little to do in his practice at first, he occupied himself with botanical studies, eventually becoming a celebrated botanist. He also kept a climatological journal. In 1772 he became physician to a hospital in Stafford. Three years later he moved to Birmingham where he became physician to the General Hospital when it opened in 1778.

An old countrywoman had recommended foxglove to Withering as "her" remedy against "dropsy" (oedema). He obviously believed her, but not uncritically: he undertook a prospective case series, collecting data for 15 years before he published his findings.

Withering based his systematic assessment of the foxglove's effects on dropsy almost entirely on patients whom he saw in private practice. Of the 163 cases that he had gathered by 1785, only seven had come from the Birmingham Hospital. He introduced the description of his cases as follows: "It would have been an easy task to have given select cases, whose successful treatment would have spoken strongly in favour of the medicine, and perhaps been flattering to my own reputation. But Truth and Science would condemn the procedure. I have therefore mentioned every case … proper or improper, successful or otherwise."[11]

Withering had thus lived up fully to Clifton's injunctions and had stepped conceptually even further, since his was a prospective study of unselected cases, thus avoiding what we would deem today to be a form of "selection bias." He also included a few numerical statements when analysing cases reported by one of his colleagues separately from his own. Withering relied on available clinical methods: close observation of the patient, assisted by quantification – counting the pulse and measuring the urinary output – as an objective check of subjective improvement.

He compared these parameters with the patients' previous condition and sometimes observed relapses on discontinuing the drug. He was reluctant to draw conclusions from such an objective inquiry: "No general deductions decisive upon the failure or success of the medicine, can be drawn from the cases I now present ... [for they] must be considered as the most hopeless deplorable that exist ... lost to the common run of practice."[12]

And he also implied a comparison with the natural incidence of death among such patients (he spoke of "cases"). Withering defended his decision to limit his descriptions to his own observations. He admitted that people might doubt the impartiality of his account but reasoned that, had he reported the cases sent to him by fellow physicians, his book would have been only seemingly free from pre-selection. In fact he worried that the critics "would ... close the book, with much higher notions of the efficacy of the plant than what they would have learnt from me ... [for] the cases [I have received] are, with some exceptions much too selected."[13] Withering thus dismissed the common practice of increasing the number of observations by adding the selected experiences of others, which would be misleading if the latter did not give all the details of their entire practice, successes and failures alike.

Withering's *Account of the Foxglove* aroused widespread interest and reaction. In terms of nosography, his approach may help explain his success in deciding which types of dropsy patients would benefit from digitalis. This differentiation was all the more remarkable as virtually nothing was known then about the pathology of different kinds of oedema. Among those who pursued research on the new drug was his acquaintance John Ferriar (1761–1815). Working at the Manchester Infirmary, opened in 1752, Ferriar initiated clinical research there. As he wrote in 1792, it was work in public hospitals that afforded "the most favourable opportunities for ascertaining with precision many facts in the history of diseases and for appreciating the value of established methods of cure ... Something may be added to the stock of science, by unwearied attention to a considerable number of patients, indiscriminately taken in a great town.[14]

Ferriar emphasized that the method "so fashionable at present of publishing single cases, appears not well calculated to enlarge our knowledge, either of the nature or cure of diseases." Indeed, however faithfully recorded and analysed a single success might be, and although the best writers since Bacon had recommended minute descriptions, these provided an insecure basis for practice. Ferriar maintained that serial observations (resulting from experiments, clinical cases, and autopsies) would become reliable only if practitioners wrote them down in a journal, regularly updated them, and included both favourable and unfavourable outcomes of a treatment. This was "absolutely necessary" if the physician wanted to avoid those false conclusions that he would obtain "if he trust[ed] to memory alone" and to "do justice to his patients." Furthermore, he had to compare such data with those of other physicians.[15]

Ferriar believed that medical writers had tended to establish theoretical (pathogenic–pathophysiological) systems embracing dogmas, and he suggested that "these gentlemen ... would do well to read Mr [John] Locke's chapters on abuse of language. A system ought to be nothing more than the arrangement of [empirical] facts, in convenient order for the memory."[16] He acknowledged his obligations to Francis Home, a former military surgeon who was then professor of materia medica at the University of Edinburgh and one of the physicians at the Edinburgh Infirmary.

Emphasizing the same points as Clifton had done sixty years earlier (without mentioning him) was one thing, but applying them was another. Ferriar did both. On the treatment of dropsy, he wrote: "I do not remember, to have seen any comparison instituted among the various methods of reducing the swelling by increasing the quantity of urine in this disorder."[17] Accordingly he presented 47 patients: 24 treated with digitalis, 10 with cream of tartar, 8 with calomel, and the others with various remedies. He presented a table with both the overall results and data relating to the four categories of "dropsy" (anasarca, ascites, hydrothorax, and combined cases), showing the numbers of patients 'cured,' 'relieved,' 'not relieved,' and 'dead.' He concluded that digitalis was the most favourable agent in general, and that cream of tartar represented the best treatment for hydrothorax (admittedly, based on only four cases).[18]

Ferriar pursued his research on dropsy well into the nineteenth century. He reported his cumulated experience in the second volume of his *Medical Histories* (1795) and published an *Essay on the Medical Properties of the Digitalis Purpurea* (1799), which recommended the use of digitalis combined with cream of tartar. In 1813, he reported on "Extract of Elaterium" – a new remedy for "dropsy." He had treated 20 selected "desperate cases" with a "nearly uniform successful" result, but noted that the observation was insecure because he had used another active diuretic along with it![19]

The case of "dropsy" illustrates some of the criteria involved in moving from Bacon's "ordinary experience," based on more or less fortuitous observation and therefore largely subjective, towards his "ordered experience," built on planned questioning and observation in a pre-established, measurable criteria and aiming at objectivity.

RATIONALISM VERSUS EMPIRICISM

Rational Deduction and Empirical Induction

As Clifton, Withering, Ferriar, and many others had done, contemporaries distinguished between two approaches to therapeutics – rationalism and empiricism – a distinction (and debate) that date back to Plato and Aristotle. The starting point for both therapeutic approaches is the patient's symptomatology. The rationalist physician explains it within a framework of pathogenic and pathophysiological theory, whence he deduces, by good argument, his therapy, which does not need testing, since his main question is theoretical: "Can this therapy work at all?" The pure empiricist physician tries out a therapy, regardless of theoretical considerations, "by guess," so to speak, and his chief question is practical: "Will this therapy work?" Trial and error, "experience" with feedback, based on the assessment of one's own observations, are therefore essential to this approach.

While an epistemic change from overwhelmingly rationalistic to empirical methods began in the natural sciences in the sixteenth century, this was by no means the case in therapeutics, as the above plans to improve medicine illustrate. Rationalism spoke of "certain" knowledge, in contrast to the "probable" results of empiricism. Certain knowledge grounded itself in ancient wisdom, if possible accorded with divine revelation, and applied scholastic–deductive logic. Probable results came from experience and experiment, according to Baconian, inductive logic. In therapeutics, the power of the traditional rationalistic concepts of "science" and "learning" – or mere routine – were understandably strong.[20] Patients might view diseases as a stroke of fate, a manifestation of God's will. The empirical approach of "trial and error" belonged to surgeons and mountebanks belonging to the lower social strata, who boasted publicly of their successes. A gentleman physician would not countenance such behavior – and indeed need not do so, since class-ridden contemporary society separated his competence from the down-to-earth consequences of his actions;[21] as a learned man, he "knew" valuable things, but also things unaccounted for in practice and wrong, as some contemporaries began to realize. How was one to judge among all these elements? The methodological recommendations of Clifton, Withering and Ferriar rejected rationalism but also hinted at some shortcomings of, and confusions arising from, traditional empiricism.

Shortcomings of Traditional Empiricism

As we have seen, some doctors realized that clinical observation was often subjective and prejudiced: haphazardly recorded, vaguely described, and small in number. Assessment of these observations was often non-existent or meaningless: based on incompletely recorded and/or selective data, it was one-sided and presented in vague terms to suit the author's own ends. Taken together, these fallacies led to "distorted truth." Individuals such as Clifton, Withering, and Ferriar strove for recognition of these fallacies and for action to "scientize" empiricism, to make it "rational." Their aim therefore was a new, methodologically guided, "rational" empiricism,[22] involving both the collection of observations and their assessment.

If records were incomplete and uncertified, they could not ground this type of "scientific" assessment. If possible, data had to be comparative, fair, and presented numerically, precisely, and intelligibly, as in commerce. One of the promoters of this method, John Millar (1733–1805), the Scottish physician of the Westminster General Dispensary in London, wrote in 1783: "detached cases, however numerous and well attested are insufficient to support general conclusions; but by recording every case in a public and extensive practice, and comparing the success of various methods of cure with the unassisted efforts of nature some useful information may be obtained; and the dignity of the profession may be vindicated from vague declaration and groundless aspersions."

Medicine thus needed demonstrations by "incontestable evidence," and Millar justified subsequent actions to take: "Error ought not to be sanctified by custom ... nor concealed by mystery and reserve; nor the test of arithmetical calculation evaded."[23]

Such a program demanded some organizational skills for producing and arranging this new type of (group) data and for handling them mathematically, i.e., new capabilities for doctors. As if he had read Clifton, Millar appointed to that end a clerk, Thomas Reide, who concluded 10 years later: "How ridiculous would it appear [for a merchant] to judge of the advantages or disadvantages of particular branches of commerce from reasoning and conjecture, whilst the result can be reduced to certainty by keeping regular accounts, and balancing them at stated periods."[24] His employer offered an analogy: "Where Mathematical Reasoning can be had, it is a great folly to make use of any other, as to grope for a thing in the dark, when you have a candle standing by you."[25]

There were networks of doctors in eighteenth-century Britain, chiefly army and navy surgeons and individuals working in new voluntary hospitals and dispensaries, pursuing these goals: be aware of prejudices and of the play of chance. Prejudice could diminish with comparison, measurement, quantitative description, and systematic, comprehensive recording. The play of chance could diminish with more observations and with the new facilities of the voluntary hospitals, as well as of the armed forces. Both institutions required feedback and reports, which could serve scientific as well as administrative purposes. As for the data, numerical analysis would be the best and most fully transparent way to achieve results "without any regard to private opinions," to paraphrase Clifton.[26]

APPLYING EMPIRICISM

Concepts for Improving Therapeutic Observations

Comparing a treatment with the natural course of disease and/or other treatment(s) – as did James Lind (1716–1794) in his prospective controlled trial of several remedies for scurvy in 1747 – addressed the inferential problems posed by basing conclusions about the effects of therapy on uncontrolled case series.[27] However, for a variety of reasons, Lind's recommendations for preventing and treating scurvy, with fresh oranges and lemons, had little impact on medical opinion in Britain, particularly on naval authorities.[28]

This situation changed when extensive data from the ships engaged in the American War of Independence (1775–1783) showed the high number of victims from scurvy despite the official policy for its prevention, which recommended sauerkraut, an infusion of malt, and vegetable soup. For the first time tables including the results of different treatments for scurvy were compiled and published. Robert Robertson (1742–1829), a Scottish naval surgeon, initiated this practice in 1760. He had kept a journal while serving as a surgeon in the Greenland whale fishery, and he continued keeping daily records during his entire tenure afloat until 1783. But more than that, he continually summarized his records in "pathological and comparative tables to show the efficacy of different modes of practice."[29] As he served in Africa, the West Indies, North America, and the Channel Fleet, good accounts of naval medicine during the American war became available from these theatres. Also, Gilbert Blane (1747–1834), who became physician to the West Indies Fleet in 1780, wrote *Observations on the Diseases Incident to Seamen,* which appeared in 1785 and was reissued in 1789 and 1799.

These books illustrated not only their authors' passion for statistics, but also their ability to draw succinct conclusions from the elaborate tables that they compiled. The new "arithmetical" clinicians sought to reduce not only "reporting bias" (in our modern terminology), but also the play of chance by increasing the observational basis (as Withering had done by allowing for time).

Other ideas aimed to systematize the assessment of such data and the presentation of results. The trust in written rather than memory-based data corresponded to the avoidance of what we term "recall bias." The quest was to compare like with like, taking account of the patients' age and sex and/or the environmental conditions in retrospective analysis and prospective studies. Comparisons had to be fair to be meaningful – a notion also inherent in the planning of prospective trials,[30] which would also minimize "allocation bias." Analysis dealt with complete records, including both successful and unsuccessful "cases," as patients came more and more to be called in this numerical culture. Numbers – success-to-failure ratios, for instance – offered a means of presenting clear evidence. As the Scot John Clark (1744–1805), a former surgeon on ships of the East India Company, wrote about his practice at a dispensary at Newcastle-upon-Tyne: "in order to determine its success from the result of general practice, it will be proper to give an account of the proportional number of patients who recovered, to those who died."[31]

All this effort intended, in James Lind's words, to "increase the certainty" of medicine. Obviously this term was incorrect, since what he meant was "increased probability." These authors were less familiar with the probability inherent in this new statistical culture than with the certainty of traditional deductive science. James Lind, for instance, conducted many therapeutic trials while physician–in-chief of Haslar Naval Hospital. He concluded in the third edition of his *Treatise of the Scurvy* (1772), "A work, indeed, more perfect, and remedies more absolutely certain might perhaps have been expected from an inspection of several thousand scorbutic patients, from a perusal of every book published on the subject, and from an extensive correspondence with most parts of the world ... but, though a few partial facts and observations may for a little, flatter with hopes of greater success, yet more enlarged experience must ever evidence the fallacy of all positive assertions in the healing art."[32]

At the same time in Edinburgh, the professor of medicine, John Gregory (1724–1773), explaining to his students the "causes that have retarded the advancement of the [medical] sciences," insisted that progress, as well as the "successful management of business in private life ... requires only an attention to probabilities ..., a quick discernment, where the greatest probability of success lies, and habits of acting, in consequence of this, with facility and vigour."[33]

But elaborating concepts and programs and putting them into practice are not the same thing! A few examples show that the new concepts *were* in fact applied.

Applying and Developing the New Concepts in Therapeutics

About 1800, experimental – that is, planned, prospective – studies were designed, implemented, and reported in surgery, internal medicine, and obstetrics. These compared, for example, the effects of immediate and deferred treatments, surgical and medical treatments, and different drugs. These studies employed either concurrent controls or successive periods of comparison, sometimes with efforts to match the comparison groups. Some masked observers, and there is at least one example of placebo treatment. At the height of their activities, about 1780, the pioneers stressed the novelty of these methods and the adoption of medical arithmetic. After 1800, their methods were more or less standard, albeit not always in their entirety, within civilian and military medicine.[34]

Efforts to diminish the play of chance, to minimize various types of bias in the design and assessment of therapeutic trials in medicine and surgery, and to apply "proto-statistical" quantification in the form of simple arithmetical calculations gradually reduced single-case reporting and encouraged the publication of ever-larger case series (see Figure 1).[35]

The treatment of bladder stones in the eighteenth and early nineteenth centuries affords a clear example. Since antiquity, surgical therapy had rested on two techniques reported in the Renaissance: incision of the bladder through the prostate or a supra-pubic approach – applied by self-trained, wandering "stone-cutters." "New" practices of the seventeenth and eighteenth centuries evolved from these two methods, particularly in France and England. In London the surgeon-anatomist William Cheselden (1666–1752), after various trials, adopted and developed the operation of "lateral" lithotomy, relying on one-sided statistics to guide his technical changes. In order to evaluate them, he considered the ages of those who recovered and those who died. He listed his 213 patients by age and gave the number of deaths for each of the eight age groups. The list showed a much lower operative mortality in children than in adults.[36]

This type of unilateral yet age-dependent assessment did not disappear completely in eighteenth-century Britain and carried over into the nineteenth. For example, Alexander Marcet (1770–1822), a Swiss-born, Edinburgh-trained physician, became a chemist at Guy's Hospital, London. His *Essay on the Chemical and Medical Treatment of Calculous*

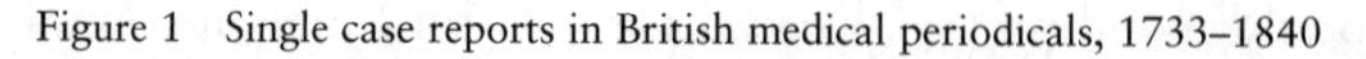
Figure 1 Single case reports in British medical periodicals, 1733–1840

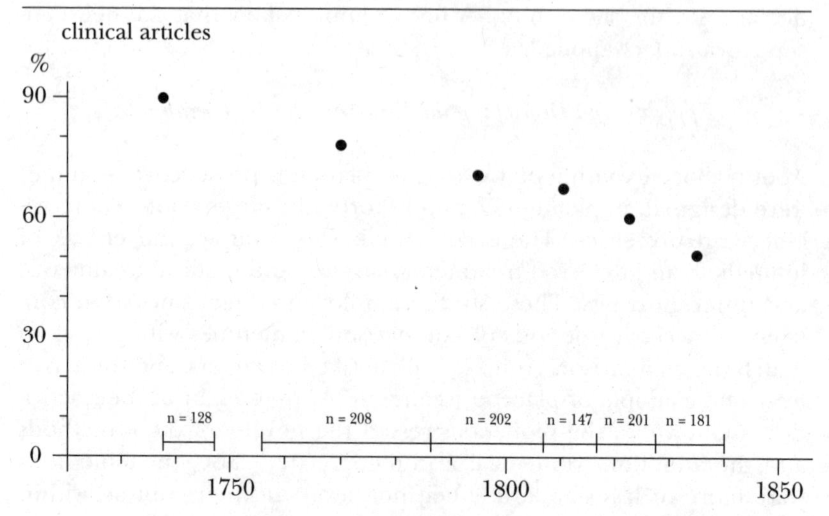

A total of 1,067 clinical articles with detailed descriptions of cases were identified in four comparable British medical periodicals published between 1733 and 1840. The number of cases in each article was registered. The graph represents the percentage of single-case reports. n = number of single-case articles per periodical evaluated for the indicated period. The periodicals were *Edinburgh Medical Essays and Observations* (1733–44); *London Medical Observations and Inquiries* (1757–84); *Memoirs of the Medical Society of London* (1787–1805); and *London Medico-Chirurgical Transactions* (1806–40). The numerical analyses appear in: U. Tröhler, "Quantification in British Medicine and Surgery 1750–1830," PhD thesis, University College, University of London, 1978, 54–8 ; H.P. Schöpflin, "Die Verwendung statistischer Methoden bei englischen Klinikern zu Beginn des 19. Jahrhunderts anhand der *Medico-Chirurgical Transactions* von 1806 bis 1840," MD thesis, University of Basle, 1996, 22.

Disorders (1817) mixed clinical arithmetic with laboratory methods, in order to "describe, and illustrate ... the characters by which the different calculi may be distinguished; to indicate the easiest analytical methods by which their chemical nature may be ascertained; and to point out the modes of medical treatment which afford the best prospect of success."[37]

Marcet was unable to find any regular records of lithotomies in Guy's and the other large hospitals of London. He therefore travelled to Norwich and looked at records collected 1772–1816 at the Norfolk and Norwich Hospital to analyse deaths associated with lithotomy, by sex and age at operation (quoting Cheselden's similar analysis), and presented them all in a table.

We should look at such data in the wider context of poorly documented claims of successful medical treatments throughout the eighteenth century. These relied mostly on patients' testimony and/or *in vitro* studies of stone dissolution, including the secret remedy of Joanna Stephens, based on a well-designed study of four patients, disclosure of which had brought this empiric £5,000 from Parliament in 1740.[38] Other observational analyses attempted to take account of the influence of confounding variables and concerned, for example, the severity of a disease (as mentioned by Withering), the place of occurrence and treatment (such as ship, hospital, or private practice), the timing and the anatomical location of an injury, and the time and the body temperature on the day of hospital admission. We find them in the evaluation of new surgical techniques, for example, for amputation, treating cataracts, use of obstetric forceps, induction of premature labour, and testing of new drugs against "fevers" and "syphilis."[39]

The treatment of "fevers" – one of the most frequent "diseases" and the focus of major therapeutic debate during the eighteenth century – became more effective through empirical research in both military and civilian medicine. In the 1770s numerical analysis of hospital reports played a fundamental role in challenging hitherto-unquestioned usage of copious bleeding, in replacing it with the use of Peruvian bark (cinchona), and in claiming the value of bleeding again a few decades later.[40] Thomas Bateman (1781–1821), physician at the London Fever Hospital, began an age-related study in 1804. His *Succinct account of the contagious fever* (1818) also contained data from the fever wards of three great general hospitals in London. He did not specify the treatments adopted in each of them, but a comparison of crude mortality statistics during comparable periods of time appeared to show that his own practice had not been particularly successful. For 1817/18 they were 1 in 13.5 in his hospital, as compared to 1 in 15, 1 in 17.5, and 1 in 19, in the others.

None the less, he asserted that such a comparison was superficial, given the different age structure of the patient populations in these hospitals: since children under 17 exhibited a lower mortality from "fevers" than adults over 50, this alone could explain the mortality differences; the adult–children ratio was two to one in one of the fever wards, but four to one in his own. Furthermore, therapeutic success depended on the early start of treatment, as had been shown numerically in the reports from an Irish fever hospital. In Bateman's hospital, however, only 124 of 678 patients had been admitted prior to the sixth day of the disease; on average his patients had entered on the eleventh day. If one also made allowance for the 11 patients already moribund on arrival and the three who died from another disease, then only 36 had died of "fever" in his hospital. This gave a "normal" ratio of 1 in 18.

These time-related variables, Bateman concluded, were probably more probable explanations of the annual fluctuations of mortality within one hospital – he himself had observed variations from 1 in 6 to 1 in 13.5 – than were the traditionally invoked seasonal epidemiological variations, the *genus epidemicus*.[41] Bateman's interpretation accorded with an ontological view of disease as fixed entities. It stood in opposition to the notion of geographical and temporal – that is, climate- and environment-dependent – variations. The idea of diseases as constant entities justified additional research into objective criteria for their definition – a further field for quantitative research (see below) and a pre-condition for adequate statistics.

Quantification and Nosography

"The want of clear and precise definition has been the cause of much confusion and disputation in medicine," explained John Gregory in 1772. Indeed in order to quantify meaningfully, the elements entering into a statistical calculation require clear definition. "It seems now to be agreed," he continued, "that it is most convenient, on the whole, to define the genera of diseases by a simple enumeration of such symptoms as are most constantly present, as are obvious to the senses, and which serve to distinguish them from others which they most resemble."[42] This systematization of diseases in terms of the predominant symptoms we call "nosology." As is the case today, there were other approaches throughout the eighteenth century. The theoretical approach classified diseases according to their pathogenic explanation; the geographical, by means of the locally and temporally limited similarity – that is, their *genus epidemicus.* The "nosological" and "geographical" systems are basically empirical, since they depend on the observation and registration of symptoms and of factors, respectively, thought to determine the climate.

As with all empirical approaches, they are amenable to quantification of various kinds: counting the symptoms and determining their frequency, on the one hand, and measuring temperatures of the air and the water, the amount of rain, and so on, on the other hand. Ever since the Hippocratic writers of antiquity, healers had taken for granted the existence of a weather–disease relationship – albeit without taking measurements.

Historians have understood the introduction of such measurement as one of the ways in which quantification entered eighteenth-century medicine. In contrast, they have thought that quantitative nosology originated in early-nineteenth-century Paris.[43] However, in actuality, in the last decades of the eighteenth century and the first of the nineteenth, a few former Edinburgh students introduced it in Britain.

One of these was Thomas Fowler (1736–1801). While a physician at the Stafford Hospital, he published a series of *Medical Reports* between 1785 and 1795 concerning the effects of various drugs tested systematically in defined diseases. On his retirement to Bath in 1791, he analysed the records of the Bath General Infirmary, kept with exemplary care for decades, in order to evaluate treatments for rheumatic diseases and compare these results with his own, based on hundreds of cases recorded during his practice at Stafford.[44]

In this studious endeavour "to render his hospital practice subservient to medical improvement," Fowler also used his numerical notes for clinical research to produce a clearer distinction between acute and chronic rheumatism. He gave precise proportional data for 87 cases of acute rheumatism and 401 of chronic rheumatism, particularly lumbago. He noted the duration of marked pain and the fatalities, analysed by age, sex, and organs. He concluded that a quarter of the acute cases (that is, accompanied by fever) had had a semi-acute onset and that three-quarters of the chronic cases were related to exposure to cold or incomplete cure of acute rheumatism.[45]

John Haygarth (1740–1827) was another former "Edinburgh man" who retired to Bath. In 1798 he decided to work on the meticulously recorded notes of 10,549 patients whom he had seen in his practice in Chester over 32 years. He had used a concise method of recording in Latin, as Clifton had recommended in 1731. Haygarth based his analysis on his private patients only because he had not had time to work up the records of the even larger number of patients he had seen at Chester Infirmary. Even so, he assembled 271 cases of herpetic or scorbutic eruption, 383 of dyspepsia, 827 of syphilis, 914 of hypochondriasis, and 470 of rheumatisms (excluding sciatica, lumbago, *"tic douloureux,"* and nodosities of small joints).

It was on the 170 cases of acute rheumatism that Haygarth wrote the first of a planned series of *Clinical Histories* (1805). He drew up abstracts of all these cases in a table with 27 columns, 11 of which concerned remedies and outcomes (recovery or death). Three of the columns dealt with the administration of Peruvian bark. Analysis of this table permitted a clear, numerical comparison of the proportional success of treatment, with or without bark, as a replacement for bleeding, including details of all 12 unsuccessful cases. Haygarth could similarly describe the clinical history of the disease and its distinctive symptomatology. Several tables gave the proportional occurrences of the disease according to sex, age, seasonal distribution, and "cause" (as diagnosed by the patients themselves). The cause was mostly exposure to cold or moisture. The average period that had elapsed before the first symptoms appeared was between 48 and 72 hours. Haygarth listed concomitant diseases in order of frequency, along with inflamed joints and/or muscles and the pulse ranges. He also noted the occurrence of pain and swelling (separately or together) and their localization in joints and muscles (separately or in both).[46]

A second example drawn from Haygarth's records concerns the "nodosity of joints," in which he described and differentiated for the first time what we now know as *arthritis deformans.* This second work showed exactly the same methodological features as the first, except for its lack of the giant, 27-column table, dropped because printing it had been "*so tedious and troublesome a business.*" Thus Haygarth applied the numerical method both for improved clinical differentiation of diseases and for the evaluation of therapy. He had also started to do such numerical research on "phthisis" (probably tuberculosis) in 1777. In 1805 he wrote: "But after I had made considerable progress in this inquiry, I found the subject too melancholy, and could not assume resolution to proceed in this investigation." Nevertheless, he was able to indicate the age and sex distributions and some of the "causes" of phthisis numerically.[47]

A truly remarkable feature of Haygarth's work was his realization that the results of his inquiries were based on probabilities, which he attempted to calculate (or rather, to estimate). In fact he had already used simple calculation of probabilities in 1784 in his *Inquiry how to prevent the Small-Pox,* and in 1801 for deciding on the mode of propagation of fevers.[48]

Similarly, William Falconer (1744–1824), yet another Edinburgh student and Haygarth's former colleague at the Chester Infirmary, described "palsy" in 1789 and "ischias" in 1805 on the basis of 100 and 556 consecutive case records, respectively.[49] Matthew Dobson (1735–1785), who also retired to Bath, employed the records of the Norwich Hospital to study the causes of bladder stone numerically.[50] Using numerical analysis of symptoms, Dobson's surgical colleague at Norwich, Edward Rigby (1747–1821), differentiated haemorrhages during pregnancy and labour – apparently independently of the previous French author, André Levret (1703–1780) – into "accidental" and "unavoidable" (with a *placenta praevia*). In the latter he recommended immediate delivery by art (turning, extraction) as the sole successful therapy, whereas one could wait for natural delivery in accidental haemorrhage.

In 1775 he based his recommendation on 36 cases; in 1789, for the fourth edition of his *Essay on the uterine haemorrhage* ...,[51] on 106 cases. These cases, collected from 1769 to 1788, broke down as follows: of 42 cases of *placenta praevia*, 31 had been delivered immediately and ended with recovery of the mother; nine were delivered late, after the onset of the haemorrhage, and they had all died, and in two there had been a spontaneous abortion of a six-month-old fetus. The 64 "accidental haemorrhages" had all spontaneously terminated well for mothers and children.

Rigby willingly acknowledged Levret's priority yet remarked that the latter had based his description on only two of his own observations.[52] His *Essay* brought Rigby European fame. It went through several English and American editions and was translated into German and French. Rigby became a fellow of the Royal Society (FRS) and of the Royal College of Surgeons (FRCS). Yet this Unitarian reformer remained attached until his death to the Norfolk and Norwich Hospital, with which he had been associated from its opening in 1771.[53]

More generally, a group of British obstetricians made great efforts to use quantification to answer questions about nosography, as well as about indications for and results of preventive and therapeutic interventions.[54] Much the same was true in the developing field of psychiatry: William Black (1749–1829), a London dispensary physician, medical historian, and vital statistician, set out to evaluate the registers of Bethlehem Asylum ("Bedlam"), near London. In his program for the improvement of medicine and surgery, he was, like so many of his fellow "arithmetic observationists and experimentalists," motivated by critical historical insight. In his *Arithmetical and medical analysis of the diseases and mortality of the human species* (1789), Black could rightly claim that his statistics were the first attempt to apply the new method of "arithmetic observation" to psychiatry: "I may with safety assert, that mine are the only numerical and certain data that ever have been published in any age or country, by which to calculate the probabilities of recovery, of death, and of relapse in every species and stage of insanity, and in every age."[55]

A parliamentary inquiry into the curability of insanity, which was initiated because King George III had fallen ill in early 1788 prompted Black's interest. In that year Black sent his first results in an open letter to the prime minister. The data's reception flattered him. He worked them over again and again for the second edition and republished them a year later in the form of nine tables; he produced an even more extended version in 1810.[56] Although Philippe Pinel later used less sophisticated statistics to study psychiatric illness, he did not, so far as I can determine, ever refer to Black's work.

As in therapeutics, numerical nosographical research dealt also with the huge issue of "fevers." Thomas Bateman (see above), for example, applied this approach to establish the diagnostic features and natural histories of different forms of fever. This served to differentiate a simple from a more severe and complicated form of "typhus." For both forms he recorded objective signs such as pulse per minute, temperature in degrees Fahrenheit, appearance of symptoms (vomiting, diarrhoea, deafness), and clinical progress (in absolute numbers out of 678 patients studied). He also drew up a percentage distribution of the various durations of the disease. In the lighter forms of "typhus," corresponding perhaps to our influenza, 60 per cent improved after a spontaneous free perspiration, and they recovered, usually quite unequivocally, without any very active assistance from medicine. The severe forms, characterized by relapses, additional respiratory symptoms, and/or inflammation of the tonsils and parotid glands, more often ended fatally.[57]

Yet another author of such numerical accounts, John Cheyne (1777–1836), deserves mention. Also a Scottish MD, he had been a surgeon in an artillery regiment from 1795 to 1799 and must thus have done much statistical reporting, prior to becoming a physician at the Hardwicke Fever Hospital, Dublin, in 1816. At any rate, he immediately set out to record all his cases.

The first of his regular reports contained the 780 cases of the year 1816–17, summarized in two tables, with emphasis on the fatal ones, all succinctly described. The next report, for 1818, illustrated even more the "admirable opportunities ... which hospitals afford of investigating disease."[58] Now Cheyne also indicated – always in appropriate tables – the relative occurrences of temperatures in fever, at intervals of one degree from 97° Fahrenheit to 109° Fahrenheit (out of 250 cases), frequencies of respiration (in 171 cases, divided into 16 groups, ranging from 20 breaths to 60 breaths per minute), and pulse rates (for 237 cases, divided into 39 groups, ranging from 52 beats to 180 beats per minute). Forty patients with a temperature of over 104° appeared in a separate table, with their pulse and respiration frequencies and their cutaneous and internal symptoms; and Cheyne recorded and analysed their "events."

Finally, Cheyne attempted to relate mortality to body temperature on the day of admission into the Fever Hospital – an extension of the Bateman study mentioned above. In fact, the mortality dropped with increase in temperature, being one in twelve (n = 83) for temperatures between 97° and 100°, one in twenty-five (n = 127) between 101° and 104°, and one in forty (n = 40) between 105° and 109°. Going into further detail, Cheyne noted an increase of pulse in parallel to that of body temperature in 23 of 32 cases, whereas respiratory frequency increased in only 9 of 22 cases with increased body temperature over 104°.

A table containing the anatomical–pathological findings of all deceased cases completed this hospital report.[59]

This work surely represented high standards of numerical nosography and outcome analysis. It sets the later but better-known contribution of the Dublin school, made by Robert Adams (1791–1875) and William Stokes (1804–1878), in proper historical perspective and antedates by a quarter-century Louis's celebrated work in Paris in the 1820s. In contrast to the latter, Cheyne's research has been largely ignored by historians, despite its remarkably early use of clinical thermometry – yet another form of quantification in clinical medicine.[60]

WILLIAM BLACK'S TEXTBOOK OF "CLINICAL ARITHMETIC"

Born in Ireland and graduated MD from Leyden, William Black settled in London. He is known as a vital statistician, especially for psychiatric problems, and as a medical historian; together with Gilbert Blane (see above), he served as physician at the General Dispensary for Poor Married Women, which opened in 1785.

Black's work illustrates and summarizes some of the major medical and social issues of clinical arithmetic, ranging from political arithmetic and demography, through methods of prevention, nosology, and the weather–disease relationship, to accounting methods in charity practice.[61] In 1789 he stated frankly: "The great utility of medical arithmetic was an accidental discovery, at least to me, about eight years ago: for in the course of many preceding years attendance on medical lectures, at different universities, I never once heard the subject mentioned. I then found in London a violent literary warfare, respecting the advantages and disadvantages of general inoculation."[62] He later wrote on inoculation himself.

The full title of his next book was *Historical Sketch of the Methods Used in Medicine and Surgery, from Their Origin to the Present Time and of the Principal Authors' Discoveries, Improvements, Imperfections and Errors* (1782). In the progressivist historical writing typical for his time, Black stressed that it had been the combination of observation, experiment, and inductive reasoning that had so far been successful in medicine. This view was in tune with Bacon, his hero, and a number of contemporary works – for instance, those of his friends from the Medical Society of London, John Coakley Lettsom (1744–1815) and John Millar (1733–1802).

Again, as Millar had done, Black concluded that, despite contradictory theories and inherent difficulties, a number of diseases were well known and distinctly described: "Amidst all the tumultuous anarchy of accessory or secondary symptoms [of fever], men of judgment can in most cases discern the true elementary type." He asserted that the examples of epilepsy, measles, smallpox, and the venereal diseases showed "that diseases, whether external or internal, whether acute or chronic, are presented to us over and over again in nearly the same form" with respect to key symptoms. This was also true for gangrene, gout, plague, scurvy, and stone. Moreover, the causes of several diseases had been elucidated. One could "even measure with tolerable accuracy, the annual waste among the human species," and in his opinion the effects of many medicines rested "upon proofs equally solid."[63]

Yet with all these good natural histories at a physicians' disposal, Black felt that "our principal defect at this day is in remedies, remedies, remedies. In the more effectual means of curing the above diseases, we have not greatly outstripped the ancients."[64] He lamented that therapy, designated the "end and essence of physick," was still dominated by fashions and that readers were "frequently bewildered in ambiguity and uncertainty"; therefore it was hardly surprising that learned writers derided therapy or classed it with necromancy and astrology.[65] Describing diseases was easier than curing them.

But Black believed that statistics would bring much-needed certainty to both nosography and therapy, if the bills of mortality were conducted on a proper and larger scale. They would demonstrate the civil and salutary state of humanity at all ages, the incidence of diseases, "the effects of diet, drink, and medical practice, the comparative salubrity and insalubrity of city, town and country air ... and their effects upon different ages ... the comparative ravages of [diseases]; we could then, independent of venerable opinions, form prognosticks upon mathematical grounds."[66]

This was necessary to distinguish the frequent from the rare diseases, the important from the unimportant, which issues the mere classification of the nosologists neglected.[67] As Black put it most suggestively later: "in medical books the extensive desolation of the most rapacious tyrants and conquerors are confounded with the uninteresting history and petty deprecations of a robber."[68]

In order to compile a reasonably distinctive list of diseases and establish valuable comparisons, Black planned to strip the systems of the nosologists – albeit necessary for order and method – of their superfluous and exaggerated ramifications. "Thank God, diseases were not so numerous as the vegetable tribe," he said, in obvious reference to nosologists' dependence on botanists.[69]

Consequently, Black's idea of using arithmetic in medicine to describe diseases and evaluate therapies, hinted at in his smallpox work in 1781, played a major role in his historical book in 1782. It became outspoken in his annual oration before the Medical Society of London in 1788, published in enlarged form in the same year, "at the unanimous request" of the society.[70] A second edition appeared in 1789 as *Arithmetical and Medical Analysis of the Diseases and Mortality of the Human Species* ... It had two main sections and contained programmatic remarks in a separate introduction. The first section, concerning the bills of mortality, provided a general demographic background, which has interested historians. The second, much larger section showed the critical but constructive application of the statistical program to individual diseases – a continuation and elaboration from the *Historical Sketch* of 1782, with new material collected in the meantime. Thus this book is a textbook rather more of clinical than of vital statistics. Black's term was "medical arithmetick."

Black's plan now envisaged the study not only of the bills of mortality, "but likewise of the collected records of hospitals, dispensaries, and individuals." And even this was not sufficient, if restricted to one geographical area and a short time frame: "We should include an interval of many years, collective numbers, large groupes of mankind, and of morbid cases."[71] As he had already departed from traditional aetiological views in his *Historical Sketch*,[72] he now took his distance from Hippocrates' prognostics, which he thought confined chiefly to fevers. He admitted: "I am aware of the imputation of heresy, in calling the aphoristick prognosticks contracted and pinioned. Without medical arithmetick it is impossible to reach the 'grandeur of generality', the sublime of medical divination ... It was necessary, in treating of morbid prognosticks, not only to ascertain the general danger, the absolute and comparative mortality by different diseases, but likewise to enter into more minute detail, and to measure the proportions of cures, incurables, and deaths."[73] Thus, through medical arithmetic, even practical branches of medicine might become as certain as any other branches, regardless of philosophy or other theoretical science. Only the prosecution of such a plan throughout Europe, and the combined information contrasted, assimilated, and harmonized, seemed sufficient to emancipate the profession from metaphysical infatuation and the sneers of conjecture.[74]

Medical arithmetic, Black believed, first emerged in James Jurin's (1684–1750) demonstrating "in numbers the comparative success under inoculation, and the natural disease." Since that time several fragmentary attempts had appeared in the miscellaneous writings of Thomas Short (1690–1772), a vital statistician. Black also mentioned the indefatigable industry of Dr Robertson of the navy and Dr Millar of London, concerning fevers in various parts of the globe and the comparative success of different febrile remedies.[73] With respect to such fevers, Black, who had in 1782 relied for their treatment on the authorities of Lind and Sir James Pringle (1707–1782),[76] now, on the evidence of numerical writers such as Robertson and Millar, had completely changed his opinion: "The false lights hung out successively by multitudes of authors, and transmitted, in some degree, through the Boerhaavean school, to steer with the antiphlogistick compass and lancet in each hand, in the generality of fevers, have been the cause of numerous shipwrecks. Even that excellent modern author, Pringle, as Dr. Millar demonstrates, must, in this instance, be followed with extreme caution."[77]

Little wonder that authors who tore monumental authorities down from their pedestals had to face rancorous opposition. This did not surprise Black, who knew the history of arts and sciences. He thought that such had been the initial reception of many other useful discoveries and of the most enlightened reformers and benefactors of humankind. The histories of the reception of Peruvian bark and of the concept of the circulation of the blood furnished him with good illustrative examples. "With respect to medical arithmetick, what time must yet revolve before ignorance and bigotry shall be enlightened, prejudices and inveterate habits done away with, envy, malevolence, and calumny silenced, I cannot determine."[78]

Black himself by no means remained simply a theoretical writer. Going through the diseases as listed in the bills of mortality, he inserted numerical comments on natural history and therapy wherever the available data made this possible. He also took the time to peruse the books of Lettsom's Aldersgate Dispensary, which kept registers at least until 1788.[79] He realized that they distinguished fevers simply according to three classes: intermittent, inflammatory, and continuous. On the basis of his own work and the data from Millar's Westminster Dispensary, from John Clark's Newcastle Infirmary (see below), from Robertson, and from others, he rejected "the supposed innumerable varieties of fevers, ... from which perplexity Sydenham could not altogether extricate himself."[80] Moreover, the numerical reports of these authors also testified to the success of treatment without bleeding.[81]

Black was enthusiastic for "medical arithmetick." None the less, he was critical of some of the available data, even of those of his friends. With hidden, yet clear reference to a literary squabble – between his friend John Millar and the prestigious Edinburgh professor Donald Monro (1727–1802), about the (lack of) success of the usual military practice in dealing with "fevers"[82] – he wrote in 1789 that critics, in contrasting the success of medical practice in different hospitals in Europe, "domestick as well as military, ... have forgotten to ascertain the diseases which were admitted or excluded, and the proportion of the former; consequently their inferences are imperfect and erroneous."[83]

As he had for fever, Black relied on the data from the Aldersgate Dispensary for a better description of true asthma, dropsy, and jaundice. Otherwise he took the data where he found them. For whooping cough, he used the records of Armstrong's Dispensary for the Infant Poor; for palsy, Charleton's data from Bath; for urinary calculi, Dobson's; and for insanity, the registers of all patients kept privately by the apothecary at Bedlam[84] (see below).

CONCLUSION: A SOCIAL REVOLUTION IN MEDICINE

About 1800 the former Manchester Hospital physician Thomas Percival (1740–1804) recommended in his *Medical Ethics* the analysis of accurate registers (as he knew them from his colleague John Ferriar) for the comparative outcome evaluation of therapeutic interventions.[85] In Manchester, Samuel Argent Bardsley (1764–1850) similarly justified in 1807 his numerical *Medical reports of cases and experiments chiefly derived from hospital practice,* as did, in Nottingham, James Clark (+1818) his statistical hospital reports, regularly printed in the *Edinburgh Medical and Surgical Journal.*[86] The same rhetoric came from within army and navy circles.

The systematic review of existing evidence, the description of diseases using numerical nosography, and the assessment of therapeutic outcomes with "protostatistical" methods met with the approval of Andrew Duncan Sr (1744–1828), editor of the *Medical and Philosophical Commentaries* (1773–95), a periodical that for some time appeared simultaneously in Edinburgh, London, and Dublin.[87]

Quantitative collection and assessment of data had obviously become common by 1800, yet the need to defend the practice regularly suggests that such empirical methods and their results had not yet received general acceptance. In fact, there existed socially as well as epistemologically motivated opposition to this "new arithmetic medical culture," propagated as it was by marginal men from Scottish and English provincial stock, frequently former army or navy surgeons, religious dissenters, engaged in charity practice in the many new voluntary hospitals and/or dispensaries of the kingdom. Rather than belonging to the prestigious Royal College of Physicians of London – the Royal College of Surgeons was founded only in 1800 – they formed more egalitarian associations, such as the Medical Society of London and provincial societies, which admitted with equal rights physicians, surgeons, and apothecaries.[88]

Defenders of the traditional hierarchies in this period of the French Revolution therefore labelled reformers "Jacobins," "democrats," or "levellers." By promoting methodically guided empiricism, "arithmetic observationists and experimentalists" also pursued social ideals, including reforming care for the poor and reforming medicine in many ways – by challenging traditional treatments with new ones, by fighting for objectification, standardization, public understanding, and what we call transparency, and even by arguing for the transformation of professional structures.[89] At the same time, they also pursued their new sorts of careers, implying a success-oriented, utilitarian meritocracy, where proven efficiency and organizational skills were more important than the status conferred by traditional notions of "science" and "profession." As one of them, William Rowley, wrote in 1804: "By their works shall ye know men, not by professions: and by a *comparative view* of the malpractices erroneously adopted, with the present improvements in curing diseases."[90]

The fact that some of these 'marginal men' built remarkable careers in public service suggests an effective empirical – perhaps 'utilitarian' – undercurrent within British society. It shaped the development of the voluntary hospital and dispensary system and led to all-purpose and specialized institutions in civilian as well as in military medicine. It encouraged counting and accounting, which were contingent on the art of reasoning through figures on matters related to government. This approach had been prefigured in the seventeenth century first by Bacon and later, as 'political arithmetic,' by John Graunt (1620–1674) and Sir William Petty (1623–1687). In medicine, this approach held true particularly for the military.[91]

The spirit of research and innovation was also at the basis of medical societies and their publications, in London as well as in the provinces, which revolutionized the exchange of observations and ideas.[92] This context allowed John Hunter, Carmichael Smyth (1741–1821), and others to develop the concept of tissue pathology.[93] These were also favourable milieux for quantification in that soldiers, sailors, and the poor were regarded rather impersonally as "lives." They could therefore be represented by impersonal numbers, and treated according to standard protocols. This casts some doubts on N.D. Jewson's often-quoted claim that the client-dominated setting of (upper-class) medicine prevented an engagement in research in eighteenth-century England.[94] There was, it turns out, a scientific community dedicated to the generation of new data and the analysis of health problems, not only in curative hospital and dispensary medicine but also in prevention. Throughout the eighteenth century there was indeed a direct link between preventive measures, statistics, and clinical medicine.[95] (See as well the essay in this volume by Rusnock.)

Of course, not everybody appreciated all of this. Applying statistical data to advance medical reform was one thing; using them for medical investigations was quite another. Medical reform could be, and often was, advocated by laymen as well as by physicians; indeed counting and accounting had long had the odour of business and commerce – not really gentlemanly activities.[96] Furthermore, as a clinical research tool, medical statistics had to vie with the other methods of the day, which were, broadly speaking, clinical observation and description, study of the medical classics, and laboratory experiment. Empiricism, speculative pathophysical theories, and laboratory experiments and their iatrochemical interpretations all supplied rationales for internal therapies during the eighteenth century.

Physicians of the 'Oxbridge' establishment and those of the London royal colleges of physicians and surgeons who staffed the great hospitals of the capital saw their "rationalism" (which supported their therapeutic certainties) as vastly superior to the "trial and error" approach of empiricism, which yielded only probable results. Consequently they gave rationalistic pathophysiology a makeover and facelift, introducing laboratory observations, measurements, the study of morbid anatomy, and experiments, such as the *in vitro* tests that were so important throughout the eighteenth century for evaluating medicines to dissolve bladder stones.[97]

As to pathological anatomy, Morgagni's *De sedibus* ... (1761) appeared in English in 1769, and Matthew Baillie's *Morbid Anatomy* in 1793. John Hunter (1728–1793), who had lectured on the subject from the 1780s on, followed with a book in 1794, and there were others.[98] Some of these hospital physicians became remarkably acute observers, and a few, perhaps the greatest clinicians that Britain has produced. Many of their observations filled the pages of medical periodicals. For these authors the presentation of facts was the primary aim; any numerical analysis of them was secondary, nearly accidental. Yet, as our summary view of four medical journals shows (Figure 1), they tended to base their work, including the definition of new disease-phenomena, on increasingly large numbers of case observations.

William Heberden the elder (1710–1801), for instance, based his famous account of angina pectoris (1772) – one of the outstanding clinical contributions of the time – on 20 case histories. His posthumously edited *Commentaries* (1802) shows that by 1782 he had recorded "nearly 100."[99] The use of larger numbers of cases may have reflected, if not the direct influence of the arithmetical program, at least a shared desire for the greater rigour and precision that Clifton had demanded earlier in the century. Other established doctors, however, insisted on the Hippocratic, individualistic notion of disease, stressing its unique nature in each patient. And busy practitioners claimed to have no time for collecting data and stuck to routine reliance on medical authorities – the main question being only whether these were ancient or modern. They still referred to classical medical authors. Indeed, it is highly likely that most doctors probably did not care about epistemological issues.

The state of scholarly medicine was thus somewhat chaotic in late-eighteenth-century Britain. The new "culture" of methodically guided rational empiricism and scepticism, aiming at a new "scientization" of medicine by objectification of observation and assessment in groups of patients, and seeking to beat biases through the use of statistics, challenged both the pathophysiologic tradition of medicine as a "science" and the equally ancient tradition of medicine as an "art," focusing on the individuality of each (upper-class) patient. It was a new culture within medicine, promoted by men with medical and social ideals and personal ambitions. It had advantages and disadvantages and carried risks as well as benefits. As William Black, one of its protagonists from the 1780s right through to 1810, put it:

> What tribunal can possibly decide truth in this clash of contradictory assertions and conjectures; or by what clue can medical wanderers find their way through the labyrinth of prognosticks and therapeuticks, except by medical arithmetick and numbers? ... Perhaps some would here answer, the best authors should decide the controversy. Who are they, ancient or modern ... ? To borrow Molière's satirical expression, Hippocrates often says Yes, and Galen flatly No. The system of medical arithmetick, although it may not shew the best mode of therapy that may hereafter be invented, it will, however, by comparison, determine the best that has yet been discovered, or in use.[100]

Three centuries after the first challenge to therapeutic theories and dogma, 'rational' empiricism based on quantification began to be practised in earnest in Britain. This new medical culture and its intellectual, social, and societal context deserve to be better known by historians. It has been too long 'obscured' by the focus on the *méthode numérique* of the Paris school about 1830,[101] which added little that was new to eighteenth-century British achievements.

NOTES

1 I thank Iain Chalmers and George Weisz for their constructive criticisms of an earlier version of this manuscript and for the latter's encouragement of its completion.

2 F. Clifton, *Tabular Observations Recommended as the Plainest and Surest Way of Practising and Improving Physick* (London: Brindley, 1731), 419–21.

3 F. Clifton, *The State of Physick, Ancient and Modern, Briefly Considered* (London: Nourse, 1732), as quoted by M. Neuburger, "Francis Clifton and William Black: Eighteenth Century Critical Historians of Medicine," *Journal of the History of Medicine* 5 (1950), 44–9.

4 Ibid., 47.

5 Ibid.

6 Ibid.

7 T. Gelfand, "A Clinical Ideal: Paris 1789," *Bulletin of the History of Medicine*, 51 (1977), 40–53, 401.

8 F.B. Hawkins, *Elements of Medical Statistics* (London: Longman et al., 1829), 2–3.

9 *Medical Observations and Inquiries* (London), 6 (1784), 400; G. Fordyce, "An Attempt to Improve the Evidence of Medicine," *Transactions of the Society for the Improvement of Medical-Chirurgical Knowledge* 1 (1793), 243–93.

10 J.K. Aronson, *An Account of the Foxglove and Its Medical Uses, 1785–1985* (London: Oxford University Press, 1985).

11 W. Withering, *An Account of the Foxglove and Some of its Medical Uses* (Birmingham: Robinson, 1785).

12 Ibid., vii–viii.

13 Ibid., ix.

14 J. Ferriar, *Medical Histories and Reflexions*, vol. 1 (London: Cadell and Davies, 1810), preface to 1st ed., xvii–xviii.

15 Ibid., xix–xxix.

16 Ibid., xxiv–xxv.

17 Ibid., 38.

18 Ibid., 97–110, 123–4.

19 Ibid., 40–1.

20 O. Temkin, *Galenism: Rise and Decline of a Medical Philosophy* (Ithaca, NY: Cornell University Press, 1973), 134–87.

21 C. Huerkamp, *Der Aufstieg der Ärzte im 19. Jahrhundert: Vom gelehrten Stand zum professionellen Experten: Das Beispiel Preussens* (Göttingen: Vandenhoeck and Ruprecht, 1985), 22–33.

22 J. Bostock, "History of Medicine," in J. Forbes et al., eds., *The Cyclopaedia of Practical Medicine*, vol. 1 (London: Sherwood et al., 1833), l–lxxii.

23 J. Millar, *Observations on the Practice in the Medical Department of the Westminster General Dispensary* (London: By Order of the Governors, 1777), 7–8.

24 T.D. Reide, *A View of the Diseases of the Army in Great Britain, America, The West Indies and on Board of King's Ships, From the Beginning of the Late War to the Present Time, Together with Monthly and Annual Returns of the Sick* (London: Johnson, 1793), xi and xiii.

25 J. Millar, *Observations on the Prevailing Diseases in Great Britain*, 2nd ed. (London: For the Author, 1798), 76.

26 U. Tröhler, *To Improve the Evidence of Medicine: The 18th Century British Origins of a Critical Approach* (Edinburgh: Royal College of Physicians, 2000), passim.

27 Ibid., 70–1.

28 R.E. Hughes, "James Lind and the Cure of Scurvy: An Experimental Approach," *Medical History* 19 (1975), 342–51; D. Harvie, *Limeys: The True Story of One Man's War against Ignorance, the Establishment and the Deadly Scurvy* (Stroud: Sutton, 2002).

29 R. Robertson, *Observations on the Diseases Incident to Seamen*, 2nd ed., vol. 1 (London: For the Author, 1804), 20.

30 I. Chalmers, "Comparing Like with Like: Some Historical Milestones in the Evolution of Methods to Create Unbiased Comparison Groups in Therapeutic Experiments," *International Journal of Epidemiology* 30 (2001), 1170–8.

31 J. Clark, *Observations on Fever, Especially Those of the Continued Type* (London: Cadell, 1780), 189–96.

32 J. Lind, *A Treatise on the Scurvy*, 3rd ed. (London: Crowder et al., 1772), v–vi.

33 J. Gregory, *Lectures on the Duties and Qualifications of a Physician 1772, Revised and Corrected by James Gregory* (Edinburgh and London: Creech and Cadell, 1805), 159, 164.

34 Tröhler, *To Improve the Evidence of Medicine*, 60–1; U. Tröhler, "Cheselden's 1740 Presentation of Data on Age-Specific Mortality after Lithotomy," in *The James Lind Library* (www.jameslindlibrary.org)

35 U. Tröhler, " 'Zwischen Argument und Erfahrung:' Die wissenschaftliche Begründung therapeutischer Entscheide im Laufe der Geschichte," in P. Rusteholz and R. Mosery, eds., *Wege zu wissenschaftlichen Wahrheiten:*

Vermutung–Behauptung–Beweis (Bern-Berlin, etc.: P. Lang, 2003), 137–64, 147–8.

36 Tröhler, *To Improve the Evidence of Medicine,* 60–1; Tröhler, "Cheselden's 1740 Presentation of Data," passim.

37 A. Marcet, *An Essay on the Chemical History and Medical Treatment of Calculous Disorders* (London: Longman et al., 1817), vii.

38 A.-H. Maehle, *Drugs on Trial: Experimental Pharmacology and Therapeutic Innovation in the Eighteenth Century* (Amsterdam and Atlanta: Rodopi, 1999), 68, 102–7.

39 U. Tröhler, "Klinisch-numerische Forschung in der britischen Geburtshilfe 1750–1820," *Gesnerus* 38 (1981), 69–80; Tröhler, *To Improve the Evidence of Medicine,* 51–7, 95–114.

40 Tröhler, *To Improve the Evidence of Medicine,* 31–51.

41 T. Bateman, *A Succinct Account of the Contagious Fever of this Country* (London: Longman, 1818), 80–1, 85.

42 Gregory, *Lectures on the Duties and Qualifications,* 168.

43 W.F. Bynum, "Nosology," in Bynum and R. Porter, eds., *Companion Encyclopedia of the History of Medicine,* vol. 1 (London: Routledge, 1993), 335–56.

44 Tröhler, *To Improve the Evidence of Medicine,* 53–4.

45 T. Fowler, *Medical Reports on the Effects of Blood-Letting, Sudorfics, and Blistering in the Cure of the Acute and Chronic Rheumatism* (London: Johnson, 1795), ix, 255–72.

46 J. Haygarth, *A Clinical History of Diseases, I. A Clinical History of the Acute Rheumatism, or Rheumatick Fever, II. A Clinical History of the Nodosity of the Joints* (London: Cadell and Davies, 1805), 6, 8, 20–7, 34, 46–9, 56, 74, 81–106, 121, 125, 156–73, 177–8.

47 Ibid., 33, 35–36, 186.

48 Tröhler, *An Arithmetical and Medical Analysis,* 92.

49 See *Memoirs of the Medical Society of London* 2 (1789), 201–26, W. Falconer, *A Dissertation on Ischias or the Disease of the Hip-Joint* (London: Cadell, 1805), passim.

50 M. Dobson, *A Medical Commentary on Fixed Air* (Chester: Monk, 1779), 148–9, 167, 170–1, 178–9.

51 E. Rigby, *An Essay on the Use of the Red Peruvian Bark in The Cure Of Intermittents* (London: Johnson, 1783), 262–4.

52 Ibid., x–xiii.

53 J.P. Marr, "Historical Background of the Treatment of Placenta Praevia," *Bulletin of the History of Medicine* 9 (1941), 258–93.

54 Tröhler, "Klinisch-numerische Forschung," passim.

55 W. Black, *An Arithmetical and Medical Analysis of the Diseases and Mortality of the Human Species,* 2nd ed. (London: Dilly, 1789), 130. The first edition

of this work was *A Comparative View of the Mortality of the Human Species at All Ages.*

56 Ibid., ii–iii; I. Macalpine and R. Hunter, *George III and the Mad-Business* (London: Allen Lane, Penguin Press, 1969), 297–9.

57 Bateman, *A Succinct Account of the Contagious Fever,* 30, 35–6, 38, 40, 48–50, 51, 57, 64, 66, 71–2.

58 See J. Cheyne, "Report of the Hardwicke Fever Hospital, for the Year Ending on the 31st March 1817," *Dublin Hospital Reports* 1 (1818), 1–116.

59 Ibid., 2: 10–14, 110–45.

60 V. Hess, *Der wohltemperierte Mensch: Wissenschaft und Alltag des Fiebermessens (1850–1900)* (Frankfurt/Main: Campus, 2000); this work does not mention Cheyne.

61 A.A. Rusnock, *Quantifying Health and Population in Eighteenth-Century England and France* (Cambridge: Cambridge University Press, 2002), 109–36.

62 Black, *An Arithmetical and Medical Analysis,* 250.

63 W. Black, *An Historical Sketch of Medicine and Surgery from their Origin to the Present Time* (London: Johnson, 1782), 228–9, 280.

64 Ibid., 280.

65 Ibid., 226–7.

66 Ibid., 254.

67 Ibid., 274.

68 Black, *An Arithmetical and Medical Analysis,* v–vi.

69 Black, *An Historical Sketch of Medicine and Surgery,* 270.

70 W. Black, *A Comparative View of the Mortality of the Human Species at All Ages* (London: Dilly, 1788), title page.

71 Black, *An Arithmetical and Medical Analysis,* v, vi–vii, 261.

72 Black, *An Historical Sketch of Medicine and Surgery,* 299.

73 Black, *An Arithmetical and Medical Analysis,* vi–vii.

74 Ibid., viii–ix.

75 Ibid., i–ii.

76 Black, *An Historical Sketch of Medicine and Surgery,* 250.

77 Black, *An Arithmetical and Medical Analysis,* 58.

78 Ibid., ii.

79 Ibid., 101.

80 Ibid., 43; Black, *A Comparative View of the Mortality,* 10–101.

81 Ibid., 100–1; Black, *An Arithmetical and Medical Analysis,* 46–7, 51–2.

82 U. Tröhler, "To Improve the Evidence of Medicine: Arithmetic Observation in Clinical Medicine in the Eighteenth and Early Nineteenth Centuries," *History and Philosophy of the Life Sciences* 10 suppl. (1988), 31–40.

83 Black, *An Arithmetical and Medical Analysis,* 42.

84 Ibid., 101–3, 108, 117, 129, 170, 178.
85 T. Percival, *Medical Ethics*, 2nd ed. (London: Jackson, 1827), 32, 36.
86 See *Edinburgh Medical and Surgical Journal* 3 (1807), 309; ibid., 4 (1808), 3, 422.
87 I. Chalmers and U. Tröhler, "Helping Physicians to Keep Abreast of the Medical Literature: Medical and Philosophical Commentaries, 1773–1795," *Annals of Internal Medicine* 133 (2001), 238–43.
88 Tröhler, *To Improve the Evidence of Medicine*, 8–9, 117–21.
89 R. Porter, *Enlightenment:. Britain and the Creation of the Modern World* (London: Allen Lane, Penguin Press, 2000), 145–55.
90 J. Millar, *Observations on the Conduct of the War: In An Appeal To The People of Great Britain* (London: For the author, 1798), 17–24, 81–4.
91 W. Rowley, *A Treatise on Putrid, Malignant, Infectious Fevers and How They Ought to Be Treated* (London: Barfield, 1804), 36.
92 Tröhler, *To Improve the Evidence of Medicine*, 8–11.
93 O. Keel, *La généalogie de l'histopathologie: Une révision déchirante, Philippe Pinel, lecteur discret de J.-C. Smyth (1741–1821)* (Paris: Vrin, 1979); O. Keel, "La pathologie tissulaire de John Hunter," *Gesnerus* 37 (1980), 47–61.
94 N.D. Jewson, "Medical Knowledge and the Patronage System in Eighteenth-Century England," *Sociology* 8 (1974), 369–85.
95 Rusnock, *Vital Accounts*, 43–70; Tröhler, *To Improve the Evidence of Medicine*, 16–17.
96 S. Shapin, *A Social History of Truth* (Chicago: University of Chicago Press, 1994), 315–17.
97 Maehle, *Drugs on Trial*, 55–125.
98 J. Hunter, *A Treatise on the Blood, Inflammation and Gun-Shot Wounds* (London: Nicol, 1794).
99 W. Heberden (the Elder), "On a Disorder of the Breast," *Medical Transactions of the Royal College of Physicians of London* 2 (1772), 59–67, 365–6; L.R. Crummer, "Robert Jackson, M.D., late inspector general of army hospitals," reprint from *Military Surgery* (Feb. 1922), 229; B. Livesley, "The Resolution of the Heberden–Parr Controversy," *Medical History* 19 (1975), 158–71, 160.
100 Black, *An Arithmetical and Medical Analysis*, vii–viii.
101 See, for example, J.H. Warner, *The Therapeutic Perspective: Medical Practice, Knowledge and Identity in America, 1820–1885* (Cambridge, Mass.: Harvard University Press, 1986), 185, 199–206; J.R. Matthews, *Quantification and the Quest for Medical Certainty* (Princeton, NJ: Princeton University Press, 1994), 3–38. Exceptions are A.M. Lilienfeld, "'Ceteris Paribus': The Evolution of the Clinical Trial," *Bulletin of the History of Medicine* 56 (1982), 1–18; T.J. Kaptchuk, "Intentional Ignorance: A History of Blind Assessment and Placebo Control in Medicine," *Bulletin of*

the History of Medicine 72 (1998), 389–433; and, most important, J.H. Warner, *Against the Spirit of System: The French Impulse in Nineteenth-Century American Medicine* (Princeton, NJ: Princeton University Press, 1998), 226–7. See also P. Stanley, *For Fear of Pain: British Surgery 1790–1850* (Amsterdam: Rodopi, 2003).

3

When the State Counts Lives: Eighteenth-Century Quarrels over Inoculation

HARRY M. MARKS

"S.F. rates best for infant mortality rate," reads a recent headline.[1] At the start of the twenty-first century, governments the world over accept mortality indices as a measure of the health of populations and as transparent evidence of medical progress (when they go down). This use of mortality data is relatively recent, dating back to the mid-seventeenth century.[2] In this paper, I discuss an early and contested use of mortality indices – Daniel Bernoulli's effort in 1760 to measure the usefulness of smallpox inoculation. Bernoulli's analysis was challenged by his fellow mathematician Jean D'Alembert in a celebrated controversy over the value of the probability calculus for judging "moral" questions.

Previous historians have read D'Alembert's critique as epistemological. According to Lorraine Daston, Michel Paty, and Eric Brian, D'Alembert uncovered deep philosophical flaws in applications of the probability calculus. I offer a complementary reading of D'Alembert that explores his political objections to Bernoulli's state-centred approach. I begin with a brief background on smallpox inoculation, followed by descriptions of Bernoulli's analysis and D'Alembert's criticisms. Then I examine some possible sources of D'Alembert's political objections. The conclusion looks at the intellectual legacy of D'Alembert's arguments.

From the early seventeenth century on, smallpox was a major cause of mortality, responsible for some 10–13 per cent of all deaths in some European countries. In 1721, Lady Mary Wortley Montagu, wife of the British ambassador to Turkey, had the Turkish folk practice of inoculation performed in England on her three-year-old child. Debate about the safety and benefits of the procedure developed in England over the next thirty years. A key concern was the mortality from the procedure itself, both among those inoculated and from secondary cases exposed to the inoculants. Although French physicians followed the British discussion, the procedure had limited support in France until 1754, when Charles de la Condamine comprehensively reviewed the European experience. La Condamine emphasized the costs to the state in allowing smallpox to proceed unchecked.[3] In the wake of his publications, it became clear that the French lacked information available elsewhere about the incidence of smallpox, the total burden of smallpox mortality, and other key points. In 1760, the mathematician Daniel Bernoulli presented a paper in support of La Condamine and inoculation to the Academy of Sciences, in the hopes that mathematical analysis could provide insight even in the absence of such empirical data.[4]

THE DEBATE

Lacking observed data about the age-specific incidence and mortality from smallpox, and with the estimated risk from inoculation in dispute, Bernoulli built what we would now call a mathematical model.[5] Starting from Edmund Halley's life table, which describes the age-specific mortality of a cohort followed from birth to adulthood (age 24), Bernoulli incorporated his calculations for the losses from smallpox at each age (Table 1).[6] He applied these figures to compare mortality in a world with and without smallpox.[7] Bernoulli offered several ways to calculate these gains (average life expectancy, total lives saved) but focused on the gain in adults – "the only ones useful to the State": "One could call the arrival of a person at their seventeenth year their 'civil birth'; I estimate this birth for all of France in the natural state at 175,000 each year, and I say that without the mortality from smallpox it would be 200,000; so that France would annually gain 25,000 people, all useful to the State."[8] As Bernoulli acknowledged, inoculation has costs, but, he argued, it would have to kill between one in nine individuals and one in eight before it did more harm than natural smallpox itself. Even a loss of greater than one in nine would be tolerable, as many of the lives lost are children, who are "useless to society," so long as a net gain in adult lives remained.[9]

Bernoulli's analysis was a brilliant, pioneering application of mathematics to estimating the value of medical treatments. While, as he recognized, some of the figures that he assumed (attack rate, fatality rate)

Table 1 Bernoulli's Life Table: Smallpox

Age	*Alive*	*At risk (w/o pox)*	*No longer at risk (exposed)*	*New cases*	*New deaths*	*Cumulative pox deaths*	*Total deaths (other)*
0	1,300	1,300	0				
1	1,000	896	104	137	17.1	17.1	283
2	855	685	170	99	12.4	29.5	133
3	798	571	227	78	9.7	39.2	47
4	760	485	275	66	8.3	47.5	30
5	732	416	316	56	7.0	54.5	21
6	710	359	351	48	6.0	60.5	16
7	692	311	381	42	5.2	65.7	12.8
8	680	272	408	36	4.5	70.2	7.5
9	670	237	433	32	4.0	74.2	6
10	661	208	453	28	3.5	77.7	5.5
11	653	182	471	24.4	3.0	80.7	5
12	646	160	486	21.4	2.7	83.4	4.3
13	640	140	500	18.7	2.3	85.7	3.7
14	634	123	511	16.6	2.1	87.8	3.9
15	628	108	520	14.4	1.8	89.6	4.2
16	622	94	528	12.6	1.6	91.2	4.4
17	616	83	533	11	1.4	92.6	4.6
18	610	72	538	9.7	1.2	93.8	4.8
19	604	63	541	8.4	1.0	94.8	5
20	598	56	542	7.4	.9	95.7	5.1
21	592	48.5	543	6.5	.8	96.5	5.2
22	586	42.5	543	5.6	.7	97.2	5.3
23	579	37	542	5.0	.6	97.8	6.4
24	572	32.4	540	4.4	.5	98.3	6.5

Source: Daniel Bernoulli, "Essai d'une nouvelle analyse ...," Académie des Sciences, *Mémoires de Mathématique et de physique* (1760), 44–45.

could be improved with more accurate data, he had demonstrated the advantages of inoculation. What objections then did fellow mathematician Jean Le Rond D'Alembert have to Bernoulli's analysis?

As historians of science Lorraine Daston and Michel Paty have emphasized, D'Alembert took issue with a fundamental concept used by Bernoulli in applying the probability calculus to social questions – namely the notion of moral expectation. After calculating the value of inoculation to the state, Bernoulli had argued that an individual's calculation of expected benefit would coincide with the state's.[10] Not so, claimed D'Alembert.

Figure 1

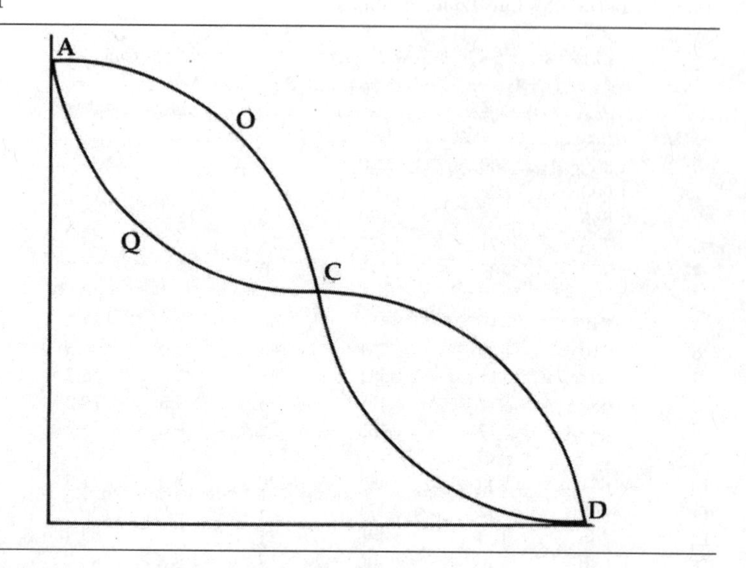

Source: Jean Le Rond d'Alembert, *Opuscules mathématiques*, vol. IV (Paris: Briasson, 1768), 93.

Suppose, D'Alembert suggested, that on average we imagine the following situation. A medical procedure offers an expected fifteen additional years of life. But what does this expectancy mean? Consider the following hypothetical example: two mortality curves with a common life expectancy. Yet the risks of dying young are much greater for curve AQCD than for curve AOCD (Figure 1).[11] Bernoulli's calculations cannot provide the desired missing data, which would tell someone which curve they were facing.[12] Bernoulli would not acknowledge that a short-term, immediate risk (death from inoculation) might matter to some individuals much more than the long-term gains of protection from smallpox, especially if that individual was deciding about the fate of his or her child: "Once it is granted that one can die from the inoculation, I would no longer dare blame a father who feared to inoculate his son. For if a son by some evil mischance is a victim, his father must forever condemn himself for having hastened the death of him whom he holds most dear. ... I grant that if he had not inoculated his son, he might someday reproach himself for having allowed the son to die of naturally occurring smallpox; but what a difference between the despair of having hastened the death of this son, and the misfortune of having allowed him to die, because one dared not run the risk of giving him smallpox."[13]

As Daston and Paty have pointed out, D'Alembert's arguments took aim at the central ambition for advocates of the probability calculus: to provide definitive, objective criteria for social decisions. This aspiration rested on the claim that the calculus offered unique and universally accepted measures of utility. D'Alembert's arguments about the subjectivity of risk, and about the inherent uncertainties of Bernoulli's calculations, undercut that claim. No doubt, as Daston argues, D'Alembert's challenge marks a defining moment in the history of the probability calculus.[14] But was this the central issue in the debate?

Debates about the notion of moral expectations provide one context for these exchanges. Yet in emphasizing epistemic issues, historians have neglected the more obvious political elements. As Bernoulli tells us repeatedly, he was calculating the benefits of inoculation to the state – an issue that permeated discussions of inoculation in France (in contrast to those in England).[15] If the rational individual's calculus coincides with the state's, so much the better, but this second issue receives little attention from Bernoulli. What about D'Alembert?

For D'Alembert, previous discussions downplayed the state: "One has confused the interest that the State in general may have in inoculation with that which particular individuals may find in it; these two interests may be quite different."[16] He posed the hypothetical case where the mortality from inoculation was one in five but where the survivors lived to 100. In such a situation, the advantage to the state was obvious, but few if any citizens would be "courageous or foolhardy" enough to take the gamble: "For each individual an interest in self-preservation is paramount; the State, by contrast, considers individual citizens impersonally, and in sacrificing one victim among five, it matters little to the State who that victim will be, so long as the other four are saved."[17] From the state's perspective, but only from that perspective, one life is pretty much like another; what matters is the net gain. Bernoulli, D'Alembert charged, counted lives as a state would.[18]

D'Alembert's critics accused him of damaging the cause of inoculation. But D'Alembert opposed neither inoculation nor quantification per se.[19] Like Bernoulli, he called for the collection of more data about inoculation.[20] He objected, rather, to a mode of quantification that required all citizens to subordinate their private calculations of inoculation's risks and benefits to those of the state.

The state, D'Alembert postulated, might have a legitimate interest in promoting inoculation but not in requiring it. It might encourage inoculation by honouring or compensating the families of those who died of the procedure; more directly, it might establish a hospital to provide inoculations to the public. Such actions served the state's purposes "to preserve by any means many hundreds of its citizens." [21] But who would avail themselves of this opportunity? Only those for whom inoculation "is really advantageous, principally men of affairs, persons of the court, and the well-off or prosperous town-dweller."[22]

Was there any group for whom the state's calculus could supplant an individual's? Only abandoned children for whom the state served as a father. Their individual lives were, D'Alembert argued, truly of equal value to the state. Even here, special precautions were necessary, to select inoculees with as much care as a father might vis-à-vis his children. The weak and infirm, those whom inoculation might kill, could not be subjected to the procedure. Doing otherwise would be to follow the "barbarous" example of Sparta, "which condemned crippled or unhealthy newborns to death."[23]

THE MEANING OF "THE STATE"

I have been arguing that D'Alembert's polemics focused as much on Bernoulli's notions of the state as on his failure to appreciate interpersonal differences in attitudes towards risk. More specifically, D'Alembert sought to delimit the sphere in which it was appropriate for a person to think (and act) like a state. Historians have largely ignored these political concerns. Even where they have noted them, as did Hervé Le Bras, they made little attempt to analyse their meaning for D'Alembert and others.[24]

But what are the sources of D'Alembert's animus against thinking like a state? Never known especially for his political writings, D'Alembert withdrew from open political action in the wake of the personal and institutional attack that followed the 1757 publication of his article on Geneva in the *Encyclopédie.*[25] Yet his writing on inoculation challenged the state, but not in conventional eighteenth-century terms about abuses of monarchical power ("despotism") or administrative corruption (the venality of offices). More fundamentally, he articulated the notion of an inherent conflict between the state's interests and the individual's.[26] This brings me to my second puzzle: what could D'Alembert have meant by "L'Etat," or "The State"?

For twenty-five years, American and French scholars have investigated and reconceptualized French political life in the decades leading up to the French Revolution. Much of this work emphasizes the emergence of an elite sphere of civil society that discussed and ultimately challenged the policies of the monarch and the court.[27] Somewhat surprisingly, "L'Etat" (The State), in contrast to "the nation" or "monarchy" and "the king," does not appear as one of the "mot-clès" in this new historiographical lexicon.[28]

Since the mid-seventeenth century, the French state had been intensifying its activities in a number of domains, including taxation, war, and, especially in the eighteenth century, the regulation of political speech. D'Alembert had a special interest in the latter two areas.[29] He admonished his patron, Frederick II of Prussia, for his occasional enthusiasm for military glory. Although he did not reject all military action, the military adventures of "great states" appalled him.[30]

Yet it was D'Alembert's estranged associate Denis Diderot who, in criticizing D'Alembert, invoked the analogy between war and smallpox inoculation. "Consider the case where 100,000 men should fight against 100,000 others, and that at some point there remain only 20,000 from each side on the field of battle? I ask M. d'Alembert if the legislator would not have the right to make him take up the sword or the musket in an instance where the defence of the State is at stake."[31] How, then, Diderot asked, could D'Alembert protest against inoculation, where an identical calculus applied? By encouraging a distinction between individual interests and the good of the nation in the inoculation controversy D'Alembert had shown himself "a fine geometer but a very bad citizen."[32] It is difficult to know how much to make of Diderot's military analogy here. Diderot disdained the military virtues in general and Louis XV's pursuit of the Seven Years' War in particular.[33] His attack came at the height of his quarrels with D'Alembert over the latter's "desertion" from the *Encyclopédie.* Perhaps Diderot, like many polemicists, reached for any argument close to hand. D'Alembert could not reply to the piece, for it remained unpublished until the nineteenth century.[34] His position – that smallpox inoculation was unlike other exercises of state power – none the less seems clear.

The sources of D'Alembert's concerns about the state seem to lie in its regulation of political speech. Episodes include its suppression of the Jesuit order in France; its suspension of the *Encyclopédie,* and debates over the meaning of loyalty and patriotism during the Seven Years' War.[35] In all three cases a particular party or faction captured the monarch's juridical or political apparatus to threaten and/or suppress its opponents, imposing a uniformity of opinion that D'Alembert found abhorrent. Because he wrote most explicitly about the suppression of the Jesuits, I concentrate on his arguments there.[36]

For D'Alembert, the suppression of the Jesuits was a world-historical event. If not on a par with the realignment at mid-century of the

Spanish, Portuguese, and Austrian empires, it reshaped Europe and the world. The Jesuits having created an empire on earth, their history was to be told like that of any mighty empire, once great and now fallen. How, D'Alembert wondered, did they exercise their "sovereign authority?"[37] What impressed D'Alembert about the Jesuits was that they governed without relying on violence. What troubled him was their suppression of individuals when the Society's corporate interests were at stake. Like the ancient Romans, D'Alembert charged, the Jesuits would subordinate (and even sacrifice) individuals in the name of the collective good. Individual minds, individual persons, had no standing with either the Romans or the Jesuits. Both put the health of the collective above all other goods.[38]

In criticizing the Jesuits, D'Alembert referred to classical political history (for example, Rome) – allusions safer and more familiar than contemporary political comment. Much of his argument is simply that of the free-thinker anxious to prevent religious groups from capturing and using the instruments of the state to suppress legitimate discussion.[39] Yet he seems deeply troubled by a society, like that of the Jesuits, in which particular individuals were of no consequence to the collective. And it is just such an imagined society that D'Alembert describes in his quarrel with Bernoulli. For D'Alembert, Bernoulli had suppressed a crucial distinction between the choices facing the individual and those facing the state.

As Elisabeth Badinter has made clear, most of D'Alembert's occasional writing related to the intellectual issues and personal alliances of the moment.[40] In the present state of D'Alembert scholarship – the first volumes of a modern critical edition have just appeared – a reading based on published texts compiled in the nineteenth century has real limitations. Any suggestion that the roots of D'Alembert's views of the state lie in his opinions on religious conscience and ecclesiology remains speculative. None the less, for a writer whose disinterest in the state's formal institutions is well-known, his critiques of corporate religious bodies remain ripe for exploitation.

LEGACIES

Neither Bernoulli's advocacy of inoculation nor D'Alembert's critique had much influence on the Paris *parlement*'s decision of 1763 to ban the procedure.[41] D'Alembert's immediate influence was on the small intellectual community that looked to the probability calculus as a way of ordering social decisions (and thereby ordering society). Thanks to Eric Brian, we know that D'Alembert's arguments posed a continuing dilemma for associates such as his protégé Condorcet.[42]

Condorcet acknowledged the force of D'Alembert's criticism, especially with regard to decisions made on behalf of others, as a parent might decide for a child. When deciding for others, Condorcet insisted, a stricter standard of justice applied: "It is not enough to believe that it will benefit the child in order to expose it to danger; this benefit must be proven. It is futile to evade the difficulty, by deciding that the interests of all should transcend it; such exaggerated patriotism is simply a dangerous illusion, capable of leading ignorant and hot-blooded individuals to commit injustice. No doubt circumstances exist where one might voluntarily sacrifice one's rights to the public good, but to sacrifice the rights of another cannot be just or legitimate."[43] Once again, we return to a political debate about which potential sacrifices could be demanded in the name of the public good. For Condorcet, no method of calculating the value of a life, much less one so crude as life expectancy, could resolve the dilemma identified by D'Alembert.

Despite the force of D'Alembert's critique for some associates, its influence proved short-lived. In inoculation and vaccination, the French lagged noticeably behind other countries in requiring such protection. Yet historians of France have yet to uncover any articulated rationales for such opposition, of the sort familiar to British historians.[44] The subsequent history of vital statistics consists largely of technical debates over the correct mathematical procedures for constructing indices such as life expectancy and mortality rates. In the nineteenth century, people assumed that such measures, correctly calculated, will reveal the underlying truths about the natural laws of sickness and health.[45] D'Alembert's apprehension about the appropriate social order for translating calculations of risk into health policy had evaporated and would not crystallize again until the late twentieth century.

ACKNOWLEDGMENTS

Thanks to Gérard Jorland, George Weisz, Lion Murard and Pierre Crépel for comments on an earlier version, and to David A. Bell for considerable advice on recent historiography. None of the above is responsible for the resulting arguments.

NOTES

1 *San Francisco Chronicle*, 7 Aug. 2002, A22.

2 Jacques Dupaquier et Michel Dupaquier, *Histoire de la démographie* (Paris: Perrin, 1985), 199–250. As the Dupaquiers argue, an interest in life

tables for calculating annuities preceded their application to questions of social condition, which generally began with the political arithmetic movement of the mid-seventeenth century. On political arithmetic, see Peter Buck, "Seventeenth-Century Political Arithmetic: Civil Strife and Vital Statistics," *Isis* 68 (1977), 67–84, and "People Who Counted," *Isis* 73 (1982), 28–45; Eric Brian, *La mesure de l'état : administrateurs et géomètres au XVIIIe siècle* (Paris: Albin Michel, 1994).

3 Genevieve Miller, *The Adoption of Inoculation for Smallpox in England and France* (Philadelphia: University of Pennsylvania Press, 1957), especially 208–10, 225–9. See also Andrea A. Rusnock, *Vital Accounts: Quantifying Population in Eighteenth-Century England and France* (New York: Cambridge University Press, 2002), 77–81.

4 Daniel Bernoulli, "Essai d'une nouvelle analyse de la mortalité causée par la petite Vérole, & des avantages de l'inoculation pour la prevenir," *Académie Royale des Sciences, Mémoires de Mathématique et de Physique* (1760), 1–43. Bernoulli's essay appeared in 1765, and D'Alembert's critique in 1761. For a detailed publication history of the treatises, see Michel Paty, "D'Alembert et les probabilités," in R. Rashed, *Sciences à l'époque de la Révolution française* (Paris: Librairie scientifique et technique Albert Blanchard, 1988), 220–6. On Bernoulli's ties to La Condamine, see Elisabeth Badinter, *Les passions intellectuelles. II Exigence de dignité* 1751–1762 (Paris: Fayard, 2002), 368–9; Rusnock, *Vital Accounts*, 81.

5 Bernoulli, "Nouvelle analyse," 8–9; for the development of the model, see 11–14.

6 Given Halley's data about survivors from other causes of mortality, Bernoulli assumed a constant attack rate and case- fatality rate for smallpox. These assumptions in turn allowed him to determine the number who died of smallpox each year, as well as the number of survivors who had not yet had smallpox and would remain at risk in the next year. See ibid., 14–18, which also discusses adjustments to the model. The resulting table is on 44–5.

7 Ibid., 18–21. For a presentation in English, see Rusnock, *Vital Accounts*, 81–4.

8 Ibid., 26. All translations are mine.

9 Ibid., 30–6, 34.

10 Ibid., 37–8.

11 Jean Le Rond D'Alembert, "On the Duration of Life," in L. Bradley, ed., *Smallpox Inoculation: An Eighteenth Century Controversy* (Nottingham: University of Nottingham, 1971), 68–72.

12 Jean Le Rond D'Alembert, "Eleventh Memoir: On the Application of the Calculus of Probabilities to Inoculation against Smallpox," in Bradley, ed., *Smallpox Inoculation*, 57–61. This memoir, read to the Académie des Sciences in November 1760, appeared in 1761 in D'Alembert's *Opuscules*

mathématiques. In his more extended treatise on inoculation, D'Alembert put slightly greater emphasis than in the 1760 memoir on the uncertainties of Bernoulli's data. See Jean Le Rond D'Alembert, "Réflexions sur l'inoculation," in *Oeuvres de D'Alembert* (Paris: A. Belin, 1821), vol. 1, 468–73 (hereafter *Oeuvres*).

13 D'Alembert, "Réflexions," 484. On intersubjective comparisons of risk, see 468–70, 486–7.

14 Lorraine Daston, *Classical Probability in the Enlightenment* (Princeton, NJ: Princeton University Press, 1988), 82–9; Paty, "D'Alembert et les probabilités." As both Daston and Paty make clear, the specific methodological and epistemological arguments over smallpox were part of a larger series of disputes over how to calculate moral expectation using the probability calculus. Eric Brian, while disagreeing with Daston's reading of D'Alembert's epistemic views on probability, similarly sets the inoculation debate within the epistemic history of probability. Brian, *La mesure de l'état,* 106–11, 124–5. Jean-François de Raymond's brief but wholly descriptive account is unusual in devoting equal space to D'Alembert's arguments about the state: see *Querelle de l'inoculation ou préhistoire de la vaccination* (Paris: Librairie Philosophique J. Vrin, 1982), 100–2.

15 Miller, *Adoption,* 226–8.

16 D'Alembert, "Réflexions," 480.

17 Ibid.

18 Ibid., 480–1.

19 See the approving remarks in Jean Le Rond D'Alembert, "Description abrégé du gouvernment du Genève," in *Oeuvres,* vol. 4, 419.

20 D'Alembert, "Reflexions," 487–9, 503.

21 Ibid., 493.

22 Ibid., 487–90.

23 Ibid., 493–4, quote at 493.

24 Despite its promising title, Hervé Le Bras's discussion similarly says relatively little about the political dimensions of D'Alembert's critique; see "D'Alembert et la querelle de l'inoculation: le sujet contre la population," in *Jean d'Alembert, savant et philosophe : Portrait à plusieurs voix* (Paris: Editions des Archives Contemporaines, 1989), 293–302. Elsewhere Le Bras sees D'Alembert as clinging to an older notion of biologically determined "individual lives," as opposed to newer statistical or demographic notions premised on social intervention. See Hervé Le Bras, *Naissance de la mortalité : l'origine politique de la statistique et la démographie* (Paris: Le Seuill, 2000), 336–42.

25 On this episode, see Ronald Grimsley, *Jean D'Alembert (1717–83)* (Oxford: Clarendon Press, 1963), 52–77; Badinter, *Les passions intellectuelles,* 298–306, 333–6.

26 On despotism, see Orest Ranum, "D'Alembert, Tacitus, and the Political

Sociology of Despotism," in *Studies on Voltaire and the Enlightenment*, vol. 191 (Oxford: Voltaire Foundation, 1980), 547–58. For a slightly later period (1770s), see Keith Michael Baker, "Science and Politics at the End of the Old Regime," and, on corruption, his "French Political Thought at the Accession of Louis XVI," both in Keith Michael Baker, *Inventing the French Revolution: Essays on French Political Culture in the Eighteenth Century* (New York: Cambridge University Press, 1990), 153–66 and 109–27.

27 In Eric Brian's commanding analysis of eighteenth-century quantification, he delineates the crucial movement of data about French population and society from the sphere of administration, where only officials could discuss (and critique) numbers, to the new sphere of "public opinion." Yet somehow he does not directly confront the question of what D'Alembert's contemporaries might have understood by "l'état," as distinct from "administrateurs." Brian's emphasis on the epistemological efforts at quantification means that he downplays juridical or political discussions of "l'état." See Brian, *La mesure de l'état*, 147–51.

28 For example, see Anne-Marie Lecoq, "La symbolique de l'état"; Édouard Pommier, "Versailles, l'image du souverain"; Hélène Himelfarb, "Versailles, fonctions et légendes"; and Pierre Nora, "Les Mémoires de l'État," all in Pierre Nora, ed., *Les lieux de mémoire* (Paris: Gallimard, 1986), 146–292, 356–400. "Nation," "public opinion," "civil society," "absolutism," and "monarchy" figure prominently in other compendia, but not "l'état." See Keith Michael Baker, ed., *The French Revolution and the Creation of Modern Political Culture*, vol. 1: *The Political Culture of the Old Regime* (Oxford: Pergamon Press 1987), 419–536.

29 On the ideological implications of the tax system, see Michael Kwass, *Privilege and the Politics of Taxation in Eighteenth-Century France: Liberté, Égalité, Fiscalité* (New York: Cambridge University Press, 2000). While present-day historians can see the links between war and the expansion of the taxation system, there is no hint of this thinking in D'Alembert.

30 On his exchanges with Frederick II, see Grimsley, *Jean D'Alembert*, 167–8. See also his chastisement of Bossuet for having failed to object to Louis XIV's wars. Jean Le Rond D'Alembert, "Éloge de Bossuet," in *Oeuvres*, vol. 2, 26. On small and large states, and the occasions when defensive wars are legitimate, see D'Alembert, "Description abrégé du gouvernment du Genève," 414–15.

31 Denis Diderot, "De l'inoculation," in *Oeuvres complètes* (Paris: Hermann, 1975), vol. 2, 360. According to Jeff Loveland, Diderot published his arguments in Grimmn's *Correspondence.* See Diderot, "Mathematics and Practice: Diderot and d'Alembert Argue Probability," *Studies in Eighteen-Century Culture* 25 (1996), 99–116. But cf. Meyer (n. 34) below. Like

other commentators on the inoculation controversy, Loveland interprets the quarrel as one about the nature of probability, not a political quarrel about the state.

32 Diderot, "De l'inoculation."

33 Edmond Dziembowski, "Un nouveau patriotisme français, 1750–1770," *Studies on Voltaire and the Eighteenth Century* 365 (Oxford: Voltaire Foundation, 1998), 116–19.

34 Jean Meyer, "Diderot et le calcul des probabilités," *Revue d'histoire des sciences* 44 (1991), 386–8.

35 For the suspension of the *Encyclopédie*, see Grimsley, *Jean D'Alembert*, 52–77. On the intensification of royalist propaganda during the Seven Years' War, see David A. Bell, *The Cult of the Nation in France: Inventing Nationalism, 1680–1800* (Cambridge, Mass.: Harvard University Press, 2001), 78–101; see also Dziembowski, *Un nouveau patriotisme français.*

36 My reading differs substantially from the standard source on the suppression of the Jesuits: Dale van Kley, *The Jansenists and the Expulsion of the Jesuits from France 1757–1765* (New Haven, Conn.: Yale University Press, 1975). In taking D'Alembert as a simple anti-clerical spokesman for the philosophes, van Kley fails to appreciate D'Alembert's ambivalence about the Jesuits and his repeated allusions to their world-historical role.

37 Jean Le Rond D'Alembert, "Sur la destruction des Jésuites," in *Oeuvres*, vol. 2, 15–8.

38 Ibid., 24–6. On the lack of violence, see 18.

39 D'Alembert makes this clear when he describes the Jansenists as a far greater threat to intellectual freedom than the Jesuits. "Sur la destruction," 67. See also the discussions in "De l'abus de la critique en matière de religion," in *Oeuvres*, vol. 1, 547–72; and "Eloge de Montesquieu," in *Oeuvres*, vol. 3, 440–66. In both, D'Alembert makes clear his intense dislike for state intervention in support of one creed or dogma over another.

40 Badinter, *Les passions intellectuelles*, vol. 2, *Exigence de dignité.*

41 Rusnock, *Vital Accounts*, 89–91.

42 Brian, *La mesure de l'état*, 124–5.

43 Marquis de Condorcet, "Eloge de D'Alembert," in *Oeuvres*, vol. 1, xxi.

44 But note possible echoes of D'Alembert in the remarks of J.-J. Paulet, a critic of inoculation, cited in Jean-Pierre Peter, "Les médecins français au problème de l'inoculation variolique et de sa diffusion (1750–1790)," *Annales de Bretagne* 86 (1979), 262. For the late nineteenth century, Lion Murad and Patrick Zylberman, "Education ou contrainte: La vaccination antivariolique en France à la Belle Epoque," *History and Philosophy of the Life Sciences* 17 (1995), 31–53.

45 For the subsequent methodological history of the life table, see Jacques et Michel Dupaquier, *Histoire de la démographie*, 242–9, 354–92; Anne M. Fagot, "Probabilities and Causes: On Life Tables, Cause of Death and Etiological Diagnoses," in Jaakko Hintikka, David Gruender, and Eduardo Agazzi, eds., *Pisa Conference on the History and Philosophy of Science: Proceedings*, vol. 2 (Dordrecht: D. Reidel, 1980), 41–104; John M. Eyler, *Victorian Social Medicine: The Ideas and Methods of William Farr* (Baltimore, Md.: Johns Hopkins University Press, 1979), 66–96.

4

Quantifying Infant Mortality in England and France, 1750–1800

ANDREA RUSNOCK

The earliest sustained calculations of infant mortality were made during the latter half of the eighteenth century in England and France as part of larger efforts to quantify mortality and to examine changes in mortality patterns. Government officials and physicians played leading roles within this new area of inquiry, often referred to as medical or political arithmetic. They introduced numerical methods for establishing how many infants died of those born within a given year and thus created a measure of infant mortality. Their calculations revealed not only high numbers of infant deaths, but also variations in infant mortality linked to both environmental and social conditions.

The emergence of infant mortality figures as a significant measure of health is generally thought to have occurred in the second half of the nineteenth century. Historians have discussed the use of infant mortality figures during this period to justify state intervention in infant welfare and family life. This paper outlines an earlier eighteenth-century tradition of calculating infant mortality that informed contemporary efforts to improve the health of babies.[1]

The high rate of mortality revealed by this eighteenth-century form of quantification contributed to a dramatic shift in public concern for infants' welfare. The signs of this shift were numerous and diverse. Parents invested more emotional and physical resources into each individual child, as evidenced by the growing number of children's toys and books, changes in naming practices, and initiatives on childhood education.[2] Calls – most famously by Rousseau – were made to mothers to breastfeed their babies rather than farm them out to wet-nurses.[3] The emergence of a humanitarian ethic that morally compelled individuals to improve the living conditions of the less fortunate – including foundlings – reflected the new emphasis on the health and well-being of infants.[4] And initiatives such as the royal sponsorship of Madame du Coudray to train French midwives underlined the state's growing interest – driven in part by its commitment to a large population as essential to national strength and prosperity.[5]

Underlying this growing concern for infant welfare were Enlightenment attitudes about change and a widespread belief in the agency of humans to bring about change. Infant lives could be saved through the education of midwives, better feeding practices (nursing by mothers or, if necessary, well-paid wet-nurses), improved maternal care, inoculation against smallpox, and ameliorated environmental conditions.[6] Both national- and local-government initiatives paralleled private charitable efforts to encourage the adoption and spread of these enlightened practices. And infant mortality figures informed these efforts.[7]

This essay focuses on English and French writers of the second half of the eighteenth century working within the tradition of medical and political arithmetic who provided some of the earliest calculations of infant mortality. The first section discusses methods of calculation in an era before governments collected vital statistics on a regular basis. Without reliable vital statistics, arithmeticians had to develop indirect methods of calculating infant mortality. The second section treats the repercussions of quantification – namely a significant shift towards environmental explanations for the large number of infant deaths. Variations in infant mortality led arithmeticians to examine contributing factors to these differences. Their investigations suggested that climate, season, geography, gender, and the level of maternal care had measurable effects on infant mortality. The final section presents two case studies in which infant mortality figures had pronounced social effects: the treatment of foundlings and the recommended age to inoculate infants against smallpox.

CALCULATING INFANT MORTALITY

Precursors

Infant mortality was first quantified by the English shopkeeper John Graunt (1620–1674). In 1662, Graunt published *Natural and Political Observations Made upon the London Bills of Mortality*. As one of the pioneering works in the history of statistics and demography, Graunt's book laid the foundation for a quantitative study of society. Graunt provided numbers for the total population of London, the mortality rates for different diseases (including plague), the ratio between the sexes, and measures of longevity. He based his calculations on the London bills of mortality, a unique source of numerical information dating back to the sixteenth century. Initially compiled to record the weekly number of burials due to plague in London, the bills, beginning in 1629, listed other causes of death as well as the number of christenings.

Graunt used this new information creatively to tally the burials attributed to diseases primarily affecting infants and children. These included "Thrush, Convulsion, Rickets, Teeth, and Worms ... Abortives, Chrysomes, Infants, Liver-grown and Over-laid."[8] From 1629 through 1636, and for 1647 through 1660, Graunt discovered that infants and children accounted for one-third of the total number of deaths per year (see Figure 1). As Graunt's table shows, he did not group infant diseases together; instead he listed causes of death alphabetically, just as they appeared in the original bills of mortality.

While Graunt identified a high number of infant deaths, he had little to say about this figure. In passing he mentioned that wet-nurses occasionally starved their charges, while children in London were less healthy because of the "Smoaks, Stinks, and close Air."[9] By contrast, he devoted several chapters of his short treatise to the plague, the dreaded disease that dominated perceptions of the mortality landscape as well as government efforts at public health.[10]

Medical Arithmetic, 1750–1800

Little notice was taken of Graunt's calculation of infant mortality until the mid-eighteenth century. After 1750, in both England and France, quantitative studies of population, mortality patterns, and other vital events multiplied. Public debates about depopulation, smallpox inoculation, and the effects of climate on health proved fertile ground for medical and political arithmetic.[11] In England, physicians such as Thomas Short (1690?-1772), William Heberden the younger (1767–1845), and William Black (1749–1829) extended Graunt's approach of analysing the London bills of mortality over time in order to calculate infant mortality, along with other vital events. These medical arithmeticians supplemented their analyses of the London bills with figures drawn from parish registers, hospital records, and dispensaries.

In France, government officials such as the *intendant* Antoine Auget, baron de Montyon (1733–1820), and his secretary, Jean-Baptiste Moheau (1745–1794), and the economist Jacques-Antoine Mourgue

Figure 1 From John Graunt, *Natural and Political Observations made upon the London Bills of Mortality* (1662)

The Table of C A S U A L T I E S

The Years of our Lord	*1647*	*1648*	*1649*	*1650*	*1651*	*1652*	*1653*	*1654*	*1655*	*1656*	*1657*	*1658*	*1659*	*1660*
Abortive and Still-born	335	329	327	351	389	381	384	433	483	419	463	467	421	544
Aged	916	835	889	696	780	834	864	974	743	892	869	1176	909	1095
Ague and Fever	1260	884	751	970	1038	1212	282	1371	689	875	999	1800	2303	2148
Apoplex and Suddenly	68	74	64	74	106	111	118	86	92	102	113	138	91	67
Bleach	-	-	1	3	7	2	-	-	-	1	-	-	-	-
Blasted	4	1	-	-	6	6	-	-	4	-	5	5	3	8
Bleeding	3	2	5	1	3	4	3	2	7	3	5	4	7	2
Bloody Flux, Scouring and Flux	155	176	802	289	833	762	200	386	168	368	362	233	346	251
Burnt and Scalded	3	6	10	5	11	8	5	7	10	5	7	4	6	6
Calenture	1	-	-	1	-	2	1	1	-	-	3	-	-	-
Cancer, Gangrene and Fistula	26	29	31	19	31	53	36	37	73	31	24	35	63	52
Wolf	-	-	-	8										
Canker, Sore-mouth and Thrush	66	28	54	42	68	51	33	72	44	81	19	27	73	68
Child-bed	161	106	114	117	306	213	158	192	177	301	236	225	226	104
Chrisoms and Infants	1369	1254	1065	990	1237	1280	1050	1343	1089	1393	1162	1144	838	1123
Colick and Wind	103	71	85	82	76	102	80	101	85	120	113	179	116	167
Cold and Cough	-	-	-	-	-	-	41	36	21	58	30	31	33	24
Consumption and Cough	2423	2200	2388	1988	2350	2410	2286	2868	2606	3184	2757	3610	2982	3414
Convulsion	684	491	530	493	569	653	606	828	702	1027	807	841	743	1031
Cramp	-	-	1	-	-	-	-	-	-	-	-	-	-	-
Cut of the Stone	-	2	1	3	-	1	1	3	4	1	3	5	6	4
Dropsie and Tympany	185	434	421	508	444	557	617	704	660	706	631	931	646	872
Drowned	47	40	30	27	49	50	53	30	43	49	63	60	57	48
Excessive drinking	-	-	2											
Executed	8	17	29	43	24	12	19	21	19	22	20	18	7	18
Fainted in a Bath	-	-	-	-	1									
Falling-Sickness	3	2	2	3	-	3	4	1	4	3	1	-	4	5
Flox[1] and small Pox	139	400	1190	184	525	1279	139	812	1294	823	835	409	1523	354
Found dead in the Street	6	6	9	8	7	9	14	4	3	4	9	11	3	6
French-Pox	18	29	15	18	21	20	20	20	29	23	25	53	51	31
Frighted	4	4	1	-	3	-	2	-	1	1	-	-	-	9
Gout	9	5	12	9	7	7	5	6	8	7	8	13	14	2
Grief	12	13	16	7	17	14	11	17	10	13	10	12	13	4
Hanged and made-away themselves	11	10	13	14	9	14	15	9	14	16	24	18	11	36
Head-Ach	-	1	11	2	-	2	6	6	5	3	4	5	35	26
Jaundice	57	35	39	49	41	43	57	71	61	41	46	77	102	76

The Years of our Lord	*1629*	*1630*	*1631*	*1632*	*1633*	*1634*	*1635*	*1636*	*1629 1630 1631 1632*	*1633 1634 1635 1630*	*1647 1648 1649 1650*	*1651 1652 1653 1654*	*1655 1656 1657 1658*	*1629 1649 1659*	*In 20 Years.*
Abortive and Still-born	499	439	430	445	500	475	507	523	1793	2005	1342	1587	1832	1247	8559
Aged	579	712	661	671	704	623	794	714	2475	2814	3336	3452	3680	2377	15759
Ague and Fever	956	1091	1115	1108	953	1279	1622	2360	4418	6235	3865	4903	4363	4010	23784
Apoplex and Suddenly	22	36		17	24	35	26	-	75	85	280	421	445	177	1306
Bleach	-	-	-	-	-	-	-	-	-	-	4	9	1	1	15
Blasted	13	8	10	13	6	4	-	4	54	14	5	12	14	16	99
Bleeding	5	2	5	4	4	3	-	-	16	7	11	12	19	17	65
Bloody Flux, Scouring and Flux	449	438	352	348	278	512	346	330	1587	1466	1422	2181	1161	1597	7818
Burnt and Scalded	3	10	7	5	1	3	12	3	25	19	24	31	26	19	125
Calenture	-	-	-	-	-	-	1	3	-	4	2	4	3	-	13
Cancer, Gangrene and Fistula	30	14	23	28	27	30	24	30	85	112	105	157	150	114	609
Wolf					-	-	-	-	-	8	-	-	-	-	8
Canker, Sore-mouth and Thrush	6	4	4	1	-	-	5	74	15	79	190	244	161	133	689
Child-bed	150	157	113	171	132	143	163	230	590	668	498	769	839	490	3364
Chrisoms and Infants	2596	2378	2035	2268	2130	2315	2113	1895	9277	8453	4678	4910	4788	4519	32100
Colick and Wind	48	57	-	-	-	-	37	50	105	87	341	359	497	247	1380
Cold and Cough	10	58	51	55	45	54	50	57	174	207	00	77	140	43	598
Consumption and Cough	1827	1910	1713	1797	1754	1955	2080	2477	5157	8266	8999	9914	12157	7197	44487
Convulsion	52	87	18	241	221	386	418	709	498	1764	2198	2656	3377	1324	9073
Cramp	-	-	3	0	0	0	0	0	01	00	01	0	0	1	2
Cut of the Stone	-	-	-	5	1	5	2	2	5	10	6	4	13	47	38
Dropsie and Tympany	235	252	279	280	266	250	329	389	1048	1734	1538	2321	2982	1302	9623
Drowned	43	33	29	34	37	32	33	45	139	147	144	182	215	130	827
Excessive drinking					-	-	-	-	-	-	2	-	-	2	2
Executed	19	13	12	18	13	13	13	13	62	52	97	76	79	55	384
Fainted in a Bath					-	-	-	-	-	-	-	1	-	-	1
Falling-Sickness	3	10	7	7	2	5	6	8	27	21	10	8	8	9	74
Flox[1] and small Pox	72	40	58	531	72	1354	293	127	701	1846	1913	2755	3361	2785	10576
Found dead in the Street	18	33	20	6	13	8	24	24	83	69	29	34	27	29	243
French-Pox	17	12	12	12	7	17	12	22	53	48	80	81	130	83	392
Frighted	1	-	-	1	-	-	-	3	2	3	9	5	2	2	21
Gout	2	5	3	4	4	5	7	8	14	24	35	25	36	28	134
Grief	18	20	22	11	14	17	5	20	71	56	48	59	45	47	279
Hanged and made-away themselves	8	8	6	15	-	3	8	7	37	18	48	47	72	32	222
Head-Ach	-	-	-	-	-	-	4	2	0	6	14	14	17	46	051
Jaundice	47	59	35	43	35	45	54	63	184	197	180	215	225	188	998

Jaw-faln	1	1	-	-	3	-	-	3	2	-	3	1	-	-	10	16	13	8	10	10	4	11	47	35	02	5	6	10	95
Impostume	75	61	65	59	80	105	79	90	92	122	80	134	105	96	58	76	73	74	50	62	73	130	282	315	260	35	428	228	1639
Itch	-	1																	10	-	-	-	00	10	01	-	-	-	11
Killed by several Accidents	27	57	39	94	47	45	57	58	52	43	52	47	55	47	54	55	47	46	49	41	51	60	202	201	217	207	194	148	1021
King's Evil	27	26	22	19	22	20	26	26	27	24	23	28	28	54	16	25	18	38	35	20	20	69	97	150	94	94	102	66	537
Lethargy	3	4	2	4	4	4	3	10	9	4	6	2	6	4	1	-	2	2	3	-	2	2	5	7	13	21	21	9	67
Leprosie	-	-	1	-	-	-	-	-	-	-	-	1	-	2	2	-	-	-	-	-	2	-	2	2	1	-	1	3	06
Liver-grown, Spleen and Rickets	53	46	56	59	65	72	67	65	52	50	38	51	8	15	94	12	99	87	82	77	98	99	392	356	213	269	191	158	1421
Lunatick	12	18	6	11	7	11	9	12	6	7	13	5	14	14	6	11	6	5	4	2	2	5	28	13	47	39	31	26	158
Meagrom	12	13	-	5	8	6	6	14	3	6	7	6	5	4	-	-	24	-	-	-	-	22	24	22	30	34	232	05	132
Measles	5	92	3	33	33	62	8	52	11	153	15	80	6	74	42	2	3	80	21	33	27	12	127	83	133	155	259	51	757
Mother	2	-	-	-	-	1	1	2	2	3	-	3	1	8	1	-	-	-	-	-	-	3	01	3	2	4	8	02	18
Murdered	3	2	7	5	4	3	3	3	9	6	5	7	70	20	-	-	3	7	-	6	5	8	10	12	17	13	27	77	86
Overlaid and Starved at Nurse	25	22	36	28	28	29	30	36	58	53	44	50	46	43	4	10	13	7	8	14	10	14	34	46	111	123	215	86	529
Palsie	27	21	19	20	23	20	29	18	22	23	20	32	17	31	17	23	17	25	14	21	25	17	82	77	87	90	87	53	423
Plague	3597	611	67	15	23	16	6	16	9	6	4	14	36	14	-	1317	274	8	-	1	-	10400	1599	10401	4290	61	33	103	16384
Plague in the Guts	-	-	-	1	-	110	32	-	87	315	446	-	253	402	-	-	-	-	-	-	-	-	00	00	61	142	844	253	991
Pleurisie	30	26	13	30	23	19	17	23	10	9	17	16	12	10	26	24	26	36	21	-	45	24	112	90	89	72	52	51	415
Poisoned	-	3	-	7															2	-	-	2	00	4	10	00	00	00	14
Purples and Spotted Fever	145	47	43	65	54	60	75	89	56	52	36	126	368	146	32	58	58	38	24	125	245	397	186	791	300	278	290	243	1845
Quinsie and Sore-throat	14	11	12	17	24	20	18	9	15	13	7	10	21	14	1	8	6	7	24	04	5	22	22	55	54	71	45	34	247
Rickets	150	224	216	190	260	329	229	372	347	458	317	476	441	521	-	-	-	-	-	14	49	50	00	113	780	1190	1598	657	3681
Mother, rising of the Lights	150	92	115	120	134	138	135	178	166	212	203	228	310	249	44	72	99	98	60	84	72	104	309	220	777	585	809	369	2700
Rupture	16	7	7	6	7	16	7	15	11	20	19	18	12	28	3	6	4	9	4	3	10	13	21	30	36	45	68	21	201
Scal'd head	2	-	-	-	1	-	-	-	2										-	-	-	-	-	-	2	1	2	-	05
Scurvy	32	20	21	21	29	43	41	44	103	71	82	82	95	12	5	7	9	-	9	-	00	25	33	34	94	132	300	115	593
Smothered and stifled		-	-	2	-	-	-	-	-	-	-	-	-	-	-	-	24	-	-	-	-	-	24	-	2	-	-	2	26
Sores, ulcers, broken and bruised limbs	15	17	17	16	26	32	25	32	23	34	40	47	61	48	23	-	20	48	19	19	22	29	91	89	65	115	144	141	504
Shot	-	-	-	-	-	-	-	-	-	-	-	-	7	20	-	-	-	-	-	-	-	-	-	-	-	-	-	07	27
Spleen	12	17	-	-	-	-	13	13	-	6	2	5	7	7	-	-	-	-	-	-	-	-	-	-	29	26	13	07	68
Shingles	-	-	-	-	-	-	-	-	-	-	-	-	1	-	-	-	-	-	-	-	-	-	-	1	-	-	-	1	2
Starved	-	4	8	7	1	2	1	1	3	1	3	6	7	14	-	-	-	-	-	-	-	-	14	-	19	5	13	29	51
Stitch				1															-	-	-	-	-	-	1	-	-	-	1
Stone and Strangury	45	42	29	28	50	41	44	38	49	57	72	69	42	30	35	39	58	50	58	49	33	45	114	185	144	173	247	51	937
Sciatica	-	-	-	-	-	-	-	-	-	-	-	-	-	2	-	-	-	1	3	-	1	6	1	4	-	-	-	-	13
Stopping of the Stomach	29	29	30	33	55	67	66	107	94	145	129	277	186	214	-	-	-	-	-	-	-	6	-	6	121	295	247	216	669
Surfet	217	137	136	121	104	177	178	212	128	161	137	218	202	192	63	157	149	86	104	114	132	371	445	721	613	671	644	401	3094
Swine-Pox	4	4	3	-	-	-	1	4	2	1	1	1	2	-	5	8	4	6	3	-	10	-	23	13	11	5	5	10	57
Teeth and Worms	767	597	540	598	709	905	691	1131	803	1198	878	1036	839	1008	440	506	335	470	432	454	539	1207	1751	2632	2502	3436	3915	1819	14236
Tissick	62	47	-	-	-	-	-	-	-	-	-	-	-	-	8	12	14	34	23	15	27	-	68	65	109	-	-	8	242
Thrush	-	-	-	-	-	-	-	-	-	-	37	66	-	-	15	23	17	40	28	31	34	-	95	93	-	-	123	15	211
Vomiting	1	6	3	7	4	6	3	14	7	27	16	19	8	10	1	4	1	1	2	5	6	3	7	16	17	27	69	12	136
Worms	147	107	105	65	85	86	53	-	-	-	-	-	-	-	19	31	28	27	19	28	27	-	105	74	424	224	-	124	830
Wen	1	-	1	-	2	2	-	-	1	-	1	2	1	1	-	-	1	-	4	-	-	-	1	4	2	4	4	2	15
Suddenly	-	-	-	-	-	-	-	-	-	-	-	-	-	-	63	59	37	62	58	62	78	34	221	233	-	-	-	63	454
																												34190	229250

(1738–1818) relied on tallies of births and deaths culled from parish registers throughout the country. The registers had been collected in response to an official request made by Controller-General abbé Joseph Marie Terray in 1772. Using these sources, French arithmeticians, like their English counterparts, were able to bring more numbers to the growing debate on infant mortality.

But one of the most difficult obstacles faced by eighteenth-century arithmeticians concerned the accuracy of their sources. Graunt was acutely aware that his calculation of infant mortality was only an estimate. He knew that not all births and deaths in London were recorded. Moreover, the "searchers" – the women who informed parish clerks of the cause of death – were not always consistent, careful, or well-informed in their assessments.[12] None the less, Graunt argued that the bills provided a rough guide to the patterns of life and death in London – but only for London. No other set of records in seventeenth- and eighteenth-century England or France contained such extensive information on the *cause* of death. Such vital statistics allowed English arithmeticians to address medical concerns more directly than their French counterparts.

A far more common source of numbers for calculating infant mortality in the eighteenth century was Church of England parish registers. In principle, these books recorded all christenings and burials, but, in practice, under-registration was common. In areas with large numbers of religious non-conformists (i.e., non-Anglicans) they were particularly inadequate. Hence the births and deaths of Jews, Catholics, Quakers, Baptists, and other dissenters were not listed.[13] Nevertheless, medical and political arithmeticians were able to quantify births and deaths for specific communities, and they frequently estimated the number of such events that were not recorded.

A comparison of William Black's and Jean-Baptiste Moheau's calculations of infant mortality nicely illustrates the strengths and limitations of each of these various sources. In 1789, Black, who received his MD from Leiden, published *An Arithmetical and Medical Analysis of the Diseases and Mortality of the Human Species.* His analysis depended extensively on the London bills of mortality. Moheau (probably with Montyon's assistance) wrote *Recherches et considérations sur la population de la France* in 1778. Moheau compiled this masterpiece in early demography from the accounts of christenings and burials made by parish clergymen and forwarded to the *intendants.* He supplemented these figures with local censuses, numbers from hospital records, and calculations from other writers.[14]

Black based his calculation of infant mortality primarily on 75 years of the London bills of mortality (1701–76) (see Figure 2). Beginning in 1728, the bills began to include age of death. This allowed Black to determine precisely the number of infant deaths. (Graunt had had to infer infant deaths from particular causes, which he assumed struck mostly, if not only, infants and young children.) Black then arranged the causes of death by category, not alphabetically, as the parish clerks and Graunt had done. At the beginning of his table, Black listed acute, febrile diseases (ague, fevers, smallpox, measles). In the middle of the first page of the chart, he grouped together stomach and intestinal diseases (vomiting, colic, gripes, flux). Diseases affecting primarily infants and children began at the top of the second page of the chart, including Abortion and Stillborn, Chrisoms and Infants ("an obsolete term, denoting the deaths in the first month after birth"),[15] convulsions, and teeth. The conclusion of Black's arrangement was plainly visible: a high number of infant and child deaths. Convulsions accounted for the greatest percentage of deaths on the bills.

By contrast, Moheau, a French government official, organized his tables according to age of death, not cause of death, reflecting the information in parish registers, which usually did not list cause of death. In one table, Moheau grouped deaths into intervals, with the smallest for the youngest ages. The first interval (*dans la première année*) contained twice as many deaths as the subsequent interval (ages 2–3). The findings echoed Black's and demonstrated the high level of infant and child mortality in France.

Both men showed the great mortality that occurred during the first year of life. Independently, they found that one in four infants died before the age of one.[16] Their explanations were remarkably similar. Each emphasized the fragility or precariousness of life in the first year. They likened the newborn's body to a young plant: weak, delicate, and vulnerable. As the child grew older, they believed, the body hardened and was able to resist changes in climate and seasons.[17]

The London bills of mortality and the English and French parish registers classified miscarriages and stillbirths inconsistently. Stillbirths and infants who died soon after birth (and before being christened) frequently did not appear in parish registers, or appeared as burials, but not christenings. Furthermore, the difference between the biological event (birth of a child) and the spiritual event (christening) became significant, not only for the numbers, but for the categories of life and death. The ambiguous status of stillbirth deeply troubled eighteenth-century arithmeticians. It was a birth and yet not a new life; it was a death without life.

Graunt and his followers worked with the popular terms "abortive" (i.e., miscarriage) and "stillborn" found in the London bills of

Figure 2 From William Black, An Arithmetical and Medical Analysis of the Diseases and Mortality of the Human Species (1789)

A CHART of all the Fatal Diseases and Casualties in London, during 75 Years; beginning from 1701, and ending with 1776.

Collected from the London Bills of Mortality, and arranged into Five separate progressive Periods of Fifteen Years each. The Total Amount of the Five Periods, or Seventy-five Years Mortality, is added together in the Sixth Column.

Diseases and Casualties	*Fifteen years, from 1701 to 1717*	*From 1717 to 1732*	*From 1732 to 1747*	*From 1747 to 1762*	*From 1762 to 1777*	*Total amount of seventy-five years Mortality from 1701 to 1777*
Ague	80	198	82	99	109	574
Fevers, malignant, spotted, scarlet and purple	50,955	53,330	57,995	45,621	48,594	256,085
Small Pox	22,219	34,448	29,462	29,165	36,276	151,570
Measles	1,972	2,618	2,858	3,099	3,319	13,866
Quinsy, Sore Throat	226	169	287	306	309	1,297
Pleurisy	384	602	811	407	321	3,525
Rheumatism	368	447	310	175	128	1,468
Gout	318	645	769	803	1,010	3,236
Consumption	42,541	49,680	66,009	61,749	68,949	288,928
Chin Cough, Hooping Cough, Cough	116	632	1,692	2,755	4,252	9,573
Asthma and Tissick	5,090	7,938	9,460	5,699	6,154	34,341
Apoplexy and Suddenly	2,228	3,013	3,287	3,271	3,353	15,152
Palsy	332	550	621	1,021	1,020	3,544
Lethargy	105	126	116	105	74	526
Meagrims	13	10	-	-	-	23
Headach	21	32	6	18	-	77
Lunatick	412	513	777	1,126	1,048	3,876
Spleen and Vapours	53	52	20	-	-	125
Rising of the Lights	1,219	1,239	197	39	10	2,074
Stoppage of the Stomach	4,139	2,557	2,286	304	179	9,465
Vomiting and Looseness	820	682	248	134	120	2,004
Cholic, Gripes, and Twisting of the Guts	13,668	11,032	3,739	1,475	796	29,710
Flux	178	200	-	252	341	971
Bloody Flux	133	248	167	94	93	745
Worms	697	662	161	115	56	1,691
Jaundice	1,261	1,798	2,032	1,729	2,089	8,909
Gravel, Stone and Strangury	789	868	700	421	429	3,205
Diabetes	37	48	19	16	5	125
Dropsy and Tympany	11,626	15,430	16,036	13,410	14,038	70,506
Livergrown	76	95	75	23	-	269
French Pox	917	1,372	1,663	997	1,016	5,965
Scurvy	63	28	14	59	42	226
Evil	1,020	919	426	197	198	2,360
Leprosy	19	53	69	39	15	195

Figure 2 (continued)

Diseases and Casualties	*Fifteen years, from 1701 to 1717*	*From 1717 to 1732*	*From 1732 to 1747*	*From 1747 to 1762*	*From 1762 to 1777*	*Total amount of seventy-five years Mortality from 1701 to 1777*
Rash	77	128	47	59	24	341
Itch	-	-	42	31	11	84
Childbed	3,560	3,894	3,412	3,005	3,186	17,057
Abortion and Stillborn	8,746	10,231	8,793	8,820	10,241	46,831
Chrisoms and Infants	850	315	606	-	-	1,771
Miscarriage	-	-	47	56	49	152
Convulsions	91,660	114,718	111,966	85,196	89,221	492,761
Headmold-shot and water in the head	609	2,374	2,013	1,022	337	6,335
Teeth	18,478	25,199	20,274	13,978	11,918	89,847
Thrush	839	1,191	1,512	1,391	1,101	6,034
Scald Head	9	15	29	22	-	75
Rickets	3,916	1,383	954	112	104	6,569
Inflammation	8	67	698	894	1,394	3,061
Imposthume	790	694	387	191	84	2,130
St. Anthony's Fire	-	73	36	63	69	241
Gangrene and Mortification	1,071	2,857	3,362	3,083	3,023	13,438
Canker	138	181	123	77	61	580
Cancer	1,041	1,059	774	682	719	2,475
Sores and Ulcers	695	485	402	253	236	2,071
Fistula	360	208	210	134	119	1,025
Bursten and Ruptures	310	309	304	163	140	1,226
Swelling and Wen	6	-	47	49	37	139
Killed by Falls, Bruises, Fractures and other Accidents	828	917	926	1,084	1,065	4,820
Self-murder	445	667	693	555	509	2,869
Murdered	132	109	147	71	77	539
Stabbed, Killed, Wounded, Shot, etc.	13	32	13	-	-	60
Executed	-	-	495	495	1,020	-
Drowned	900	1,193	1,444	1,718	1,781	7,043
Burnt	90	54	90	127	132	493
Scalded	15	36	45	51	40	191
Stifled, Suffocated and Smothered	16	34	62	90	68	276
Overlaid	814	1,180	1,293	414	95	3,799
Found dead	386	547	668	336	133	2,082
Grief	-	267	-	87	77	421
Frightened	-	14	8	13	2	45
Surfeits	684	131	59	31	27	133
Starved	-	17	96	53	57	223
Excessive Drinking	19	267	678	189	69	1,222
Bleeding	80	69	57	70	114	397
Poisoned	-	7	7	24	10	40
Bit by Mad Dogs and Cats	-	3	14	15	6	38
Bedridden	-	104	-	56	105	265
Aged	27,333	34,708	30,058	25,109	22,032	139,248

mortality. Graunt doubted whether the searchers had accurately distinguished between the two terms and questioned their use of "infant." While many people considered an infant to be a child under the age of one, Graunt emphasized the ability to speak: "For, I say, it is somewhat to know how many die usually before they can speak, or how many live past any assigned number."[18]

In the mid-eighteenth century, Thomas Short, a physician who practised in Sheffield, modelled his extensive analysis of the London bills of mortality from the early seventeenth century until 1750 on Graunt's work. Short argued that the eighteenth-century bills did not regularly record abortives and stillbirths but did not explain this supposed change in recording practices, which he thought accounted for the decrease in reported infant deaths between 1700 and 1750.[19]

By 1800 William Black had reassessed the classification and meaning of abortives and stillborn, as well as the addition of miscarriages as a category in the London bills. Black was affiliated with the General Dispensary for Poor Married Women in London, where he had observed that miscarriages were most common between the third and fifth months of pregnancy. Because of this relatively early onset, such events would not appear in the bills. "In all probability," Black concluded, "a very great majority of the registered abortives and stillborn in London, had arrived at or near the full period of uterine maturity."[20]

Today demographers and epidemiologists have refined the category of infant mortality into perinatal, neonatal, infant, and child mortality, in order to define more precisely the causes for premature death.[21] In the eighteenth century, physicians tried to make sense of these ambiguous events. Only near-full-term miscarriages or stillbirths were, in Black's view, "thought deserving of formal interment" and hence would be recorded in a church document of burials. Black continued: "To carry a diminutive embryo, a Lilliputian in miniature, to a churchyard, and to bury it with funeral pomp and obsequies, would be ridiculous."[22] None the less, Black thought that the bills should record stillbirths. So, too, did Moheau. In his discussion of a model register that would list causes of death, Moheau placed *enfans mort-nés* as the first type of natural death.[23]

DEVELOPING ENVIRONMENTAL EXPLANATIONS

While Black and Moheau stressed infants' biological weakness to account for the large number of deaths, they also pointed to variations in mortality, which suggested other causes. Their late-eighteenth-century project to quantify infant mortality thus contained an inherent paradox: arithmeticians established a universal figure (25 per cent of all infants born perished) – Black "endeavoured to establish the mortality of the human species at different ages" – yet documented quantitative differences in infant mortality rates depending on geography, season, gender, and social class.[24]

Geography was the single most investigated factor. Arithmeticians considered numerous variations – urban versus rural environments, mountainous versus swampy villages, and cold versus warm climates. Moheau, for example, noted that infant mortality was greater in Sweden than in France, which fact he ascribed to Sweden's cold, harsh climate.[25] Such environmental reasoning reflected a resurgence of Hippocratic ideas.[26] Airs, waters, and places seemed determinative for patterns of health and illness.

All arithmeticians agreed that cities were more deadly to infants than the countryside. Many blamed air quality: Graunt had attributed a higher number of infant and child deaths in London to "smoaks, stinks, and close Air." To demonstrate the ill effects, Black compiled a set of tables listing mortality figures for different ages from several European cities (London, Vienna, Berlin) as well as from small parishes in England, Switzerland, and Brandenburg. These tables clearly showed greater infant mortality in large cities.[27] "Here," Black observed, "is an astonishing disparity between the prospects of city and country life, in the early stages of puerile existence. Infants in cities resemble tender plants excluded from fresh air, or fish confined to stagnant water; and [they] perish before they can acquire a solidity and seasoning to endure the adulterated quality of the surrounding element."[28]

Air quality was dependent not only on geography, but also on the time of year. Arithmeticians in both England and France focused on seasonal changes in infant mortality. Moheau, for example, calculated monthly variations in mortality among three age groups (0–15 years of age, 15–60, and over 60). Infants and children died in greater numbers in early autumn, and adults, in winter and early spring.[29]

Jacques-Antoine Mourgue, a writer from the south of France, reached different conclusions. Mourgue compiled observations on the number of births, marriages, and deaths, along with meteorological reports from Montpellier, for the years 1772–92. These numbers appeared initially in *Histoire et Mémoires* (1780, 1781) of the Société Royale de Médecine, and later in a short *Essai de Statistique* (1800). Mourgue constructed a set of tables, including one that listed the number of deaths at each age for the twenty-year period by month, (see Figure 3). From this table Mourgue concluded that winter (November, December, January, and February) was normally the most

Figure 3 From Jacques-Antoine Mourgue, *Essai de Statistique* (*an* 9).

NÉCROLOGE OU NOTICE
DES AGES DES PERSONNES MORTES PARMI LES HABITANS
DE MONTPELLIER,
pendant vingt-une années consécutives, de 1772 à 1792 inclusivement,
réduit en mois collectifs

	de la naiss. à nn an.		*de 1 à 5 ans.*		*de 5 à 10 ans.*		*de 10 à 20 ans.*		*de 20 à 30 ans.*		*de 30 à 40 ans.*		*de 40 à 50 ans.*		*de 50 à 60 ans.*		*de 60 à 70 ans.*		*de 70 à 80 ans.*		*de 80 à 90 ans.*		*de 90 à 100 ans.*		*Totalité*	
Mois.	*garç.*	*filles*	*garç.*	*filles*	*garç.*	*filles*	*garç.*	*filles*	*hom.*	*fem.*	*hom.*	*fem.*	*hom.*	*fem.*	*hom.*	*fem.*	*hom.*	*fem.*	*hom.*	*fem.*	*hom.*	*fem.*	*hom.*	*fem.*	*hom.*	*fem.*
Janvier.	502	229	119	125	31	31	18	22	51	49	40	48	62	50	65	67	75	79	74	105	38	77	9	21	881	605
Février.	265	210	114	107	44	32	23	16	44	35	31	43	54	40	67	68	72	73	53	65	52	78	5	21	824	788
Mars.	234	204	143	129	39	34	20	23	59	43	36	47	44	61	69	58	81	69	64	82	52	64	3	24	804	838
Avril.	217	139	130	135	40	57	21	23	45	51	52	46	46	42	66	58	81	70	56	68	29	44	6	10	789	723
Mai.	194	126	156	129	35	35	24	32	43	46	34	41	47	41	53	49	55	59	44	61	34	50	5	7	724	676
Juin.	228	184	178	180	37	42	15	23	25	41	41	39	49	32	63	54	45	57	47	62	26	68	3	10	757	792
Juillet.	531	262	336	352	51	51	28	23	38	35	40	53	64	60	74	57	75	69	66	67	31	56	3	9	1137	1074
Août.	351	256	417	417	73	62	32	46	53	37	39	50	55	61	68	61	76	69	62	73	35	60	4	13	1265	1206
Septembre.	229	255	364	440	82	87	25	32	47	50	55	59	62	42	75	63	76	90	62	80	30	56	2	10	1179	1264
Octobre.	256	234	355	572	70	89	28	45	51	57	46	70	64	67	77	69	104	83	59	70	44	73	5	15	1139	1244
Novembre.	300	246	276	280	64	63	32	50	45	45	63	49	60	56	74	84	88	93	82	80	55	73	6	18	1145	1115
Décembre.	306	256	204	195	49	47	31	25	42	50	48	56	64	59	75	64	87	79	85	90	60	103	8	16	1059	1040
	3283	2601	2772	2841	615	610	297	340	525	557	525	601	671	612	826	752	915	890	754	903	466	802	56	174	11703	11663
Totalité.	5384		5613		1225		637		1060		1126		1283		1578		1805		1657		1268		230		23366	

deadly for infants, while spring was the most healthful. Years when smallpox epidemics raged in Montpellier were exceptional: smallpox was then most likely to strike in July, August, and September, and Mourgue noted that children between the ages of one and four were particularly vulnerable.[30]

William Heberden, an English physician who studied the London bills of mortality for the entire eighteenth century, along with records from various London hospitals, constructed an extensive set of tables to show weekly variations in mortality (see Figure 4). These tables appeared in his *Observations on the Increase and Decrease of Different Diseases and Particularly of the Plague* (1801). Heberden's tables had a column for deaths under the age of two immediately adjacent to the total number of deaths for that week. Thus, the high level of infant mortality and the weekly variations were immediately apparent. His inclusion of deaths attributed to certain diseases (especially smallpox) revealed the impact of acute diseases on the number of infant deaths.

This new method of tabular display incorporated a growing awareness of how diseases interacted with each other to affect mortality patterns. From his tables, Heberden concluded that "Under two years of age, there die most either in January February and March, or else in September and October," thus confirming Moheau's analysis.[31] Heberden attributed the autumnal increase to "bowel complaints [which] are most prevalent in persons of all ages." "[A]nd when it is considered how large a part they constitute of the diseases of infants, it seems by no means improbable that the general cause should be capable of producing this particular effect."[32]

Gender also influenced infant mortality. Many arithmeticians had calculated that males died at greater rates than females at all ages. Moheau did not give a reason for this, although he ascribed greater mortality rates for adult men to their professions and passions.[33] Black showed that more male infants died than females, and that there were more abortives and stillbirths among males than females. But Black, like Moheau, limited his explanation to the conditions that adult men faced.[34] Mourgue's figures from Montpellier indicated that one-fifth more boys than girls died before the age of one, a difference that proceeded from the "impatience and vivacity that, all things being equal, causes accidents among boys that girls are not exposed to."[35] Percival noted that gender differences in mortality were notable "especially in the earliest stages of [life]," when nearly one-half more males than females were stillborn.[36] He ascribed this finding to the larger size of the male fetus, which led to more difficult births.[37]

In addition to these explanations, eighteenth-century arithmeticians looked to moral causes. Physical and moral factors joined in

Figure 4 From William Heberden, *Observations on the Increase and Decrease of Different Diseases and Particularly of the Plague* (1801).

Weekly Bills of Mortality

1767	*Whole Number. buried.*	*Under two Years.*	*Above sixty Years.*	*Apoplexy, Palsy, Suddenly.*	*Childbed and Mis-carriage*	*Con-sump-tion.*	*Fever.*	*Colic, Flux, Gripes, Looseness.*	*Measles.*	*Small Pox.*
6 Jan.	391	113	69	6	7	93	51	0	4	43
13 Jan.	532	144	92	11	5	120	87	0	10	38
20 Jan.	519	129	100	16	6	126	63	2	1	42
27 Jan.	503	136	94	12	4	107	81	1	1	33
3 Feb.	468	127	84	8	2	107	76	2	0	31
10 Feb.	446	108	72	6	3	96	79	0	2	25
17 Feb.	439	137	80	5	3	101	80	1	0	18
24 Feb.	413	111	67	7	3	102	61	0	0	24
3 Mar.	404	134	69	7	4	96	59	1	1	22
10 Mar.	416	144	67	9	3	86	62	0	0	21
17 Mar.	457	140	73	9	5	90	86	0	0	20
24 Mar.	439	148	64	10	5	105	65	0	0	27
31 Mar.	432	162	71	5	3	86	59	1	1	24
7 Apr.	472	177	70	2	8	88	79	1	1	25
14 Apr.	392	126	53	7	3	75	72	2	3	16
21 Apr.	419	137	60	3	4	90	70	1	1	35
28 Apr. -	519	205	58	10	6	109	73	5	2	28
5 May	462	167	79	8	2	90	69	1	1	29
12 May	441	158	65	4	1	78	61	0	3	49
19 May	448	153	70	6	3	96	69	1	3	39
26 May	422	142	75	2	3	87	75	0	2	36
2 June	385	139	56	7	2	80	62	0	0	39
9 June	408	142	66	3	5	84	61	0	3	41
16 June	423	146	57	3	4	68	72	0	2	38
23 June	431	146	56	6	1	87	57	1	1	48
30 June	457	149	78	7	4	84	70	2	2	51
7 July	476	129	81	5	4	86	95	1	1	49
14 July	358	128	37	4	3	61	71	3	0	29
21 July	398	131	54	8	3	81	71	1	0	46
28 July	399	120	73	3	5	57	83	1	1	42
4 Aug.	339	102	40	7	3	64	53	4	1	47
11 Aug.	407	136	59	8	4	77	71	1	1	51
18 Aug.	350	108	43	3	2	59	70	1	1	58
25 Aug.	371	160	51	2	0	52	68	3	0	44
1 Sept.	352	140	43	5	0	60	40	6	1	43
8 Sept.	384	138	37	6	4	60	67	4	0	54
15 Sept.	338	144	36	4	2	48	56	2	1	47
22 Sept.	358	145	56	5	2	57	52	1	0	55
29 Sept.	388	165	42	3	1	62	70	4	1	42
6 Oct.	444	184	43	4	1	99	62	9	0	54
13 Oct.	469	177	57	4	3	75	78	2	4	44
20 Oct.	437	196	57	10	2	69	64	6	2	54
27 Oct.	396	134	49	3	4	61	73	0	1	64
3 Nov.	564	229	69	2	4	96	91	1	5	64
10 Nov.	450	176	55	7	1	72	78	0	0	59
17 Nov.	446	157	52	6	2	77	83	1	0	67
24 Nov.	487	173	54	2	2	80	84	0	2	61
1 Dec.	544	176	82	6	7	110	110	3	3	57
8 Dec.	475	160	67	13	5	93	91	0	1	48
15 Dec.	613	206	80	6	4	101	113	1	2	109
22 Dec.	495	157	62	4	5	76	7	0	2	74
29 Dec.	441	195	63	5	2	94	77	2	2	61

cities where foul air and debauched behaviour combined to wreak havoc on health. The numerical evidence compiled by Black, and confirmed by other arithmeticians, showed clearly that infants born in the countryside had a far greater chance of survival than their urban brothers and sisters. These quantitative conclusions confirmed widely held beliefs (especially among moralists) that cities were unhealthy, unwholesome, and wicked. Though widely accepted as fact, the contrast between the diseased city and the healthy countryside was neither obvious nor straightforward.[38] The city held perils for infants, but so too did the ignorance associated with country life.[39] No wonder writers such as Richard Price suggested a third possibility: "Moderate towns, being seats of refinement, emulation, and arts, may be public advantages. But *great* towns ... become checks on population of too hurtful a nature, nurseries of debauchery and voluptuousness."[40]

As Price's comments reveal, weak morals as well as physical hardships were the sources of disease and death. Black too ascribed the high number of infant deaths to numerous causes, many of which involved human agency. For example, disease could result from ill treatment by the mother or nurse: "the ligatures, bandages, and pins too tight, and tormenting the infant," or "from errors of the mother or nurse in food, drink, rest, exercise, excretions, passions of mind, from ill temper, hystericks, addiction to raw spirituous liquors and drunkenness, diseases, fasting too long before the infant sucks."[41] Mourgue looked into the causes of infant deaths (much like Black) and concluded that this "distressing mortality must be attributed less to the influence of climate and seasons" and more to "the fault of working class mothers." Because these women did not work at home, he reasoned, they did not nurse their infants often or long enough, and the infants died of exhaustion from crying, tears, and lack of care.[42]

This focus on social status was not unique to Mourgue. Many arithmeticians considered how social class affected the health of infants and children. Moheau demonstrated that the number of infants born who died before the age of 10 was smaller among *rentiers* (those collecting dividends, interest, or rent and generally considered privileged) than among the general population; this suggested that higher social standing increased an infant's chances of survival.[43] And Percival offered similar figures comparing poor children with "those in a higher station" from the parish of Dunmow in Essex.[44] Percival decried the ill effects of factory work on children: "It is a common but injurious practice in manufacturing countries, to confine children, before they have attained a sufficient degree of strength, to sedentary employments, in places where they breathe a putrid air, and are debarred the free use of their limbs." Percival denounced child labour. People generally "spare their horses and cattle, till they arrive at a due size and vigour." Similar treatment of children, he declared, should be in order.[45]

THE IMPACT OF QUANTIFICATION AFTER 1750: TWO CASE STUDIES

Foundlings

One especially vulnerable group of infants was foundlings. Mothers abandoned these babies, more often than not illegitimate, shortly after birth. Institutions to care for foundlings dated back to the Middle Ages, and church charity supported most of them. During the eighteenth century, the treatment of foundlings became a concern for enlightened efforts to improve the lives of the unfortunate. In England, secular charities supported by subscription emerged to care for foundlings. In France, the state increasingly took responsibility for abandoned infants.[46]

All commentators on infant mortality agreed on the dismal fate of foundlings. Moheau, for example, compiled numbers from the hospitals in Clermont, Rouen, and Tours and demonstrated that average mortality among abandoned infants was 25 per cent higher than infant mortality among the general population – "a frightening disproportion."[47] Other records confirmed this finding. New charitable medical institutions in London, such as the Foundling Hospital (1739) and the British Lying-In Hospital (1749), issued reports to their subscribers; these frequently contained numerical accounts of the women and infants cared for.[48] At the Foundling Hospital during its first fifteen years between 40 and 50 per cent of all abandoned infants died.

This shockingly high level forced its governors to shift from feeding the infants by hand at the hospital to sending them to wet-nurses in the countryside for the first three years of life. Further policy changes followed. After a series of mysterious deaths of infants sent to wet-nurses, the governors changed the nurses' payment schedule from one lump sum at the beginning to yearly instalments, with a bonus for keeping an infant alive one year.[49]

Concerns, even fears, about the care given by wet-nurses were widespread. The administrators of the Hôpital Général in Montpellier surveyed the fate of 610 children sent to wet-nurses during the years 1767–77. They discovered that 433 (70.9 per cent) of these infants had died, and they attributed at least some of the deaths to neglect brought on by the poor wages that wet-nurses received.[50] Financial constraints, however, prevented them from raising wet-nurses' wages. Presumably, conditions did not improve.

These institutional records revealed horrifically high rates of mortality, much greater than the one out of four stated by Black and Moheau. Because the hospital figures were so high, efforts were made or at least considered to improve the health and preserve the life of foundlings. Quantifying the number of deaths of foundlings thus promoted specific policy changes in their treatment. Correspondingly, growth in the number of foundling and maternity hospitals and the importance of accountability for such charitable institutions made new sources of numbers available to arithmeticians quantifying infant and maternal mortality.

Smallpox Inoculation

Infant mortality figures also affected the practice of smallpox inoculation. From its introduction in England in the 1720s, the practice of inoculation had been evaluated numerically. This first arithmetical analysis of a medical procedure compared the risks of dying from inoculated and from natural smallpox. Over the course of the eighteenth century, calculations of the risks and benefits of inoculation became increasingly refined to address not only risks to the individual, but potential gains to the state (in population growth).[51]

Physicians generally thought that children should be inoculated after teething at the age of two or three years.[52] Their reasoning reflected the view of infants as particularly weak and vulnerable – as Black and Moheau had argued. Percival, an ardent supporter of inoculation, endorsed this opinion in his 1789 treatise: "if we regard only the state of the body," then the best ages for inoculation were 2–4 for healthy children and 3–6 for delicate children, because "the powers of nature are then sufficiently vigorous." But, he continued, "other considerations, besides the state of the constitution, demand our attention."[53]

What Percival had in mind was the risk that infants faced in contracting smallpox. He had collected information from parish registers and calculated mortality figures for Manchester and surrounding villages. He also investigated the relationship between age and smallpox mortality. He compiled two tables that recorded information on age of death due to smallpox in two locales. The figures showed clearly that the largest number of deaths from smallpox occurred between 18 and 36 months. Percival concluded, "The risque of receiving the natural smallpox by infection appears to be very great during the second year of life." Accordingly, "the inoculation of healthy and vigorous children, at the *age of two or three months,* seems to be advisable, especially in large towns."[54]

Percival shared his tables with the physician John Haygarth, who conducted similar inquiries in the northern town of Chester. Haygarth took an active interest in inoculation and in the use of mortality figures to guide medical policy. He found that, in 1774, 202 individuals died from smallpox and that 51 of these deaths were infants under one year of age.[55] Although it is difficult to know the extent to which Percival's recommendations took hold, his more precise calculations of infant mortality firmly established the vulnerability of infants to smallpox.

CONCLUSION

Eighteenth-century efforts to quantify infant and child mortality paradoxically both confirmed and questioned the inevitability of the high number of deaths. Calculations confirmed that in general one out of four infants died within the first year of life. At the same time, quantification enabled arithmeticians to identify variations in infant mortality that depended on geography, season, social status, and gender. Their tables made infant mortality visible, and after 1750 the figures increasingly suggested that the high number of deaths among infants was not the divine will of Providence, but a product of human actions and environmental conditions. Quantification enabled arithmeticians to identify, calculate, and publicize high rates of mortality that helped spur reform.

ACKNOWLEDGMENTS

I would like to thank the organizers and participants of the conference. I also thank the members of the Research Network for Women in the Humanities, especially Catherine Sama and Marie Schwartz, for their helpful suggestions on revision. Finally, I am indebted to Paul Lucier.

NOTES

1 On infant mortality in the nineteenth century, see David Armstrong, "The Invention of Infant Mortality," *Sociology of Health and Disease,* 8 (1986), 211–32; Joshua Cole, *The Power of Large Numbers: Population, Politics, and Gender in Nineteenth-Century France* (Ithaca, NY: Cornell University

Press, 2000); Richard A. Meckel, *Save the Babies: American Public Health Reform and the Prevention of Infant Mortality, 1850–1929* (Ann Arbor: University of Michigan Press, 1998).

2 J.H. Plumb, "The New World of Children," in Neil McKendrick, John Brewer, and J.H. Plumb, eds., *The Birth of a Consumer Society: The Commercialization of Eighteenth-Century England* (London: Hutchinson, 1983), 286–315.

3 Valerie A. Fildes, *Breasts, Bottles and Babies: A History of Infant Feeding* (Edinburgh: Edinburgh University Press, 1986); Sara Matthews Greco, "Breastfeeding, Wet Nursing and Infant Mortality in Europe (1400–1800)," in *Historical Perspectives on Breastfeeding* (Florence, Italy: UNICEF, 1991), 15–62; George Sussman, *Selling Mother's Milk: The Wet Nursing Business in France, 1715–1914* (Champaign: University of Illinois Press, 1982).

4 Thomas W. Laqueur, "Bodies, Details, and the Humanitarian Narrative," in Lynn Hunt, ed., *The New Cultural History* (Berkeley: University of California Press, 1989), 176–204.

5 Nina Rattner Gelbart, *The King's Midwife: A History and Mystery of Madame du Coudray* (Berkeley: University of California Press, 1998); Michel Foucault, *The History of Sexuality*, vol. I: *An Introduction*, trans. Robert Hurley (New York: Pantheon Books, 1978); Andrea Rusnock, "Biopolitics and the Mathematics of Population: Medical and Political Arithmetic in the Eighteenth Century," in William Clark, Jan Golinski, and Simon Schaffer, eds., *The Sciences in Enlightened Europe* (Chicago: University of Chicago Press, 1999), 49–68.

6 Walter Radcliffe surveyed efforts to reduce infant mortality, especially in Britain, during the eighteenth century: "The Problem of Infant Mortality prior to 1800," *Community Health* (Bristol), 1 (1970), 276–82.

7 John McManners, *Death and the Enlightenment: Changing Attitudes to Death among Christians and Unbelievers in Eighteenth-Century France* (Oxford: Clarendon Press, 1981).

8 John Graunt, *Natural and Political Observations Made Upon the London Bills of Mortality* (London, 1662), 29.

9 Ibid., 33, 56.

10 Laurence Brockliss and Colin Jones discuss the preoccupation with plague mortality over other types of mortality in *The Medical World of Early Modern France* (Oxford: Clarendon Press, 1997), 66–7.

11 Andrea A. Rusnock, *Vital Accounts: Quantifying Health and Population in Eighteenth-Century England and France* (Cambridge: Cambridge University Press, 2002).

12 Richelle Munkhoff, "Searchers of the Dead: Authority, Marginality, and the Interpretation of Plague in England, 1574–1665," *Gender and History* 11 (1999), 1–29; T.R. Forbes, "The Searchers," *Bulletin of the New York Academy of Medicine* 50 (1974), 1031–8.

13 E.A. Wrigley and R.S. Schofield, *The Population History of England: A Reconstruction* (Cambridge, Mass.: Harvard University Press, 1981), 15–32. For France, see Guy Cabourdin and Jacques Dupâquier, "Les sources et les institutions," in *Histoire de la population française*, vol. 2: *De la Renaissance à 1789* (Paris: Presses Universitaires de France, 1988), 9–50; Alain Bideau, Jacques Dupâquier, and Hector Gutierrez, "La mort quantifiée," in ibid., 222–43.

14 For evaluations of Moheau and Montyon's contributions to demography, see the excellent collection of essays appended to the recent edition of his book: *Jean-Baptiste Moheau, Recherches et considérations sur la population de la France* (1778), new edition annotated by Eric Vilquin (Paris: Presses Universitaires de France, 1994). All cited page numbers refer to this edition.

15 William Black, *An Arithmetical and Medical Analysis of the Diseases and Mortality of the Human Species* (London, 1789), 222.

16 Black, *An Arithmetical and Medical Analysis*, 34; Moheau, *Recherches et considérations*, 166.

17 Moheau, *Recherches et considérations*, 166; Black, *An Arithmetical and Medical Analysis*, 220–1.

18 Graunt, *Natural and Political Observations*, 29.

19 Thomas Short, *A Comparative History of the Increase and Decrease of Mankind in Several Countries Abroad According to the Different Soils, Business of Life, Use of the Non-Naturals, &c.* (London, 1767), 19.

20 Black, *An Arithmetical and Medical Analysis*, 211–12.

21 For a recent discussion of the registration of stillbirths in Britain, see Nicky Hart, "Beyond Infant Mortality: Gender and Stillbirth in Reproductive Mortality before the Twentieth Century," *Population Studies* 52 (1998), 215–29.

22 Black, *An Arithmetical and Medical Analysis*, 212.

23 Moheau, *Recherches et considérations*, 183.

24 Black, *An Arithmetical and Medical Analysis*, 35.

25 Moheau, *Recherches et considérations*, 154.

26 James Riley, *The Eighteenth-Century Campaign to Avoid Disease* (New York: Macmillan, 1987); David Cantor, ed., *Reinventing Hippocrates* (Aldershot: Ashgate, 2002).

27 Black uses figures from the clergymen Johann Peter Süssmilch and Jean-Louis Muret; Black, *An Arithmetical and Medical Analysis*, 32–3.

28 Ibid., 20.

29 See William Coleman, "Inventing Demography: Montyon on Hygiene and the State," in Everett Mendelsohn, ed., *Transformation and Tradition in the Sciences: Essays in Honor of I. Bernard Cohen* (Cambridge: Cambridge University Press, 1984), 221–2.

30 Jacques-Antoine Mourgue, *Essai de statistique* (Paris, 1800), 28.

31 William Heberden, *Observations on the Increase and Decrease of Different Diseases and Particularly of the Plague* (London 1801), 50.
32 Ibid., 51.
33 Moheau, *Recherches et considérations*, 165, 168.
34 Black, *An Arithmetical and Medical Analysis*, 14–15, 24.
35 Mourgue, *Essai de statistique*, 25.
36 Thomas Percival, *Observations on the State of Population in Manchester* (1789), 65; reprinted in B. Benjamin, ed., *Population and Disease in Early Industrial England* (Farnborough, Hants: Gregg, 1973).
37 Certain environments were shown to be more deadly than others. Rusnock, *Vital Accounts*, 163–7.
38 See Marie-France Morel, "City and Country in Eighteenth-Century Medical Discussions about Early Childhood," in Robert Forster and Orest Ranum, eds., *Medicine and Society in France* (Baltimore, Md.: Johns Hopkins University Press, 1980), 48–65; originally published in *Annales ESC* 32 (1977), 1007–24.
39 For examples of the treatment of infants in rural France, see Gelbart, *The King's Midwife*, 59, 115.
40 Richard Price, "Observations on the Expectations of Lives, the Increase of Mankind, the Influence of Great Towns on Population, and Particularly the State of London with Respect to Healthfulness and Number of Inhabitants," *Philosophical Transactions* 59 (1769), 119.
41 Black, *An Arithmetical and Medical Analysis*, 223.
42 Mourgue, *Essai de statistique*, 26–7.
43 13 per cent of infants born to rentiers died before the age of 10, while in the general population, 51 per cent died. Moheau, *Recherches et considérations*, 172–3; also see Coleman, "Inventing Demography," 223.
44 "The ratio of deaths, during the last five years," Percival wrote in 1789, "has been, of the poor children 1 in 45½; of those in a higher station 1 in 37½." Percival, *Observations on the State of Population in Manchester*, 67.
45 Ibid., 41–2.
46 Rachel Fuchs, *Abandoned Children: Foundlings and Child Welfare in Nineteenth-Century France* (Albany: State University of New York, 1984); Ruth K. McClure, *Coram's Children: the London Foundling Hospital in the Eighteenth Century* (New Haven, Conn.: Yale University Press, 1981).
47 Moheau, *Recherches et considérations*, 172–3; also see Coleman, "Inventing Demography," 222.
48 On London charitable institutions, see Donna T. Andrew, *Philanthropy and Police: London Charity in the Eighteenth Century* (Princeton, NJ: Princeton University Press, 1989).
49 See Andrew, *Philanthropy and Police*, 61–2.
50 Colin Jones, *Charity and Bienfaisance: The Treatment of the Poor in the*

Montpellier Region, 1740–1815 (Cambridge: Cambridge University Press, 1982), 103–7.

51 Rusnock, *Vital Accounts,* chaps. 2–4.

52 Deborah Brunton, "Pox Britannica: Smallpox Inoculation in Britain, 1721–1800," PhD thesis, University of Pennsylvania, 1990, 75.

53 Thomas Percival, "Essay on the Small-Pox and Measles" (1789), reprinted in B. Benjamin, ed., *Population and Disease in Early Industrial Britain* (Farnborough, Hants: Gregg, 1973), 77. Percival had published another essay on this topic supporting the inoculation of children above the age of three: *On the Disadvantages which attend the Inoculation of Children in Early Infancy* (London, 1768).

54 Percival, "Essay on the Small-Pox and Measles," 76.

55 Cited in ibid., 77.

PART TWO

Quantification and Instrumentation

5

Medical Statistics at the Paris School: What Was at Stake?

ANN F. LA BERGE

Classic stories, such as the well-known controversy over medical statistics in Paris in the 1830s, function as points of reference, part of a common academic tradition to which everyone can refer. This is convenient and comforting, as a consensus of recognition emerges. But such stories can also function as black boxes, so well known that they become part of an agreed-on narrative. It is important to reconsider these classic stories in light of changing historiographical concerns and new ways of thinking about quantification historically and in present-day medical science and public health.

This article focuses on one of these classic stories – the debate over medical statistics at the Académie de médecine in Paris from April to June 1837. The debate started when Benigno Risueño d'Amador (1802–1849), professor of general pathology and therapeutics at the Faculté de médecine in Montpellier and a corresponding member of the Académie, travelled to Paris to read an essay on the calculus of probability applied to medicine.[1] His main argument was that the calculus of probability was an inappropriate tool for the natural and medical sciences, where variation was the norm and the variables were too numerous to be controlled. He feared that quantifying medicine would make medical practice impersonal, that reducing patients to numbers would objectify them and would deprive physicians of their judgment and authority. He raised many other objections, but his principal concern was that quantification would lead to dehumanization in medicine and the rationalization of medicine and society.

In this article I reconsider the controversy over medical statistics at the Paris School to ask: what was at stake for those who defended medical statistics and for those who critiqued it? A brief review of the 1837 debate provides the starting point from which to explore this question. Although historians have analysed this debate within the context of the history of statistics and medicine, I seek to broaden the analysis by addressing more specifically the role of medical technologies at the Paris School.[2] I next look at numerists' defence of their methods. In my analysis of what was at stake, I suggest that Risueño d'Amador used medical statistics as a way to argue more broadly about society and culture, as a way to articulate his fear of modernity.

THE CONTEXT OF THE 1837 DEBATE

The debate over medical statistics took place during the era in which Paris clinical medicine was world-renowned. At the Paris School (École clinique de Paris) widespread interest in applying statistics to medicine dated from the 1820s with the work of Pierre Louis, whose "numerical method" showed that bloodletting, a popular therapy at the time, was less successful than had been thought.[3] His work challenged the principal therapy of François Broussais's "physiological medicine," which relied on bloodletting to reduce inflammation and suggested instead that the numerical method could be a scientific way for physicians to evaluate therapeutic effectiveness.[4] Louis's work opened the way for major discussions of the application of statistics to clinical medicine. Medical statistics might join other technologies, such as scalpels, stethoscopes, and microscopes, in the research arsenal of Parisian physicians.

The institutional infrastructure of Paris medicine provided a setting in which medical statistics might have wide applicability, since thousands of patients and diseases were available for observation and quantification. [5] The hospitals were the physicians' laboratories, housing the patients on whom Parisian physicians and surgeons perfected their skills.[6] Physicians considered public-hospital patients objects of scientific study, both while alive and after death.[7] Public hospitals were a main site for the research, teaching, and practice of medical science at the Paris School. The royal academies provided a forum for the debate and discussion of new research methods and therapies as well as for the practice of medicine and science more generally.[8]

The debate on medical statistics took place within the framework of the larger debate ongoing in Paris among mathematicians and philosophers over the applicability of mathematics to social and moral issues. This debate over mathematical imperialism occurred in 1835–36 between S.D. Poisson – P.S. Laplace's successor in probability theory – and A.L. Cauchy. Laplace had argued, and Poisson continued the tradition, that the calculus of probability could be profitably applied to almost every area of human endeavour, including medicine. For example, in 1835 Poisson had asserted before the Académie des sciences that his "law of large numbers" had universal application, as did probability theory. Cauchy and other mathematicians opposed Poisson, favouring a more restricted view of the mathematical enterprise and contending that there were some areas beyond the scope of probability theory. Cauchy emerged as the leading proponent of the restricted view of mathematics. He argued that mathematical analysis did not apply to all the speculative sciences and suggested: "Let us eagerly pursue the study of the mathematical sciences without letting them extend beyond their domain; and let us not imagine that we can approach history through mathematical formulas or sanction morality with algebraic theorems or integral calculus."[9]

So it was within the framework of this larger mathematical-philosophical controversy that Risueño d'Amador examined the application of the calculus of probability to medicine. In so doing he generalized his argument to include Louis's numerical method under the rubric "calculus of probability." This strategy opened the way for a discussion of his broader concerns about medicine and society.

The prelude to the 1837 debate was a discussion on the application of statistics two years earlier at the Académie des sciences, occasioned by the publication of a book by Dr. J. Civiale on cutting for the stone. Civiale had used numerical data gathered from leading European surgeons to show that the older method, lithotomy, had a mortality rate of 1 in 5, whereas with his technique, lithotrity, the mortality rate was only 1 in 42. Discussion of this book allowed the reporter, physician François-Joseph Double from Montpellier, to discuss the application of the calculus of probability to medicine.[10] Double, a graduate of Montpellier's Faculté de médecine and a well-known Hippocratist,[11] praised Civiale's book, using his numerical data on the two surgical methods to raise larger questions about the application of the calculus of probability to medicine. He pointed out that statistics was now in vogue and that some physicians wanted to apply statistics to therapeutics. In the case under discussion, he explained, employing statistics was an attempt to apply the calculus of probability. What should physicians think of it? And here Double, coming out of the same Montpellier medical tradition as Risueño d'Amador, made a point that prefigured the latter's argument two years later. "In the matter of statistics ... the first concern is above all to lose sight of man taken individually ... He must be stripped of his individuality in order to eliminate everything that this individuality might accidentally introduce into the question." He contrasted the goals of statistics with those of the practice of medicine: "In applied medicine … the problem is always individual ... it is always a single person with all his idiosyncrasies that the physician must treat. For us the masses remain completely outside the question."[12] Referring to Poisson's law of large numbers, widely discussed in Paris at the time, Double explained that with the calculus of probability one approached more closely to the truth when the observations encompassed a large number of facts or individuals. But, he argued, these laws had nothing to do with an individual.

Double contended that in practical medicine the facts are not numerous enough for the calculus of probability. Medical facts, he suggested, are not limited by the nature of things; nor can the physician ever know or assemble all the facts. Along with the few facts published by physicians, there exist thousands lost in the obscurity of the clinic. Practically, he argued, most medical facts escape calculation, comparison, and control: from all these lost facts, which elements, which results, would one introduce into this medical arithmetic? No one would dare say, he contended; medicine was not amenable to the application of the calculus of probability because it was too complex, with too many variables to be controlled. Double would play an important role in the 1837 debate as well, and Risueño d'Amador would reiterate many of the same points that Double had articulated.

The 1837 debate also took place within the larger context of an ongoing dialogue on therapeutic medicine. Contemporaries and historians have considered therapeutics to be one of the weak areas of Paris medicine, and studies in the 1830s suggested that the most successful therapy was no therapy at all. Paris became known for its so-called therapeutic nihilism. Shortly before the statistics debate (which began in April 1837) there had been a discussion at the Académie de médecine in which Gabriel Andral had concluded for the commission investigating the efficacy of bloodletting as a therapy: "I have seen all treatments succeed and all treatments fail." By this Andral meant that numbers were not facts divorced from values, but rather were used for rhetorical and ideological purposes to justify conflicting treatments. For Andral it was not clear that numbers were any more certain than any other kind of observational data.[13] Risueño d'Amador's essay was part of the ongoing discussion about the role of therapeutics at the Paris School.

MEDICAL STATISTICS AT THE ACADÉMIE DE MÉDECINE

Risueño d'Amador began his essay by locating the roots of the numerical method in the calculus of probability of Condorcet and Laplace. Both had been mathematical imperialists, he asserted, claiming that the calculus of probability could be fruitfully applied to almost every area of human endeavour, including medicine.[14] He disagreed, arguing that mathematicians' probability "was only the theory of chance" and that to invoke it in medicine was to renounce the goal of medical certainty to which Parisian physicians subscribed.[15]

Risueño d'Amador challenged the numerists on their scientific method. Translating ideas into numbers was their method of doing science, he asserted: "They count and believe that by counting they are doing science."[16] He argued that it was anti-scientific to apply the calculus of probability to medicine: "Its incorporation into medicine is anti-scientific, abolishing, as it does, true observation; and substituting for action of the spirit and for individual genius of the artist, a uniform, blind, and mechanical routine."[17]

Coming from Montpellier, a stronghold of neo-Hippocratic medicine, Risueño d'Amador stressed the skill of the physician necessary to understand both patient and disease.[18] He believed that the numerical method threatened the authority of the physician, who was above all an artist, with judgment developed by years of experience. He protested the efforts of Parisian physicians to objectify disease. Medicine, he contended, dealt with individual patients, and the doctor–patient relationship was critical. Patients should not lose their individuality, nor should diseases be divorced from patients: "for Monsieur Louis," he charged, "the disease is everything, the patient nothing."[19] The neo-Hippocratic physician, in contrast, diagnosed and treated disease within the context of the individual patient.[20]

For Risueño d'Amador, the traditional methods of medical research and practice – reasoning, induction, observation, and experiment – were far superior to the "uniform, blind, and mechanical routine" of calculating. Physicians had their own rich tradition; there was no need to apply mathematics to medicine. Medicine, after all, was both art and science; but the calculus of probability would deprive medicine of some of the richness of its tradition, the certainly of its knowledge: "Medicine," Risueño d'Amador charged, "will no longer be an art, but a lottery." He argued that the calculus of probability did not deal in reality, but in illusion. The numerical method could not be trusted, he asserted, because it wasn't real; it was rather a mathematical creation. Mathematical abstractions were inappropriate for medicine, a science grounded in observation and experiment.[21]

The application of statistics to the natural and social sciences – which included medicine – was problematic because of the epistemological and methodological problems posed by variability and variation, Risueño d'Amador maintained. He emphasized that all diseases have a history and change through time; the same diseases change character, vary in intensity, appear, and disappear from the pathological horizon, and then reappear. The pathological picture of an individual or an epidemic was also changing. Variability was the first law of nature, of life, of disease, he asserted. The numerical method, however, could not encompass or address this variability, he contended, but rather attempted to "fix" disease at a point in time. The numerical method, he charged, was an attempt to fix, order, make static, and constrain. It was a system in which variability had no place.[22]

Risueño d'Amador was also suspicious of the general tendency to make medicine a "social science," an approach that he considered anti-historical. He contrasted the numerical method with the historical, which, he contended, was the traditional way of studying diseases – the classic case-history and epidemiological approach. We recall the importance that nineteenth-century physicians attached to understanding the patient's history in order to prescribe individualized therapies. Everything about the patient's past and present – his or her environment and way of life – was valuable for diagnosing a medical problem and prescribing the appropriate therapy.[23]

Risueño d'Amador contrasted the numerical method with the traditional medical approach, which focused on the individual patient. He explained that when confronted with a new case the physician informs himself, classifies, compares with past cases; if he encounters a problem that he has not met before, he gives it individual attention. Numbers, he argued, would be useless. What could they tell you about the individual patient? The physician tries, tests, invents, follows his hunches; he has to practice the art of medicine, that is, finely tuned judgment, as well as the science. The physician is interested in more than the number of times a therapy has worked. He wants to know circumstances and conditions – the therapeutic context – in which a therapy has worked.[24] Risueño d'Amador was most upset by what he saw as the abandonment of the case-history approach. Physicians should shun the numerical method, then, because it would objectify, quantify, and depersonalize the patient, dramatically altering the practice of medicine to the disadvantage of both patient and physician.[25]

Nor was medicine analogous to the physical sciences, Risueño d'Amador asserted. He portrayed the numerical method as another attempt to use the physical sciences as a model for medicine.[26] The underlying hope of some physicians was that laws of disease might emerge to correspond to Newton's universal law of gravitation. They based their hope on a misunderstanding of nature, according to Risueño d'Amador, for the idea was to endow nature with a certainty and regularity that it did not possess.[27] Systems such as the numerical method were attempts to constrain nature, to establish certainty where none existed. Just as certainty in medicine was not possible, neither was uniformity. Risueño d'Amador denied any uniformity in pathology and therapeutics, concluding with conscious irony: "Make it so there is uniformity in pathological facts, identity in therapeutics, fixity in all. Do the contrary of what exists and thus you will have inevitably displaced the basis of medical science, and established [inadvertently], for the profit of humanity, its indecisive character."[28]

As a professor of therapeutics, Risueño d'Amador worried especially about what the numerical method would mean for therapeutic medicine. He did not foresee improvement. If probability theory were employed to assess the effectiveness of therapies, he argued, the majority would prevail: what then would happen to the minority? Suppose the physician counted to determine the efficacy of a therapy, and it became clear that in most cases the therapy was harmful or ineffective. What about the minority for whom it worked? If a particular medication appeared to be safe in the majority of cases, what would happen to the minority for whom it was hazardous? He suggested that the numerical method would not benefit each individual patient. If a standardized, rationalized approach replaced individualized therapies, he feared that the minority would suffer.[29]

In the final analysis, Risueño d'Amador saw the numerical method as Bentham's utilitarianism applied to medicine.[30] Disease would replace the patient as the focus of the physician's attention, swallowing up the patient in Poisson's "law of large numbers." Therapies would be prescribed en masse, without consideration for individual differences.[31] The result, Risueño d'Amador asserted, would be standardized, impersonal medicine – detrimental to both physician and patient.

Thus Risueño d'Amador challenged the rhetoric of the numerists who claimed that their method was scientific and would help physicians acquire positive knowledge, by arguing that the numerical method was anti-scientific, that it was just one more medical system. He also contended that the numerists were basing their notions on a false idea of science; they hoped for certainty, whereas the basic nature of the natural and social sciences was uncertainty. Furthermore, the numerical method was dangerous for patient and physician alike. Its application threatened to change the practice of medicine by depriving patients of individual care and treatment and preventing physicians from exercising individual genius and judgment. Instead, he argued, the focus on the individual patient would give way to a standardized, utilitarian approach, dehumanizing to both patients and physicians.

THE NUMERISTS DEFEND THEIR METHOD

Once Risueño d'Amador had finished what seemed to many Parisian physicians a diatribe against progress and positive knowledge and a misunderstanding of the numerical method, the numerists defended medical statistics. Pathologist Jean-Baptiste Bouillaud affirmed the necessity of counting and measuring in medicine and the value of using statistics to assess therapies. Citing Laplace, he explained that in order to recognize the best treatment, the physician should test each therapy on the same number of patients, keeping all circumstances exactly the same.[32] A.F. Chomel challenged Risueño d'Amador's concerns that the numerical method would change the practice of medicine and the doctor–patient relationship. He argued that the physician who counted did not treat patients any differently from one who did not count. He further asserted that the numerical method did not introduce mathematics into medicine, constrain medicine, or impose a precision that medicine lacked. Rather, he defended the numerical method as one of the most certain means of destroying errors and arriving at truth.[33]

Pierre Louis declared the goal of medical statistics to be "as rigorous as possible determination of general facts."[34] He claimed that without numerical analysis no science of medicine was possible, for counting was an essential part of the observational science of medicine. He pointed out that terms such as "more," "less," "rarely," and "frequently" had no real value: did they mean 10, 15, 20, or 80 out of 100? Only the numerical method could provide the precision necessary to make medicine a science.[35] Louis disputed Risueño d'Amador's charges that the numerical method meant ignoring individual differences, arguing instead that it clarified them. For example, if the physician found wide variations in frequency or duration of illness among his patients, he would have to figure out why. Unless he had counted, he might not have known of these differences. Counting, he argued, isolated individual variations, bringing them to the physician's attention. The numerical method was a way of achieving more certain knowledge, of arriving at precision. Addressing Risueño d'Amador's concern that the numerical method excluded the minority, Louis argued that counting allowed physicians to identify and address exceptions and minorities. The numerical method, Louis contended, was a way of perfecting physicians' observations.[36]

Both Louis and J. André Rochoux denied any distinction between the physical and natural sciences, asserting that physiological phenomena were subject to invariable natural laws. Rochoux boldly declared, "Statistics is stronger than a Faculty, stronger than an Academy, than all the academies in the world. In a word, medical statistics is true; it is an answer to everything."[37] Meanwhile, François Guéneau de Mussy used a different strategy by denying the novelty of medical statistics, placing it within the observational tradition. He claimed that physicians had always counted and would always count, asserting that the numerical method was nothing new. The only novelty was its large-scale application.[38]

Finally, Pierre Rayer saw the whole debate as much ado about nothing. He maintained that anatomy and physiology had already incorporated counting, that taking weight, height, and vital statistics was a common medical practice. So Rayer argued that the utility of the numerical method was not in question; what was controversial was its application in pathology and therapeutics. Rayer defended the use of the numerical method in both these areas, placing it squarely within the experimental, observational tradition.[39]

ANALYSIS: WHAT WAS AT STAKE?

The overarching concern for all participants in the medical statistics debate was the kind of medicine that would prevail at the Paris School and elsewhere. More specifically, both numerists and critics wanted to determine if there was a scientific way to evaluate therapeutic efficacy. Underlying these issues were broader considerations about the nature of disease and the reality of medical power. And, finally, participants sought to determine the role of technologies at the Paris School.

At stake for leading Parisian physicians was the scientific and international status of Paris medicine: the primacy of the clinic and the development of a clinical science. Parisian physicians sought to identify approaches that would enrich and perpetuate their clinical tradition. The numerists argued for a forward-looking clinical science, making full use of available technologies, while the critics saw this Parisian orientation as harmful to the best tradition in medicine: their own Montpellier tradition of vitalist, neo-Hippocratic medicine.

The day-to-day practice of medicine was at stake for the critics of medical statistics but was a less important issue for the Parisian numerists. Leading Parisian physicians worked in both public hospitals, which exemplified Risueño d'Amador's concerns, and private practice. The realities of public-hospital medicine in Paris contrasted sharply with the private practice of medicine, as Jacalyn Duffin has shown in her study of the public and private patients of René Laennec.[40] Risueño d'Amador feared public medicine, which he saw as standardized, rationalized, and utilitarian, while applauding private medicine, which, he believed, allowed the physician to employ the traditional Hippocratic approach, in which the doctor–patient relationship figured prominently. At stake for the critics, then, was how quantification might alter the day-to-day practice of medicine and the doctor–patient relationship.

A major consideration was that the introduction of medical technologies could threaten the professional status of physicians. Both Double and Risueño d'Amador worried that application of medical technologies such as medical statistics might lessen medicine's stature, depriving physicians of their socioprofessional status, and reduce medicine as a learned profession to a craft. The microscope, being introduced into Paris medicine at the same time as medical statistics, seemed also to threaten the physician's status. In the 1840s and 1850s clinician and microscopist Hermann Lebert took offence, for the same status reasons, at being labelled a microscopist. He wanted to be not a mere "micrographer" but rather a clinician who practised microscopy.[41]

Within this dispute about the kind of medicine that would prevail, the debate focused on therapeutic efficacy, especially on clinical trials. Paris medicine had made important strides in diagnostic medicine, but this was not the case with therapeutics. Technologies such as the scalpel, the stethoscope, and, most recently, the microscope, had improved diagnosis, but they did little to improve therapeutics. Physicians sought to identify the best way to test the efficacy of therapies. There were no ethical or professional standards in place except for what was considered customary and usual.[42] The numerists hoped that the numerical method might be the instrument that could provide clear and factual answers to therapeutic questions. Critics viewed it as a troublesome technology that would cause more problems than it would solve and would threaten the fundamentals of the private practice of medicine.

Changing understandings of the nature of disease underlay the concerns about what kind of medicine to practise and what kind of therapies to prescribe. Would traditional views of disease as imbalance – the cornerstone of Hippocratic medicine – prevail? In a recent article Charles Rosenberg has argued that the nineteenth-century change in notions of disease was as revolutionary for medicine as was the work of Newton, Darwin, and Freud in their respective domains.[43] Rosenberg has called this shift the "specificity revolution." The view of disease specificity articulated in 1830s' Paris, which would mature later in the century, assumed the existence of specific disease entities outside patients' bodies. This approach, as Risueño d'Amador suggested, would separate diseases from patients in order to study and treat them. In the older paradigm, the physician moved between the art and science of medicine, as Risueño d'Amador expressed it, or, in Rosenberg's terms, between the idiosyncratic and the generalizable.

Work at the Paris School in fields as diverse as pathological anatomy, pathological physiology, and medical chemistry was leading physicians toward the notion of stable disease entities. Much of this "specificity revolution" would occur before the 1860s, antedating the era of the germ theory of disease, with which it is often associated. Thus the controversy over medical statistics was taking place at the beginning of the process of conceptual change that transformed not only the practice of medicine and the doctor–patient relationship, but also medical research and teaching. By the 1860s in Paris, as Joy Harvey has shown in her study of the clinic during the Second Empire, for both teachers and students of medicine at the Parisian hospitals, diseases were objectified, disembodied, suitable for study as individual entities. Drawing from the weekly medical gazettes, Harvey showed how hospitals numbered and identified beds by disease, so that students knew precisely where to go to observe the disease of their choice.[44] The goal of the "specificity revolution" was to transcend the subjective, the local, the idiosyncratic, in order to embrace the universal, to strive for the replicability of disease entities, regardless of culture. This approach was completely at odds with Risueño d'Amador's understanding of Hippocratic medicine and his view of society.

The debate over medical statistics was part of a long-standing struggle between Montpellier and Paris for medical dominance. For critics Double and Risueño d'Amador, the reputation and survival of Montpellier medicine was at stake. The locus of medical power had moved from Montpellier in the eighteenth century to Paris in the nineteenth. But Montpellier physicians were reluctant to accept their diminished position. Underlying the debate was the keen resentment of Paris medicine by Montpellier physicians, such as Risueño d'Amador, even though he readily accepted some of its principal orientations.

The background of this sense of loss related not just to a specific type of medicine, but also to institutional realities, as Elizabeth Williams has shown. According to Williams, Risueño d'Amador and Double preached the Montpellier gospel of vitalistic Hippocratism that she calls the medical science of man. Since the eighteenth century there had been a continuing struggle between the Paris and Montpellier faculties. Revolutionary reforms had invigorated the Paris Faculté de médecine, which emerged by the 1810s as a center of medical learning and power. Physicians at the Faculté, at the hospitals, and in other institutions of Paris medicine were constructing the Faculté as the leading medical school in France and Paris as the leading medical center in the world.[45] According to Williams, one way for Parisian physicians to increase their own reputation was to compare the Paris School with provincial medical schools, such as Montpellier. In fact, the status of Montpellier had already decreased during the French Revolution, when legislation had changed it from an autonomous "university" with its own charter to a "faculty" subordinate to the larger administrative structure known as the Université de France. During the first half of the nineteenth century, Montpellier had to endure regular taunts from Parisians about its decline.

With their reputation at stake, Montpellier physicians wanted to improve their position vis-à-vis Paris by contrasting their own orthodoxy – that is, their vitalistic Hippocratism – with what they considered the overweening materialist orientation of Paris medicine. With the goal of reclaiming some of their lost authority and power, they emphasized their Hippocratism. In the 1840s, physician and professor Jacques Lordat (under whom Risueño d'Amador studied medicine) defended Montpellier medicine against Parisian professors who wanted to shut down the Montpellier Faculté de médecine. The sharply drawn contrasts continued as Parisian physicians identified their medicine as progressive and scientific, in contrast to Montpellier's, which they portrayed as backward-looking, unscientific, and subordinated to religious orthodoxy.[46] It seemed as if the Montpellier Hippocratists could at best hope to keep alive their tradition – a major goal that related, as Risueño d'Amador saw it, not only to medicine, but to a way of life, a worldview. The technology of medical statistics provided him with a "way in" to discuss his broader social concerns.

The role of medical technologies at the Paris School was a subject of continuing debate in the early nineteenth century. Research physicians embraced technologies such as the scalpel, the organization of the clinic, and the stethoscope, but medical statistics and microscopy provoked controversy. Technologies can be tools for controlling and managing information and people. The numerical method was a technology to manage and control therapeutic data, but also patients and physicians, at least according to the critics. Numbers are a technology of communication and representation.[47] Numbers are also rhetorical tools.[48] Technologies can also be tools of transformation, and it was this point that the critics emphasized.[49] Risueño d'Amador and Double saw more clearly than the numerists the transformative nature of medical statistics. They argued that the numerical method was not just an extension of the observational method, not just business as usual, as some of the numerists contended. Rather, the introduction of quantification threatened to change the fundamentals of medicine. More than the numerists, Risueño d'Amador understood that numbers embodied the values of order, precision, rationalization, standardization, and control. These were important values at the Paris School, but they challenged the Montpellier medical tradition.

It would be a mistake, however, to see Risueño d'Amador as an opponent of scientific medicine or of clinical science just because he took a critical stance vis-à-vis medical statistics. In 1836 he had published a prize-winning essay for the Académie de médecine on the history of pathological anatomy that praised pathological anatomy, medical chemistry, and pathological physiology as valuable tools. He saw all these research orientations leading towards a vitalistic neo-humouralism that he identified not only with Montpellier but also with some leading Parisians, including Gabriel Andral.[50] He saw vitalistic neo-humouralism – his term for pathological physiology – as the direction in which medicine was moving, and he applauded this orientation. Criticizing the organicism of some pathological anatomists as not going far enough in uncovering disease, he was supportive of Andral and the "eclectics." So we cannot label him as anti-scientific and anti-progressive, while viewing the numerists and the Paris School as progressive and scientific. Rather he feared the particular, value-laden technology of medical statistics, with all its consequences for the practice of medicine.

Risueño d'Amador recognized the transformative nature of technologies to alter not only the practice of medicine but also the wider society. He saw the introduction of medical statistics as part of an ongoing revolution in worldview, a point that he elaborated in a lecture in 1844 at Montpellier. This inaugural lecture at the Faculté emphasized local culture and indigenous knowledge as a way of defending his type of medicine.[51] Changes in medicine reflected social changes – in this case the quantification of French – and modern – society. Widely accepted in Paris among leading physicians and bureaucrats was the modern administrative state, exemplified by the increasing efforts since early in the century to gather statistics at the national and local levels, with the goal of rationalizing and standardizing French society.[52] Risueño d'Amador argued against the quantification of individuals, which he thought would dehumanize society. He defended not only a view of disease and a kind of medicine but also a way of life.[53]

Risueño d'Amador's criticism of what the numerical method meant for clinical medicine, patients, and physicians mirrored larger social concerns being voiced by contemporary social critics in response to socioeconomic forces such as industrialization and urbanization. Both conservatives – social Catholics, such as Alban de Villeneuve-Bargemont – and socialists argued that industrialization deprived workers of their humanity.[54] Even some liberals – moral economists such as Louis-René Villermé – voiced concern that lack of paternalism on the part of factory owners would dehumanize workers, turning them into "machines à produire."[55]

In opposition to these trends, Risueño d'Amador championed local knowledge and indigenous culture, now under threat;[56] he argued for a way of life that he thought was being undermined by modernity.[57] There existed a widespread perception among urban physicians and reformers that several social groups, including many workers, the poor, and hospital patients, were being dehumanized and that urban society was sick. Pathology was not limited to organs and tissues, but applied to large portions of French society as well. Risueño d'Amador's critique, then, suggests broader political and social concerns related to power, authority, social order, and the place of individuals within that order.

We also need to consider briefly the rhetorical dimensions of the controversy as well as the notion of scientific debate as a key feature of nineteenth-century science and medicine. Participants invoked the rhetoric of science, the rhetoric of Hippocrates, including a more general rhetoric of hostility to medical "systems," and the rhetoric of numbers. J. Rosser Matthews has discussed in detail the rhetoric of science, or the use of science as a tool of legitimation.[58] Both sides justified their position by arguing that they were pursuing scientific goals, that they had the best understanding of science, that their way was scientific, while the opponents' was anti-scientific. For the Parisian numerists, science implied certain or at least reliable knowledge. It also meant the empirical, observational method as they understood it. Risueño d'Amador did not disagree with this notion of science. But he employed anti-system rhetoric to argue that the numerical method represented just one more medical system and that working deductively within a given system was anti-scientific. He argued for inductivism, for observation, which he portrayed as Hippocratic and hence free of system. In so doing, he employed the rhetoric of Hippocrates – a common strategy at the Paris School and elsewhere, which identified Hippocratic medicine with the best, the purest tradition in medicine.

Systematizers of every stripe could be and were portrayed as having departed from this tradition. Hippocratic medicine, as variously understood and used rhetorically, stood for the most scientific and the best medicine. Parisian physicians also used the rhetoric of Hippocrates to support a variety of medical orientations, as I have shown elsewhere.[59]

Numerists subscribed to the rhetoric of numbers: that is, the notion that numbers stood in for value-free facts, facts beyond dispute. Numbers also functioned as representations, not only in and of themselves but especially when arranged in columns and tables. As such, they became pictorial representations, which could stand in for words, be more factual, more scientific, and more convincing.[60] Many physicians remained unconvinced by numerical data, however, as illustrated not only by Double and Risueño d'Amador's arguments, but also by the controversy over puerperal fever at the Académie de médecine in the 1850s discussed in Gérard Jorland's essay in this volume.

Finally, the notion of academic debate as scientific practice deserves brief mention. Both George Weisz and I have shown elsewhere that the academies functioned as sites for the practice of science and medicine.[61] As part of the cultural analysis of science, I have argued that debates are in effect duelling by other means.[62] The practice of science at the academies was a masculine endeavour in which gentlemanly codes of honour prevailed just as they had earlier, as studies of seventeenth-century scientists and academies have shown.[63]

CONCLUSION

In this paper I have argued for the importance of reconsidering classic stories in the history of science and medicine – in this case, the 1837 debate over medical statistics. My goal was to examine the controversy provoked by the introduction of statistics into medicine in order to determine what was at stake for both sides. A new look at this justly famous controversy has revealed the principal issues that were at stake. The main point of contention was the kind of medicine to practise. Related issues included how best to test the efficacy of therapies, the nature of disease, medical power, and the role of technologies both in medicine and in the larger society.

In the end there were no winners in this academic debate. Each side represented a valid way of looking at medicine and disease, and both approaches existed in tension throughout the nineteenth century in France. Despite Risueño d'Amador and famous detractors such as Claude Bernard, quantification in medicine proved to be fruitful. After 1850 the development of medical instrumentation to measure physiological events led to the quantification of pathological processes: the EKG, the sphygmomanometer, the calibrated thermometer, and a variety of laboratory tests to quantify and assess bodily fluids. By the end of the century physicians were finding more and more ways to quantify patients' bodies.

NOTES

1 *Bulletin de l'Académie Royale de Médecine* (*BARM*) 1 (1836–37), 622–806. Benigno Risueño d'Amador had been elected a corresponding member of the academy in December 1836. His essay on pathological anatomy was recognized in 1836 and appeared in the *Mémoires de l'Académie de Médecine* in 1837. The debate began in April 1837. Risueño d'Amador died in 1849.

2 John Rosser Matthews, *Quantification and the Quest for Medical Certainty* (Princeton, NJ: Princeton University Press, 1995). See also Terence D. Murphy, "Medical Knowledge and Statistical Methods in Early Nineteenth-Century France," *Medical History* 25 (1981), 301–19; Theodore M. Porter, *The Rise of Statistical Thinking, 1820–1900* (Princeton, NJ: Princeton University Press, 1986), 152–62; Gerd Gigerenzer et al., *The Empire of Chance: How Probability Changed Science and Everyday Life* (New York: Cambridge University Press, 1989), 45–8.

3 Pierre Louis, *Researches on the Effects of Bloodletting* (Boston: Hilliard, Gray, 1836); cited in Matthews, *Quantification*, 154.

4 On Broussais, see the classic article by Erwin Ackerknecht, "Brousssais or a Forgotten Medical Revolution," *Bulletin of the History of Medicine* 28 (1953), 320–43; see also Michel Foucault, *The Birth of the Clinic: An Archaeology of Medical Perception*, trans. A. Sheridan Smith (New York: Vintage Books, 1975), chap. 10; Michel Valentin, *François Broussais: Empereur de la médecine* (Dinard: Association des Amis du Musée du Pays de Dinard, 1988); Jean-François Braunstein, *Broussais et le matérialisme: Médecine et philosophie au XIXe siècle* (Paris: Méridiens-Klincksieck, 1986); Jacalyn Duffin, "Laennec and Broussais: The 'Sympathetic' Duel," in Caroline Hannaway and Ann La Berge, eds., *Constructing Paris Medicine* (Amsterdam: Rodopi, 1998), 251–74.

5 One estimate by Apollinaire Bouchardat was about 53,000 patients a year. Cited in Erwin Ackerknecht, *Medicine at the Paris Hospital, 1815–1848* (Baltimore, Md.: Johns Hopkins University Press, 1967), 15, 18. See also Dora B. Weiner, *The Citizen Patient in Revolutionary and Imperial Paris* (Baltimore, Md.: Johns Hopkins University Press, 1993).

6 Jacalyn Duffin, "Private Practice and Public Research: The Patients of R.T.H. Laennec," in Ann La Berge and Mordechai Feingold, eds., *French*

Medical Culture in the Nineteenth Century (Amsterdam: Rodopi, 1994), 118–48; Foucault, *Birth of the Clinic*, chap. 5.

7 Russell Maulitz, *Morbid Appearances: The Anatomy of Pathology in the Early Nineteenth Century* (New York: Cambridge University Press, 1987).

8 George Weisz, *The Medical Mandarins: The French Académie de Médecine in the Nineteenth and Early Twentieth Centuries* (New York: Oxford University Press 1995), 73–83.

9 Ivo Schneider, "The Probability Calculus in the Nineteenth Century," in Lorenz Kruger et al., eds., *The Probabilistic Revolution*, 2 vols. (Cambridge, Mass.: MIT Press 1987), vol. 1, 192–210; Cauchy's quotation, 200.

10 *Comptes rendus hébdomadaires des séances de l'Académie des Sciences* (*CRHAS*), 5 (Oct. 1835), 167–77; 19 Oct., 247–50; 26 Oct., 280–1 (Paris: Bachelier, 1835). Mathematician Siméon-Denis Poisson was also a member of the commission.

11 Ackerknecht, *Paris Hospital*, 26, 58, 187; Weisz, *Medical Mandarins*, 24; on the Montpellier medical tradition, see Elizabeth Williams, *The Physical and the Moral: Anthropology, Physiology, and Philosophical Medicine in France, 1750–1850* (New York: Cambridge University Press, 1994). For the eighteenth-century background, see Elizabeth Williams, *A Cultural History of Medical Vitalism in Enlightenment Montpellier* (London: Ashgate, 2003), and also "Hippocrates and the Montpellier Vitalists in the French Medical Enlightenment," in David Cantor, ed., *Reinventing Hippocrates* (London: Ashgate, 2001), 157–77.

12 *CRHAS*, 173, for both quotations.

13 Louis Peisse, *La médecine et les médecins: philosophie, doctrines, institutions, critiques, moeurs et biographies médicales*, 2 vols. (Paris: Baillière, 1857), vol. 1, 149–50; cited in vol. 1, 150; originally in *Bulletin de l'Académie de Médecine*, 28 March 1837.

14 Medical journalist Louis Peisse recalls just how the debate began and lists the main participants. See Peisse, *La médecine*, I, 134. Peisse was not a physician but a medical journalist who wrote a regular column for the *Gazette médicale de Paris*; Schneider, "The Probability Calculus," 193–210.

15 *BARM*, 624.

16 Ibid., 623.

17 Ibid., 634.

18 Peisse, *La médecine*, vol. 1, 232–5; Williams, *The Physical and the Moral*, 20–3.

19 *BARM*, 640.

20 On the varieties of Hippocratic medicine, see Cantor, ed., *Reinventing Hippocrates*; on the uses of Hippocrates in early nineteenth-century France, see Ann La Berge, "The Rhetoric of Hippocrates at the Paris School," in Cantor, ed., *Reinventing Hippocrates*, 178–99 and Peisse, *La médecine*, vol. 1, 236.

21 *BARM*, 624–32; quotations, 624.

22 Ibid., 641–7.

23 John Harley Warner, *The Therapeutic Perspective: Medical Practice, Knowledge, and Identity in America, 1820–1885* (Cambridge, Mass.: Harvard University Press, 1986), 58–80. See also Charles Rosenberg, "The Therapeutic Revolution: Medicine, Meaning, and Social Change in Nineteenth-Century America," in Charles Rosenberg, *Explaining Epidemics and Other Studies in the History of Medicine* (New York: Cambridge University Press, 1992), 9–31.

24 *BARM*, 638–9.

25 Ibid., 634–7.

26 See, for example, Jean-Baptiste Bouillaud, *Essai sur la philosophie médicale* (Paris: de Just Rouvier and E. Le Bouvier, 1836), vii.

27 *BARM*, 676.

28 Ibid., 677.

29 Ibid., 634–5.

30 Ibid.

31 Ibid., 640. On Poisson's "law of large numbers," see Ian Hacking, *The Taming of Chance* (New York: Cambridge University Press, 1990), chap. 12.

32 *BARM*, 699–70. The citation given for Laplace is *Essai philosophique sur le calcul des probabilités*, 35.

33 *BARM*, 719–30.

34 Ibid., 730.

35 Ibid., 732.

36 Ibid., 733–47.

37 Ibid., 751.

38 Ibid., 757–67.

39 Ibid., 778, 787–8.

40 Duffin, "Private Practice." See also her book, *To See with a Better Eye: A Life of R.T.H. Laennec* (Princeton, NJ: Princeton University Press, 1998).

41 On Lebert, see Ann La Berge, "Dichotomy or Integration? Medical Microscopy and the Paris Clinical Tradition," in Hannaway and La Berge, eds., *Constructing Paris Medicine*, 275–312, and also "Medical Microscopy in Paris, 1830–1850," in La Berge and Feingold, eds., *French Medical Culture*, 296–326.

42 See, for example, Joan Sherwood, "Syphilization: Human Experimentation in the Search for a Syphilis Vaccine in the Nineteenth Century," *Journal of the History of Medicine* 54 (1999), 364–86. See also Alex Dracobly, "Ethics of Experimentation on Human Subjects in Mid-Nineteenth-Century France: The Story of the 1859 Syphilis Experiments," *Bulletin of the History of Medicine* 77 (2003), 332–66.

43 Charles Rosenberg, "The Tyranny of Diagnosis: Specific Entities and Individual Experience," *Milbank Quarterly* 80 (2002), 237–60.

44 Joy Harvey, "Faithful to Its Old Traditions? Paris Clinical Medicine from the Second Empire to the Third Republic (1848–1872)," in Hannaway and Ann La Berge, eds., *Constructing Paris Medicine*, 313–36.
45 Ann La Berge and Caroline Hannaway, "Paris Medicine: Perspectives Past and Present," in Hannaway and La Berge, eds., *Constructing Paris Medicine*, 1–69.
46 Ibid. Also see Williams, *The Physical and the Moral*, 140.
47 Theodore Porter, *Trust in Numbers: The Pursuit of Objectivity in Science and Public Life* (Princeton, NJ: Princeton University Press, 1995), vii. The term he uses is "strategies of communication."
48 Hacking, *Taming of Chance*, 85. Hacking argued that in this era statistics were "tools of rhetoric, not science."
49 See, for example, Langdon Winner, *The Whale and the Reactor: A Search for Limits in an Age of High Technology* (Chicago: University of Chicago Press, 1986) and David Nye, *Electrifying America: Social Meanings of New Technology* (Cambridge, Mass.: MIT Press, 1990).
50 "Influence de l'anatomie pathologique sur la médecine," *Mémoires de l'Académie Royale de Médecine* 6 (1837), 313–493.
51 Benigno Risueño d'Amador, *La vie du sang au point de vue des croyances populaires* (Montpellier, 1844).
52 See, for example, Marie-Noëlle Bourguet, *Déchriffrer la France: La statistique départementale à l'époque napoléonienne* (Paris: Editions des Archives Contemporaines, 1988), chap. 1; Ann F. La Berge, *Mission and Method: The Early Nineteenth-Century French Public Health Movement* (New York: Cambridge University Press, 1992), chap. 2.
53 Risueño d'Amador, *La vie du sang.*
54 Alban de Villeneuve-Bargemont, *Economie politique chrétienne*, 3 vols. (Paris: Paulin, 1834).
55 Louis-René Villermé, *Tableau de l'état physique et moral des ouvriers employés dans les manufactures de coton, de laine, et de soie*, 2 vols. (Paris: Renouard, 1840), vol. 2, 55.
56 Risueño d'Amador, *La vie du sang.*
57 Matthews, *Quantification*, 147–8.
58 Ibid.
59 La Berge, "Rhetoric of Hippocrates."
60 Mary Poovey, *A History of the Modern Fact* (Chicago: University of Chicago Press, 1998); Barbara Maria Stafford, *Artful Science: Enlightenment Entertainment and Eclipse of Visual Education* (Cambridge, Mass.: MIT Press, 1994).
61 Weisz, *Medical Mandarins*, 73–83 and chap. 7; Ann F. La Berge, "Debate as Scientific Practice in Mid Nineteenth-Century Paris: The Controversy over the Microscope," *Perspectives on Science: Historical, Philosophical, Social* 12 (2004), 424–53.

62 La Berge, "Debate"; Robert Nye, *Masculinity and Male Codes of Honor in Modern France* (New York: Oxford University Press, 1993).

63 Steven Shapin, *A Social History of Truth: Civility and Science in Seventeenth-Century England* (Chicago: University of Chicago Press, 1994); Mario Biagioli, *Galileo Courtier: The Practice of Science in the Culture of Absolutism* (Chicago: University of Chicago Press, 1993).

6

Standardizing Body Temperature: Quantification in Hospitals and Daily Life, 1850–1900

VOLKER HESS

One of the first quantifying techniques in medicine, the thermometer, entered hospitals only in the mid-nineteenth century and found its way from there into everyday life at the end of the century.[1] Fever measurement was thus the first instrumental technique to incorporate the principles of modern medicine in three respects. First, the measurement translated traditional modes of judgment based on assessing the tactual heat or the patient's feelings into an abstract number. Second, by defining the normal ranges of a physiological function, the data distinguished between the healthy and the sick in a way that became characteristic of the quantifying approach of modern medicine.[2] Third, by discretely demarcating borderlines, fever measurement established a new way of dealing with illness inside and outside of the hospital.[3] In a sense, body temperature became standardized in triplicate – as a procedure for measurement, as biological nature, and as a social value.

It is not my intention, however, to recount this story in the epistemological framework of Canguilhem or as part of a normalizing discourse à la Foucault.[4] Instead, I concentrate on the practices through which quantitative methods were established and deployed in the hospital and in daily life. I wish to demonstrate that the instrumental quantification of morbid states took on very different meanings that we cannot understand simply in terms of Foucault's concept of normalization. Normalization is often too easily attributed to the intrinsic effects of measurement and the quantitative appropriation of the individual. By contrast, I intend to show for the German case that, in order to account for the complexity of historical processes, one must distinguish between different stages in the standardization of instruments and measurement practices on the one hand and Foucault's normalization on the other.

Hence, I first consider the standardization of measurement practices. Then I analyse the objectivity of the body subjected to those practices and their meanings for the patients. Finally, I look at technical standardization in terms of the introduction of fever measurement in day-to-day practice, emphasizing the social recognition and stabilization implied in instrumental quantification.

STANDARDIZING THE PRACTICE OF MEASUREMENT

Replacing qualitative thinking was the first step in standardization. Although there were – even by modern standards – reliable thermometers dating back to the late seventeenth century,[5] physicians and scientists remained sceptical well into the mid-nineteenth century as to whether the thermometer recorded the natural heat of life or the unnatural warmth of fever.[6] At the turn of the seventeenth century, the orderly measurements that Anton de Haen (1704–1776) had taken in the Vienna Citizen Hospital seemed to contradict Hippocratic doctrine. As one contemporary remarked, "de Haen was certainly able to observe sensitive heat – without inborn heat necessarily being likewise constituted."[7] Today, we can barely imagine the qualitative diversity once involved in distinguishing a caustic, dry, or burning heat – to say nothing of a so called cold fever. This wealth of heat qualities disappeared through the introduction of instrumental measurement, which translated the subjective experience of illness into the visible extension of a mercury column and thereby reduced the sensory qualities to the discrete quantities that one could read from a scale.

Medical historiography has often portrayed objectifying quantification as an inevitable consequence of scientific measurement.[8] Indeed, mid-nineteenth-century thermometry first gained a foothold in the hospital as part of the scientific turn of medicine, when clinicians tried hard to mimic the laboratory methods and disciplinary identity of contemporary physiology. The transformation of hospitals from social asylums into institutions of medical care provided ample space for such efforts. In large city hospitals, such as those in Berlin or Leipzig, clinicians managed within a few years to determine the 'normal range' of human body temperature. One of them was Carl August Wunderlich (1815–1877), the professor of the internal ward in Leipzig. In 1868, having taken the temperatures of thousands of patients and accumulated reams of data in less than ten years, he proudly published the "fundamental rules" in fever diseases based on the behaviour of inner heat.[9]

However, neither Wunderlich nor his colleagues justified their definitions of physiological norms. Nor did nineteenth-century clinicians pay much heed to statistics (in the narrow sense) and calculations of the distribution or the standard deviation.[10] As long as the data were obtained using scientific measurement techniques they were taken to offer an objective representation of the state of the human body.

But this historiographical perspective neglects the "normalization" of fever measurement in hospitals. It appears as though measurement merely brought hidden nature to light. That was why biological norms – unlike other social or technical norms – expressed in the form of normal values seemed particularly sacrosanct. In the case of body temperature, however, this biological nature of the normal range was a very artificial product. The reproduction of measurements independent of place, time, and measurer was not as simple as we might think in today's world of digital and ear thermometers. The classic minute maximum thermometer emerged only after establishment of the new method.[11] Without it, surveying body temperature was an extremely laborious and time-consuming venture that often lasted more than half an hour. Taking scientific – i.e., systematic – measurements involved not fitting the instrument to the patient, but vice versa. The Berlin clinician Ludwig Traube (1818–1876) first described this management of the patient's body in 1851 and called it the "method of measurement":[12]

> First of all the patient is placed as horizontally as possible on his back ... The arm is then brought toward the trunk so that it rests as tightly as possible along the length of the trunk. As soon as it touches the trunk, it is bent to a right angle at the elbow and the lower arm is passed by the thermometer and placed on the stomach. The upper arm, which now rests tightly on the trunk is then fixed in this position with a chaff-pillow, which is pressed against the arm horizontally by means of a nearby heavy object, such as a chair. After ten minutes the level of the mercury column is recorded and from then on every five minutes, until the column finally remains at a constant height for a period of five minutes. Usually this will be the case only after a period of 25 to 35 minutes, occasionally even longer. One of the main ways to ensure that a constant level is reached quickly is doubtless the careful closure of the armpit.

In effect, patients participated in producing an objective representation of their biological 'nature.' The choreography of this new body technique[13] depended on patients who practised and learned such sequences of controlled movement. The disciplined posture thereby made possible the controlled and reducible measurements. In turn, these measurements shaped the 'normal' ranges. One may ask why hospital patients were willing to offer up their bodies to these ends. Why did they willingly adapt themselves in such a manner so as to guarantee the necessary fit between themselves and the instrument? Why did they subject themselves to this procedure of measurement? Why did they offer their body to the curiosity of the physician? And what benefit did they derive from the objectification of their bodies? In order to answer these questions, we must first look at the historical background of the hospitals in which this body technique of temperature measurement arose.

THE BODY'S OBJECTIVITY

For a long time, the German hospital was primarily a coercive institution for poor relief. In recent years, however, empirical studies have uncovered important nineteenth-century developments.[14] By the first half of the nineteenth century, the growing proportion of insured patients had already transformed the traditional poor house into an institution of medical treatment,[15] while poor patients shifted to complementary forms of ambulant care.[16] The hospital clientele came increasingly from the lower class, especially the 'labouring poor.' In the Charité Hospital in Berlin, the proportion of so-called self-payers increased from 30 per cent in 1834 to 70 per cent in 1868.[17] These people had to pay for health insurance through workers' unions or hospital subscriptions, and they came to consider hospitalization not as an arbitrary act of mercy or bountiful philanthropy, but rather as a service purchased by their own contributions.

Academic physicians had little interest in hospitals before the early nineteenth century because of their orientation towards traditional bedside treatment.[18] Although the social transformation of hospitals gave them access to very interesting acute 'patient material,' it also presented them with a new type of patient they considered unworthy of their attention. And those patients had expectations and claims that physicians were ill prepared to handle. The contrast between the new clinical practice and traditional bedside treatment could hardly have been greater.[19] In traditional medicine, patients and physicians hailed from the same socioeconomic class and shared the same conceptions of the world and of themselves, as well as a common concern for the human body and the civic ideals of a healthy life and regular behaviour. In hospitals, however, patients were not civic patrons who honoured the physician, but instead workers, journeymen, or menial labourers with room and board paid for by insurance companies.

While the structure of the traditional consultation aimed at helping patients to cope meaningfully with their disease experience, the primary interest of hospitalized patients could well be the rapid restoration of fitness to work. In the eighteenth century, examination of patients was the essential element in the interaction that excavated subtle perceptions and hidden feelings.[20] In the nineteenth-century hospital, however, the patient's voice became useless to the physician. As a widespread handbook of clinical medicine remarked, the patient's "descriptions usually concern only various feelings, combined with speculations about the origin of the illness. If the patients are able to relate the temporal course of their complaints, one can learn something about the actual condition of their bodies from these rather confused reports. One must learn to understand the vernacular and to translate these vague reports into the language of medical reality."[21]

The academic arrogance and social alienation associated with this viewpoint are unmistakable. The educated doctor and the uneducated, proletarian hospital patient hailed from different social worlds no personally negotiated discourse about complaints and sickness could bridge. For the doctor at the bedside and for clinical scientists in general, hospital patients remained largely mute. Their speech seemed vague, confused, and full of sensations – in a word, subjective. But this judgment involved more than simply social exclusion. It points to the central function of objectifying measurement in the doctor–patient relationship. The rules of traditional bedside medicine never governed hospital patients, because they were never able to participate in the learned and enlightened discourse that characterized examination in private practice. While measurement could not alter a patient's social standing, it did replace muted speech with a technology that granted the body an 'objective voice.' This objective body, brought into the hospital by the voiceless, lower-class patient, now comprised the language of medical reality. The objective measurements configured the body as the object of reference in the interaction between doctor and patient.

One can suppose that patients were well aware of the problems of communication. Because verbalization was insufficient to communicate illness and its severity, measurement also offered patients a form of communication based on the objective language of their bodies. If Wunderlich, as I have suggested, spent more time on his rounds visiting the fever curves rather than the patients themselves,[22] then the *bon mot* seems not as farfetched as its author may have intended; the well-drawn curve was perhaps more communicative than any story told by a case history.

The objective body, which spoke in an obvious, exact, and undeniable manner, superceded the eloquent patient. And the sense and meaning of illness emerged not in enlightened conversation, but through negotiation in a practice, which actively involved patients in fitting themselves to the instrument. For the patient, the objective body comprised not only the means and basis of the interaction, but also the reference point from which to derive the illness's meaning.

The sole verbal statements about this communicative function came from physicians. For example, the clinician Felix Niemeyer confessed publicly in 1869 that he would "often hide the body temperature from hospital patients for reasons of humanity, because the patients had learned *first hand* that high temperatures decreased their prospects of recovery."[23] In this way, the bodies' objectivity, articulated in measurable numbers, opened up new forms of perception and experience that patients too shared.

However, the patients imposed their body's objectivity not only in the course of ward rounds. The body became the object of all medical interest. Hospital staff pondered, cleansed, nursed, and fed it – and in the 1860s, its recovery was a question no longer of subjective well-being, but of quantifying practices such as daily weight control. In the records of the Leipzig hospital, one can find the case of a young craftsman, whose "status was, much improved ... after a treatment of six weeks, the appetite and all functions [were] good, liveliness fully returned and weight had increased at first slowly, then more quickly."[24] As the reports on weight control over the next ten weeks prior to discharge indicate, the objectified body remained the reference point for doctor–patient interaction.

As the complaints of the Leipzig city fathers demonstrate, the new form of care was not simply the side effect of a new clinical treatment. Concerned about rising costs, they noticed that disbursement for patients' food was increasing in comparison with other costs – despite the falling price of bread. Analysing the details showed the reason for the cost increase: physicians had ordered more and more special rations instead of the regular meatless food.[25] The hospital rightly boasted about its food and catering, and it "did everything the physicians deemed necessary without protest or delay."[26] And some patients even mentioned in their autobiographies that they had spent the "best time" of their lives in hospital.[27]

It would be wrong to explain patients' conduct simply as a response to the 'reward system' of institutionalized care. This would ignore the expectations and claims brought about by the transformed hospital. Patients usually received back the costs of the hospital stay, but sick pay rarely compensated for lost wages. Each hospitalization meant a loss of income and required individuals to weigh the conflicting interests of medical treatment and financial security. Thus the patient might feel even better 'understood' by an interaction based on the moral economy of the objective body.

Clinical measurement did not simply *translate* physical distress and need into medical language. It *reduced* them as well to 'purely medical' phenomena. Hospitals could hardly be expected to be able to treat the 'proletarian disease' and misery but they could deal with the abnormal heat or excessively low weight of an objective body. Quantifications might also operationalize needs and demands from the patients' perspective in a way that fulfilled their expectations of good care and treatment because they resulted in an immediate action. The scales measured physical need as "underweight" and translated it into a therapeutic diet. And the thermometer inscribed physical illness into readable fever curves and rewrote it in the form of therapeutic concepts. The clinical quantifications not only endowed patients with bodies of therapeutic relevance, but also freed them from all family needs, doubts, and justifications by recognizing only 'objective facts.'[28]

In the second half of the nineteenth century, the objective body acquired a value of its own in three respects. First, medical practices such as measuring temperature or weight became entirely adequate body techniques from the patient's point of view because they combined into a meaningful relationship their own worries about the sick body and physicians' specialized knowledge and interests. Not only did quantification meet the expectations placed in medical expertise and competence, but it also assured that the situative and adequate application of that expertise would depend on patients' body techniques.[29] Hence, body training in the regular procedure of measurement ensured the controlled and regulated application of the medical power that new forms of knowledge production had generated.

Second, clinical quantification configured the objective body as a social point of reference. One may today mourn the fact that the patient's subjective speech does not receive due consideration; but in the historical context of the nineteenth century, minimizing doctor–patient communication might have offered a chance to compensate somewhat for pre-existing social inequalities in the treatment situation. Furthermore, the enlightenment discourse about "excavating" subtle perceptions and hidden feelings turned out to be extremely fuzzy and subjective and was ultimately disavowed and condemned as unscientific. The practice of quantification made the bodies of lower-class patients both scientifically objective and socially normal.[30]

Third, debates have arisen in the context of cultural history. Scholars have emphasized that the often-obsessive self-observation so characteristic of the enlightened discourse of bedside medicine served to facilitate an understanding and an internalization of the values of scientific objectivity and social normality. These values distinguished bodies of the bourgeois from those of the nobility and the lower classes. The fragile nature of bourgeois bodies – corresponding to their delicate social status – required diligent observation, careful control of internal motions, and constant concern about harmful influences.[31] If examination of patients had once centred on body care, on which the aspiring middle class had based its hegemony, then what was the meaning of measured and objectified hospital bodies? Quantification also established a conscious and controlled interaction with the body. The precision of the measurement was based on the precision of the body. Only control could subject its physical nature to scientific objectification and deem it 'normal.' Ultimately, over the course of the nineteenth century, this body's scientific qualities and meanings became generally normative. Its objectivity also legitimated claims to political and social equality at a time when the hierarchically divided class society was changing into a complex and functionally arranged industrial society. In this context, quantifying measurement established a point of social reference beyond the economic and social class divide.[32]

TECHNICAL STANDARDIZATION

Real standardization of body temperature began when fever measuring gained general acceptance. At the end of the nineteenth century, 'normal ranges' of temperature embedded themselves in the daily life experience of illness as measuring instruments entered into the private household. If we can believe contemporary physicians, faith that temperature measurement could distinguish between morbidity and health greatly facilitated this process. Furthermore, in private practice the sick person had quickly learned to derive "reassurance from the temperature measurement." As Wunderlich proudly pronounced, it had become "customary that patients, asked how they felt, answered by stating their temperature."[33] Laypersons also soon measured themselves.

And to the extent that patients began to verify their actual well-being with instruments, the physiologically defined normal temperature acquired a normative meaning, which it had not previously had in the laboratory or hospital. One remarkable episode appears in Jens Lachmund and Gunnar Stollberg's recent study of patients' autobiographies. Lilly Braun (1865–1916), socialist and feminist, noted in her diary about 1900: "I was so weak and scorching! I crept to the bedroom with my last ounce of strength and place a fever thermometer under the arm: 39½ [degrees Celsius] – I called for Berta and sent for the doctor."[34] But aligning the subjective experience of illness with measurable normality does not fully explain why a normative definition of health entered daily life. What led ill persons to view this alignment as self-evident? And why did they trust the measured quantities? An initial clue surfaces in gauging and calibrating of thermometers – practices that opened the way for the instrument to move into daily life.

From the late eighteenth century on, the calibration of thermometers had posed no serious problems. In contrast to measuring lengths and volumes, temperature scales related to the physical properties of water – and these were easy to reproduce everywhere as long as one accounted for air pressure. Consequently, nineteenth-century clinicians could and had to gauge their own instruments. All the instruments were employed, even if "the manufacturer's calibration was incorrect." Only the "uniform calibration" of the scale, which could be "carefully compared with a normal-thermometer," was important.[35] Usually each hospital had one or two so-called normal thermometers with which people matched the clinical instruments. Such local standardization turned out to be sufficient for limited application within hospitals. Outside, however, accuracy at a personal level required specifying the manufacturer of the instruments and the clinician conducting the readings. This seemed to be sufficient for the dissemination of fever measurement as clinical practice.

Until the early twentieth century, states did not base efforts to calibrate thermometers on public health or hygiene policy; instead, they responded to issues relating to industrial production and trade. The official certificates granted by the Imperial Physical-Technical Institute (Physikalisch-Technische Reichsanstalt) attested to the quality of manufacturers' products as tested by an independent, scientific agency and thereby promoted sales.[36] The technical standardization of the fever thermometer was part of the processes of industrial competition, whereby strict standards could help ensure transparent construction, function, and material quality. Official certification – on paper or etched on the glass tube – vouched for the instrument's integrity.

Implementing technical standardization in the medical world of hospitals also had important social components. This we can see in the reports that the Prussian ministry of culture requested from the medical administration districts in 1907.[37] At first, the ministry wanted to know the benefits that use of officially certified thermometers had brought to public hospitals. Second, it was keen to find out what hospital directors and local medical officials thought about state-controlled standardization. Throughout the empire – from Swabian Sigmaringen to Upper Silesia – local officials did not necessarily support government policy in this domain. Comparing the reliability and the precision of standardized and unstandardized instruments, they saw no benefit from official calibration. Nor did they perceive any technological advantages to state-certified calibration as opposed to self-calibration: "[T]he competition of the manufacturers among themselves resulted in more diligent production of instruments," as experience had shown. The results of officially certified instruments were "not at all favourable."[38] Some reports "recommended no general enforcement."[39]

Agreement with or objection to the draft edict related not to technical concerns about precision or reliability. The decisive arguments flowed from other considerations. Even opponents did not dispute "the progress ... that state certification will bring."[40] However, expert opinions were usually rather hazy about what constituted progress. They stressed again and again the "reliability" of official instruments and their "desirable uniformity," although these benefits had not emerged in practice. So it was not any qualitative gain, but the so-called guarantee of reliability, that was crucial. Thus, officially certified measurement seemed to imply not instrumental accuracy, but rather authoritative safety. It was not so much the metric correctness of the measuring but rather some sort of general reliability that state sanction ensured and guaranteed.

The reports showed the significance of the state guarantee in three respects. First, they articulated independent expertise in the form of demands that state-employed physicians use state-certified standards. The certification took on the function of a state guarantee for the objectivity of medical opinion in the same way as trade associations and insurance companies required certified thermometers for the reports of medical examiners. Here objectivity meant official justification and assessment free from any personal inclinations. Second, for use of thermometers by unqualified staff and lay personnel, only state-certified, technical quality control could guarantee competence and reliability – at least in the eyes of the medical officials. While state regulation appeared superfluous or counter-productive in hospitals, it was necessary for everyone involved with thermometers outside the medical profession. Official certification seemed to guarantee the safety and validity of the measurement that – from the physicians' perspective – only the professional authority of their own guild could legitimate.

Third, official certification granted social status to the measurements. It validated the measurement independent of the technical quality of any single instrument. There was also no longer need for medical confirmation if a certified instrument indicated a temperature that the enclosed instructions defined as "high fever." State guarantees granted an official status to such terms and meanings. Therefore state certification served a social function, transporting professional authority from an originally medical practice to an impersonal and independent standard.

At three levels state-ordered certification replaced locally authorized standards in hospitals with statewide standardization. Within the profession, it legitimated medical expertise; outside the profession, it sanctioned the work of general practitioners vis-à-vis academic physicians. And in the public sphere, it guaranteed that everyone could measure fever without regard for professional expertise.

Despite medical officials' objections, state certification began in 1910. As a consequence of technical, industrial standardization, the normalized body temperature, created in hospitals, could now acquire greater social influence. The most obvious example occurs in the instructions of the Imperial Physical-Technical Institute enclosed with the certified thermometer describing the meaning of high readings. Those instructions allowed lay people to participate in the privileged objectivity of measurement.

Physicians were not enthusiastic about this development, although they were partly responsible for the increasing popularity of thermometers. One of them presented horror scenarios in which "a kind of meteorological station would be set up in the home of a feverish person or a number of instruments would wander promiscuously into all the accessible body openings of male and female clientele."[41] Such apprehensions surfaced most outspokenly in the illustrated mass press. There readers learned that "amicable doctor–patient relations" were impossible if patients tried "to control or even to master" the physician by acquiring medical knowledge.[42]

One author complained bitterly about the "unauthorized appropriation" of medical competence. After the introduction of antifever drugs, some patients, with a certain satisfaction, told their doctor that an hour earlier the thermometer still showed almost 38 degrees Fahrenheit but that now the temperature had dropped to 37. The measurement permitted the patients to form their own judgment about their illness – something that physicians did not always like. Some doctors tried in vain in the mass press to inform the lay public that a "small deviation from the ordinary level was often the cause of wholly unfounded concern."[43] This was, however, no longer an esoteric one available only to physicians. If the mercury column rose above the red mark, then the illness was officially certified. At this level of social interaction, measurement registered a standardized meaning.

Technical standardization supported an inner standardization, of the definition and understanding of disease, most notably in the health insurance industry. The organizational structures developed in this sphere facilitated emergence of uniform standards of behaviour that were just as important for the labour movement as for the state or industrialists. Health insurance schemes (Kassen), to which factory workers or former guild members contributed for their own benefit, made it incumbent on all contributors to behave in a financially responsible manner if they wished to enjoy the practical solidarity of their colleagues. In spite of rigid rules set down in the statutes of Kassen, there was no need for sanctions or pressure in smaller ones, where everybody knew everyone else. Mutual control could form the backbone of insurance schemes because everybody had an interest in low payments and adequate reserves.[44]

Physicians received a major place in this care structure. Only they could determine whether to grant or deny benefits.[45] Their professional judgment could unlock sick pay. Yet their judgments were anything but independent. Working for insurance plans put them in a "most unfortunate" position.[46] They always had to deal with the suspicion of simulation of illness, which most company regulations threatened to punish in draconian fashion and which was implicit in the procedures verifying sickness.[47] None the less, at the turn of century the handbooks for health-plan doctors constantly reminded them not to treat the patient unjustly "as a simulator or hypochondriac."[48] They even insisted "that any member seeking medical help first and foremost be viewed as an ill person." In questionable cases, physicians should, like judges, always rule "in favor of the patient."[49]

Doctors often did not do this. Health-plan patients frequently complained about unjust treatment.[50] Some physicians in turn felt that patients were being presumptuous whenever they did not behave as indigents receiving medical care as an act of charity. Thus conflicts arose time and again, ignited by self-confident patients who, because they paid insurance premiums, made claims to services that, in the eyes of physicians, should be only for private patients. Newspapers accused health-insurance plans of awakening expectations by raising the mere "possibility of treatment." Whole "classes of the population" had acquired a "consciousness and a feeling for all manner of suffering that they had previously never taken notice of."[51]

Within this matrix, technical standardization and official certification exercised a social impact. They served as an independent authority that could resolve conflicts impartially and objectively, irrespective of the individuals involved.[52] State-certified objectivity could serve as a corrective force for social control. If, according to the labour health library, workers had a "certified standardized thermometer" at home, then an abnormal temperature relieved the sick from the moral pressure that the solidarity of the health-insurance community imposed. It also granted the worker the right to go on sick leave. An abnormal temperature justified physicians' actions in the face of penny-pinching insurance company boards. It likewise shielded them from workers' expectations – regardless of whether they simulated their complaints or, more probably, dissimulated them. Standardized measurement balanced mutually conflicting interests, obligations, and values in this way.[53]

Moral education and the internalization of Protestant virtues did not minimize the conflict for the persons concerned. On the contrary, things became rather more complicated for everyone caught up these conflicting motivations – care for the needy body, the threat of the family sinking into poverty, and behaviour that conformed with the social world of the labour community.

CONCLUSION: TECHNOLOGIES OF QUANTIFICATION

The quantification of body temperature was not a necessary result of technological advance that simply progressed as an instrumental objectifying practice from the laboratory to daily life via the hospital. It was also not an inevitable result of the inherent forces of medical science driven towards progress by curiosity and the urge to know. The technology of quantification was no black box that could move from one space of knowledge to another. Each shift related to a specific labour of assimilation: to the hospital, where patients adapted to new body techniques, and to daily life, where state decree standardized instruments.

Consequently, despite long-existing technical and scientific preconditions, fever measurement established itself only after the 1850s. It did so in two steps: in the transformation of the hospital before 1900 and in the daily life of most people soon afterwards. Quantifying body temperature grew out of a specific social space and was linked to specific social practice.

To say this is hardly new. Fever measurement, however, shows that the usual model of normalization which sees quantification as an essential element of modern biopolitics cannot fully explain the technology of quantification. Without a doubt, quantifying and objectifying forged the biological, social, and cultural bodies we have today. However, other social practices also imparted these technologies. Embedded in a set of actions, they produced and related meanings that historians overlook if they understand quantification as *only* a disciplinary and regulative technique. Thus the body technologies that gave data their scientific value did not simply secure the coherent use of medical power. Quantification provided the patient with a body, whose objectivity lay outside the social restrictions and the social exclusion of traditional forms of interaction. Even state certification was not necessarily in the interests of medical experts. Rather, it contributed to their regulation. It ensured that, within the social asymmetry of the system of sickness insurance, patients could exert some social control over medical authority.

No doubt the quantification of body temperature is only one example of a new social technology. But the standardizations that prepared the way for quantification in the hospital and in daily life did not simply serve to document, measure, control, and regulate the individual. They also somehow allowed the individual to regulate and control this social technology.

NOTES

1 On this and many of the arguments presented in the article, see Volker Hess, *Der wohltemperierte Mensch: Wissenschaft und Alltag des Fiebermessens (1850–1900)* (Frankfurt am Main: Campus, 2000).

2 Stanley Joel Reiser, *Medicine and the Reign of Technology* (Cambridge: Cambridge University Press, 1977), chap. 5.

3 Georges Canguilhem, *Essai sur quelques problèmes concernant le normal et le pathologique*, 2nd ed. (Paris: Société d'Editions les Belles Lettres, 1950).

4 Michel Foucault, *Surveiller et punir: La naissance de la prison* (Paris: Gallimard, 1975), and especially his later work, *Histoire de la sexualité, vol. 1: La volonté de savoir* (Paris: Editions Gallimard, 1976), on which the recent discourses about "normalization" build. See, for example, Jürgen Link, *Versuch über den Normalismus: Wie Normalität produziert wird*, 2nd ed. (Opladen: Westdeutscher Verlag, 1997).

5 W.E. Knowles Middleton, *A History of the Thermometer and Its Uses in Meteorology* (Baltimore, Md.: Johns Hopkins Press, 1966). In the 1660s the first closed thermometers were produced, and after 1700 there were many trials to determine fix points and scales of graduation. See also Audrey B. Davis, *Medicine and Its Technology: An Introduction to the History*

of Medical Instrumentation (Westport, Conn.: Greenwood Press, 1981), 61–85.

6 It was "remarkable," as Gershon-Cohen mentioned, "how the thermometer comes in and out of prominence in physics and medicine without achieving a permanent niche in medical practice in spite of being fostered by some of the learned men in science and medicine." See J. Gershon-Cohen, "A Short History of Medical Thermometry," *Annals of the New York Academy of Sciences* 121 (1964), 4.

7 Kurt Sprengel, *Die Apologie des Hippokrates und seiner Grundsätze* (Leipzig: Schwickert, 1789), 165.

8 See, for example, Reiser, *Medicine and the Reign of Technology.*

9 Carl Reinhold August Wunderlich, "Remittierende Fieber mit Phlyetenideneruption," *Archiv für Heilkunde* 5 (1864), 57–77, and "Vorlegung einiger Elementarthatsachen aus der praktischen Krankenthermometrie und Anleitung zur Anwendung der Wärmemessung in der Privatpraxis," *Archiv für Heilkunde* 1 (1860), 385–416.

10 William Coleman, "Experimental Physiology and Statistical Inference: The Therapeutic Trial in Nineteenth-Century Germany," in Lorenz Krüger, Gerd Gigerenzer, and Mary S. Morgan, eds., *The Probabilistic Revolution* (Cambridge: Cambridge University Press, 1987), 201–26.

11 See Karl Ehrle, "Ueber den Quecksilberthermometer mit permanenter feiner Luftblase, für die Körperwärmebeobachtung am Krankenbette, für physiologische und pharmakologische Versuch," *Deutsches Archiv für klinische Medizin* 7 (1870), 345–55.

12 Ludwig Traube, "Ueber die Wirkungen der Digitalis, insbesondere über den Einfluß derselben auf die Körpertemperatur in fieberhaften Krankheiten," *Annalen des Charité-Krankenhauses zu Berlin* 1–2 (1850–51), 622–91; 12–120, 119ff.

13 See Marcel Mauss, "Die Techniken des Körpers (Les techniques du corps, 1934)," in Wolf Lepenies and Henning Ritter, eds., *Soziologie und Anthropologie* (München: Hanser, 1975), 199–220.

14 For an overview, see Alfons Labisch and Reinhard Spree, eds., "Einem jeden Kranken in einem Krankenhause sein eigenes Bett," in *Zur Sozialgeschichte des Allgemeinen Krankenhauses in Deutschland im 19. Jahrhundert* (Frankfurt am Main: Campus, 1996).

15 See Johanna Bleker, "To Benefit the Poor and Advance Medical Science: Hospitals and Hospital Care in Germany, 1820–1870," in Manfred Berg and Geoffrey Cocks, eds., *Medicine and Modernity: Public Health and Medical Care in Nineteenth and Twentieth Century Germany* (Washington, DC: German Historical Institute, 1997), 17–33.

16 See Ragnhild Münch, *Gesundheitswesen im 18. and 19. Jahrhundert: Das Berliner Beispiel* (Berlin: Akademie-Verlag, 1995).

17 See Hess, *Der wohltemperierte Mensch.*

18 The best example is the debate on the establishment of the Berlin University, in which physicians such as Hufeland argued for a small teaching clinic separated from the Charité hospital. Along the lines of the *theatrum nosologicum,* they argued that the prospective physician learned not from the quantity of observation but from the quality of exemplary study.

19 Claudia Huerkamp, "Das unterschiedliche Verhalten von Arzt und Patient in der Krankenhauspraxis und der privaten ärztlichen Praxis im 19. Jahrhundert," in Peter Schneck and Hans-Uwe Lammel, eds., *Die Medizin an der Berliner Universität und an der Charité zwischen 1810 und 1850* (Husum: Matthiesen, 1995), 254–68.

20 See Jens Lachmund and Gunnar Stollberg, "The Doctor, His Audience, and the Meaning of Illness: The Drama of Medical Practice in the Late 18th and Early 19th Century," in Jens Lachmund and Gunnar Stollberg, eds., *The Social Construction of Illness: Illness and Medical Knowledge in Past and Present* (Stuttgart: Steiner, 1992), 38–51.

21 Paul Uhle and Ernst Wagner, *Handbuch der allgemeinen Pathologie,* 5th ed. (Leipzig: Wigand, 1872), 23ff.

22 Adolf Strümpell, *Aus dem Leben eines deutschen Klinikers: Erinnerungen und Beobachtungen* (Basel: Vogel, 1925), 66–7.

23 Felix Niemeyer, *Ueber das Verhalten der Eigenwärme beim gesunden und kranken Menschen: Ein populärer Vortrag* (Berlin: Hirschwald, 1869), 43 (emphasis added).

24 Wunderlich, "Remittierende Fieber mit Phlyetenideneruption," 62ff.

25 For details, see Hess, *Der wohltemperierte Mensch,* 215–18.

26 Gustav Biedermann Guenther, "Ueber das Jacobshospital in Leipzig," *Leipziger Tagblatt und Anzeiger* 89 (1846), 829–31.

27 Barbara Elkeles, "Arbeiterautobiographien als Quelle der Krankenhausgeschichte," *Medizinhistorisches Journal* 23 (1988), 353, and "Der Patient und das Krankenhaus," in Alfons Labisch and Reinhard Spree, eds., *"Einem jedem Kranken in einem Hospitale sein eigenes Bett": Zur Sozialgeschichte des Allgemeinen Krankenhauses in Deutschland im 19. Jahrhundert* (Frankfurt A.M.: Campus, 1996), 361ff. See also Jens Lachmund and Gunnar Stollberg, *Patientenwelten: Krankheit und Medizin vom späten 18. bis zum frühen 20. Jahrhundert im Spiegel von Autobiographien* (Opladen: Leske & Budrich, 1995), especially 151–78.

28 V. Hess, "Die moralische Ökonomie der Normalisierung: Das Beispiel Fiebermessen," in Werner Sohn and Herbert Mehrtens, eds., *Normalität und Abweichung: Studien zur Theorie und Geschichte der Normalisierungsgesellschaft* (Opladen: Westdeutscher Verlag, 1999), 222–43.

29 See Per Maseide, "Possibly Abusive, Often Benign, and Always Necessary: On Power and Domination in Medical Practice," *Sociology of Health and Illness* 13 (1991), 545–61.

30 See V. Hess, "Messen und Zählen: Die Herstellung des normalen Menschen als Maß der Gesundheit," *Berlin Wissenschaft Geschichte* 22 (1999), 266–80.

31 See Michael Stolberg, "'Mein äskulapisches Orakel!' Patientenbriefe als Quelle einer Kulturgeschichte der Krankheitserfahrung im 18. Jahrhundert," *Österreichische Zeitschrift für Geschichtswissenschaft* 7 (1996), 385–404.

32 The political impact of science in general and of quantification and objectification in particular was evident in the liberal-democratic movement of 1848 and in subsequent decades, See the detailed study by Constantin Goschler, *Rudolf Virchow. Mediziner – Anthropologe – Politiker* (Cologne: Böhlau, 2002), especially part 3: "Szientismus und liberale Utopie."

33 C.R.A. Wunderlich, "Vorlegung einiger Elementarthatsachen aus der praktischen Krankenthermometrie und Anleitung zur Anwendung der Wärmemessung in der Privatpraxis," *Archiv für Heilkunde* 1 (1860), 416.

34 Lily Braun, *Memoiren einer Sozialistin,* cited in Gunnar Stollberg, "Haben messende Verfahren die Lebenswelt der Patienten kolonisiert? Überlegungen auf der Basis von Autobiographien," in Volker Hess, ed., *Normierung von Gesundheit: Messende Verfahren der Medizin als kulturelle Praktik der Medizin um 1900* (Husum: Matthiesen, 1997), 133.

35 Wunderlich, "Vorlegung einiger Elementarthatsachen aus der praktischen Krankenthermometrie."

36 See David Cahan, ed., *An Institute for an Empire: The Physikalisch-Technische Reichsanstalt 1871–1918* (Cambridge: Cambridge University Press, 1989).

37 See *Geheimes Staatsarchiv Preußischer Kulturbesitz,* Rep. 76 VIII B, Nr. 1731 (Berichte über Krankenanstalten und Prüfung der Thermometer).

38 Ibid., Report of the Medical Councilor, Aachen, 27 Nov. 1907.

39 Ibid., Report of the Medical Councilor, Stralsund, 18 Dec. 1907.

40 Ibid., district government Cologne, 30 Dec. 1907.

41 Johann Hermann Baas, *Medizinische Diagnostik,* 2nd ed. (Stuttgart: Enke, 1883), 66.

42 Fr. Dornblüth, "Aerzte und Publicum," *Gartenlaube* (1884), 478–80, 527–8.

43 Carl Posner, "Fieber und Fiebermittel," *Gartenlaube* (1909), 13.

44 Ute Frevert, *Krankheit als politisches Problem 1770–1880: Soziale Unterschichten in Preußen zwischen medizinischer Polizei und staatlicher Sozialversicherung, vol. 62: Kritische Studien zur Geschichtswissenschaft* (Göttingen: Vandenhoeck & Ruprecht, 1984), 215.

45 Ibid., 214.

46 Justus Thiersch, *Der Kassenarzt: Eine Darstellung der Gesetze für Versicherung der Arbeiter und ihre Bedeutung für den practischen Arzt* (Leipzig: Barth, 1895), 62.

47 Ignaz Zadek, *Die Arbeiterversicherung* (Jena: Fischer, 1895), 33; Marlene Ellerkamp, *Industriearbeit, Krankheit und Geschlecht, Zu den sozialen Kosten der Industrialisierung: Bremer Textilarbeiterinnen 1870–1914, Kritische Studien zur Geschichtswissenschaft* (Göttingen: Vandenhoeck und Ruprecht, 1991).

48 Jacob Wolff, *Der praktische Arzt und sein Beruf, Vademecum für angehende Praktiker* (Stuttgart: Enke, 1896), 97.

49 Karl Jaffé, "Stellung und Aufgabe des Arztes auf dem Gebiete der Krankenversicherung," in Moritz Fürst, ed., *Handbuch der Sozialen Medizin*, vol. II (Jena: Fischer 1903), 139.

50 Ibid., 139.

51 E. Düring, "Der Hausarzt," *Gartenlaube* (1910), 35.

52 Theodore M. Porter, *Trust in Numbers: The Pursuit of Objectivity in Science and Public Life* (Princeton, NJ: Princeton University Press, 1995).

53 Hess, "Die moralische Ökonomie der Normalisierung."

7

Les multiples usages de la quantification en médecine : Le cas du diabète sucré

CHRISTIANE SINDING

Si le terme de quantification en médecine évoque souvent les essais cliniques et les statistiques, il ne faut pas oublier qu'il y a bien d'autres usages de la mesure et des nombres dans le domaine médical, qu'il s'agisse de la recherche ou de la pratique clinique. Dès le XIXe siècle, par exemple, Claude Bernard (après Broussais) fut un défenseur ardent de la conception quantitative de la maladie, qui seule selon lui permettait de donner à la médecine des fondements scientifiques. Plus généralement, on retrouve l'opposition entre quantitatif et qualitatif tout au long de l'histoire de la médecine. Cette opposition est par exemple à l'œuvre dans l'opposition entre "réductionnistes" et "holistes" ou dans la critique des essais cliniques randomisés par certains médecins. Par ailleurs, la médecine dite "scientifique" s'est construite au carrefour de plusieurs types de savoirs hétérogènes. Il n'est donc pas étonnant que les travaux historiques sur la maladie permettent de mettre au jour différents types de mesure et de quantification à l'œuvre dans la construction des entités morbides. À partir d'un exemple historique concret, celui du diabète sucré, je voudrais indiquer quelques pistes de réflexion sur cette hétérogénéité des usages médicaux de la quantification et me demander, pour terminer, s'il est possible d'esquisser une théorie unitaire de la mesure en médecine.

LA QUANTIFICATION DANS LA DÉFINITION ET L'ÉVALUATION DE LA GRAVITÉ DE LA MALADIE

Claude Bernard fonde sa conception de la maladie sur l'exemple du diabète sucré. Il paraît donc intéressant de s'interroger sur les différents statuts de la mesure dans cette maladie. Broussais, le premier, avait proposé de définir de façon quantitative la maladie en l'assimilant à un excès ou un défaut d'excitabilité des tissus. Exploitant ses propres travaux sur le diabète sucré, Claude Bernard défend une conception similaire : établissant, contre une partie des médecins de l'époque, qu'il y a du sucre dans le sang des sujets sains, il en constate l'élévation des taux dans le sang et les urines des diabétiques. Il se prévaut de ces découvertes pour asseoir le principe de l'identité du normal et du pathologique, lesquels ne diffèrent que de façon quantitative, et propose une conception de la maladie purgée de toute notion qualitative et de toute valeur esthétique ou morale. Les conséquences théoriques et pratiques de cette doctrine sont capitales puisqu'elles aboutissent à identifier santé, normalité et moyenne statistique, et permettent de faire de la maladie un objet de science, réparable par des techniques appropriées : les fondements de la médecine moderne sont ainsi posés. Cette conception bernardienne de la maladie permet aux premiers spécialistes du diabète d'en construire un tableau clinique dominé par des signes "cardinaux" quantifiables : polyurie (émission excessive d'urines), polyphagie (augmentation de l'appétit), hyperglycémie (élévation de la glycémie) et glycosurie élevée (présence de sucre dans les urines en quantités abondantes). Avec la mise en évidence de la fonction glycogénique du foie, Claude Bernard esquisse une théorie de la transformation des aliments dans l'organisme. Dans le cas du sucre apporté par l'alimentation, celui-ci est stocké dans le foie sous forme de glycogène puis libéré sous forme de glucose en fonction des besoins de l'organisme. Ces processus de transformation des aliments seront désignés sous le nom de "métabolisme intermédiaire" (MI). Comme l'a montré Frederic Holmes, le diabète sucré fournit un modèle de prédilection pour les spécialistes du MI. Les corps cétoniques que l'on trouve dans l'urine des diabétiques avaient attiré l'attention de chercheurs qui souvent étaient – ou avaient été – des cliniciens qui pensaient que les problèmes pratiques posés par le diabète et les problèmes théoriques posés par l'étude du MI étaient étroitement liés. Or, à la fin du XIXe siècle, les spécialistes du MI font un large usage de la mesure et de la quantification en étudiant "les quantités de graisses, de glucides et de protéines consommées; l'équilibre entre les éléments pénétrant l'organisme et ceux qui sont rejetés à l'extérieur par la respiration et les excrétions; la relation entre les échanges matériels et énergétiques du corps; et les effets de conditions variables de nutrition, repos ou exercice, âge, santé et maladie sur toutes ces relations. Dès le début du XXe siècle, les méthodes de mesure dans ce domaine étaient extrêmement perfectionnées et il existait un important corpus de connaissances accumulées[1]."

Très tôt, le but premier des cliniciens qui s'occupent de diabète est de réduire la glycosurie et, quand on peut la mesurer, la glycémie. On pense dès la fin du xixe siècle que la gravité de la maladie est parallèle à l'élévation de l'hyperglycémie, qu'on essaie donc de faire baisser par tous les moyens. Dans un premier temps, seul un régime alimentaire permet d'obtenir ce résultat. Pour évaluer l'état des diabétiques, les cliniciens hospitaliers utilisent le modèle nutritionnel et métabolique très quantifié des spécialistes du MI. Ils quantifient l'apport alimentaire des malades, calculent l'équivalent calorique des trois grandes classes d'aliments (protides, glucides, lipides), mesurent de nombreuses substances excrétées dans les urines et les selles des patients. La mesure du quotient respiratoire, de réalisation plus longue, se pratique sur quelques patients dans les services spécialisés[2]. Les cliniciens déterminent aussi la "tolérance en hydrates de carbone" de chaque patient, c'est-à-dire la quantité maxima d'hydrates de carbone (glucides) que chacun peut consommer sans que du sucre apparaisse dans les urines. Ils reportent tous ces résultats sur des tableaux standardisés qui permettent une véritable mise en fiche quantifiée du statut métabolique de chaque patient[3]. De même, leur thérapeutique, essentiellement fondée sur la mise au point de régimes alimentaires, variables suivant les lieux et les praticiens, est localement standardisée. On voit donc que, lorsque l'insuline arrive sur le marché en 1922–23, les cliniciens spécialistes du diabète ont développé une véritable *culture de la quantification* qui leur permet d'évaluer plus facilement l'effet de l'insuline en termes d'efficacité sur le métabolisme des sucres et aussi de l'adapter aisément à chaque cas, en tenant compte des caractéristiques métaboliques de chaque individu[4]. En effet, quand l'insuline devient disponible, on mesure les différents paramètres métaboliques avant et après insuline, notamment la "tolérance en hydrates de carbone". La quantité de glucides supplémentaires que l'insuline permet de consommer sans que du sucre apparaisse dans les urines indique le "pouvoir de combustion" du nouveau médicament : en divisant le nombre d'unités d'insuline injectées par le nombre de calories supplémentaires consommées, on obtient la valeur d'une unité en grammes de sucres.

QUANTIFICATION ET GESTION DE L'INCURABLE EN MÉDECINE

À partir de 1909, Frederik Madison Allen (1879–1964), un médecin du Département de santé publique de la Harvard Medical School, entreprend un travail expérimental de trois ans sur des animaux pour mettre au point un régime alimentaire destiné aux diabétiques. À la suite de ces expériences, il conclut que seul un régime hypocalorique sévère peut faire baisser la glycosurie et la glycémie de ces animaux[5]. Il applique ce régime aux malades diabétiques et affirme que les patients soumis au "régime de famine", comme on le désigne très vite, échappent en partie aux complications infectieuses de la maladie et à l'acidocétose ; ils se sentent mieux et peuvent vivre ainsi quelques mois, voire quelques années. Mais les patients affamés cherchent sans cesse à échapper à cette diète, de sorte que le personnel soignant doit se livrer à une activité policière pour débusquer les "tricheurs" et traquer la nourriture cachée, souvent apportée par la famille. Dans un article paru peu avant la découverte de l'insuline (1922), Allen stigmatise les "mauvais" diabétiques rendus largement responsables des complications qu'ils présentent. En analysant la cause des décès observés sur une série de patients soumis à son régime, il explique qu'un certain nombre d'entre eux sont dus à des "degrés divers d'infidélité au traitement[6]." Il reproche aussi aux médecins d'avoir tendance à sacrifier le futur du patient à la facilité d'un présent plus agréable.

Les vues d'Allen trouvent un écho important chez le plus respecté des spécialistes américains du DM sucré à l'époque, Elliot P. Joslin, qui depuis 1915 prend les diabétiques en charge au Massachusetts General Hospital pour leur appliquer le "régime de famine". On trouve chez Joslin la même moralisation du traitement que chez Allen, bien que l'un et l'autre justifient leur méthode thérapeutique par des raisons d'ordre scientifique[7]. En 1919, Joslin écrit un manuel destiné aux médecins et aux patients diabétiques dans lequel certaines recommandations prennent la forme d'un véritable catéchisme[8]. L'exaltation du courage, de la volonté et de la discipline fait donc partie intégrante des programmes de contrôle du diabète. Chris Feudtner estime que Joslin jouait auprès de ses malades le rôle d'un "directeur moral" (*moral manager*) autant que d'un expert scientifique[9]. Il voit dans cette attitude un mélange d'idiosyncrasie – convictions religieuses fortes et goût des citations bibliques – et de conceptions partagées par les médecins de cette époque, qui voient la lutte contre la maladie, comme un combat moral personnel davantage que comme une question technique. En même temps la maladie permet de tester le caractère du malade : "Il s'agit d'une maladie qui permet de tester le caractère d'un patient, et pour la supporter avec courage, en plus de la sagesse, il doit posséder honnêteté, contrôle de soi et courage[10]."

Dès la naissance de ce qu'on appellera plus tard la "diabétologie", la dimension morale est donc constitutive des pratiques médicales de surveillance et de soins. Une rigueur morale est exigée qui n'est sans doute pas séparable de la rigueur scientifique, quasi-mathématique,

que les spécialistes du diabète mettent en œuvre quotidiennement. Mesure et quantification sont les maîtres mots des interventions médicales. Le patient doit régulièrement surveiller ses urines pour mesurer la glycosurie et faire mesurer ses taux de glycémie. Il doit peser ses aliments et doser savamment la composition des repas, pris de préférence à heure fixe. Enfin, il doit pratiquer de l'exercice physique, sans excès ni mollesse. Nous sommes bien dans la fabrique des corps disciplinés chère à Foucault[11]. Pour Feudtner, ce dispositif de surveillance des malades aide Joslin à faire face à cette maladie, toujours mortelle en quelques mois ou années, et pour laquelle on n'a en vérité aucune arme vraiment efficace avant 1922. Peser, mesurer, quantifier, examiner quotidiennement ses urines : pris dans cet engrenage, malades et médecins ont sans doute l'impression d'œuvrer pour contenir l'évolution de la maladie. On peut rapprocher cette attitude de celle analysée par Ilana Löwy en cancérologie. Elle suggère que les essais cliniques de l'interleukine – molécule extrêmement toxique et rapidement soupçonnée d'être peu efficace – chez les malades atteints de cancers évolués relèvent d'un "éthos de l'action" qui permet au médecins et aux malades de faire face plus facilement à ces situations[12].

LA STANDARDISATION DE L'INSULINE ENTRE PHYSIOLOGISTES ET CLINICIENS

Les quelques historiens qui se sont intéressés à l'histoire de la standardisation des médicaments avant les années 1970 sont presque toujours des physiologistes ayant une expérience dans ce domaine. Tout naturellement, ils ont présenté les travaux de standardisation des médicaments comme une œuvre de physiologiste, négligeant totalement l'apport des cliniciens et le va-et-vient inévitable et nécessaire entre les physiologistes et les cliniciens. Dans le premier article publié sur les effets cliniques de l'insuline, les chercheurs de Toronto avaient déterminé la quantité d'extrait à injecter de façon très grossière, d'après son effet sur les chiens pancréatectomisés, et exprimé la quantité d'extrait injecté en centimètres cube (cc) sans autre précision[13]. Dans cet article, les auteurs décrivent les effets thérapeutiques sur un seul des patients testés, Leonard Thomson. Les effets de quinze injections de 4 à 15 cc d'extrait sont représentés sur 48 jours pour la glycosurie des 24 heures mesurée sur ce patient, avec une représentation plus détaillée (toutes les deux heures) pour trois jours consécutifs. Deux autres courbes montrent l'effet d'une injection sur la cétonurie et la glycémie. Un tableau général reprend l'ensemble des données pour ces quatre variables. Dans le corps de l'article, les auteurs observent simplement que les extraits donnés le 11 janvier "n'étaient pas aussi concentrés que ceux utilisés plus tard". À ce premier stade de l'application clinique, les chercheurs apprécient donc les effets de l'insuline de façon largement qualitative et directement sur les patients.

La découverte de l'effet hypoglycémiant et convulsivant de l'insuline chez le lapin par le biochimiste Bertram Collip, arrivé à la rescousse des chercheurs de Toronto, permet d'imaginer un dispositif de dosage biologique de la nouvelle hormone qui sera utilisé jusqu'au début des années 1970. Dans un premier temps, l'équipe canadienne suggère de considérer comme unité d'insuline la quantité d'extrait – toujours mesurée en cc – qui provoque chez le lapin normal une chute du taux de glycémie à 45 % de son taux de départ[14]. Ce chiffre est choisi parce que ce taux de glycémie provoque presque toujours des convulsions chez l'animal. Les physiologistes mettent donc une observation clinique en rapport avec une mesure biologique pour construire leur dispositif de dosage de l'insuline.

Mais des difficultés de toutes sortes apparaissent, liées d'une part au fait que les chercheurs travaillent dans un contexte de grande instabilité, et d'autre part aux problèmes propres à la standardisation biologique. Contexte d'instabilité : les chercheurs doivent tout à la fois mettre sur pied des laboratoires et des colonies d'animaux, définir l'unité d'insuline et mesurer ses effets physiologiques, développer une méthode d'utilisation clinique, assurer une gestion financière de l'ensemble et résoudre des problèmes de brevet. Problèmes liés à la standardisation : les historiens de la standardisation d'un système de mesure, quel qu'il soit, connaissent bien la chaîne infinie des calibrages successifs qu'exige toute standardisation[15]. C'est pourquoi l'équipe de Toronto, qui avait d'abord confié la production de l'insuline à une petite entreprise locale, les laboratoires Connaught, doit bientôt faire appel à la compagnie Eli Lilly, installée à Indianapolis. Déjà relativement importante quand Toronto la contacte, cette entreprise fait partie des compagnies qui affichent leur volonté de développer une recherche scientifique de qualité et d'agir de façon éthique. Une standardisation rigoureuse figure au premier rang de ses objectifs[16]. Le directeur de la compagnie, J.K. Lilly, avait engagé en 1919 Henry A. Clowes, britannique de naissance, comme directeur de recherche. Ce scientifique compétent joua un rôle majeur dans la production industrielle de l'insuline.

Pour la standardisation de l'insuline, chaque élément du dispositif, de l'animal au dosage de la glycémie, en passant par l'insuline elle-même, est constamment réévalué. De plus, les premières décisions sont souvent revues en fonction de l'expérience acquise. On constate d'abord, aussi bien dans les laboratoires Lilly que dans ceux de Connaught, que l'apparition des convulsions produites par l'injection d'insuline varie d'un animal à l'autre. Le Comité de l'insuline de l'Université de Toronto, créé pour gérer les problèmes liés à la commercialisation du nouveau médicament, décide alors de standardiser les animaux eux-mêmes, en fixant leur poids à 2 kg et en stipulant qu'ils doivent être à jeun depuis 24 heures. Bientôt, on s'aperçoit que la réponse convulsive varie dans le temps suivant l'animal : le Comité décide alors qu'il convient de mesurer les taux de sucre dans le sang 1½ heure, 3 heures et 5 heures après l'injection.

Cette première construction de l'unité d'insuline par les physiologistes procède donc par essais et erreurs. Les premiers résultats cliniques incitent rapidement le Comité de l'insuline à la modifier. Les cliniciens observent en effet que certains patients ont besoin de moins d'une unité d'insuline et expliquent que la manipulation de fractions d'unités est difficile pour les infirmières et les patients. Le 30 décembre 1922, le Comité décide de diviser l'unité originale par 5, et l'on appelle cette nouvelle unité "l'unité clinique" par opposition à l'unité originale qui est nommée "unité physiologique". De 1922 à 1923, outre le problème de rendement, qui est d'ordre à la fois économique et clinique, les problèmes majeurs auxquels Lilly doit faire face sont la détérioration et la toxicité de la préparation injectée, et bien sûr la standardisation, qui devient plus fiable au fur et à mesure que les autres problèmes se résolvent.

Or, Henry Clowes se fie peu aux tests faits sur les animaux. Il attend avec impatience les rapports réguliers des cliniciens pour avoir des informations sur la qualité de l'insuline produite. Le 8 janvier 1923 il écrit à Macleod : "La vérité est que je crois que nous devrons nous reposer presque entièrement sur les tests menés dans les hôpitaux sur des cas humains[17];" et deux mois plus tard, le 14 mars 1922 : "Nous ne sommes certainement pas en position d'affirmer qu'une méthode absolument fiable de standardisation de l'insuline est disponible. Nous sommes encore très dépendants de grandes séries de tests conduits par les cliniques qui coopèrent[18]."

Clowes s'entoure rapidement d'un petit comité clinique informel et constitue un excellent réseau de cliniques et d'hôpitaux américains, pièce primordiale de son dispositif. Dans ce comité, on note la présence d'Elliot Joslin et de Frederik Allen : ils sont au premier rang des interlocuteurs réguliers de Henry Clowes et leur avis prime sur tout autre quand il s'agit des problèmes cliniques posés par l'utilisation de l'insuline. Parmi les non-médecins qui travaillent sur l'insuline, Clowes est sans doute un de ceux qui comprend le mieux la nature du travail médical et cette caractéristique, jointe à son sens de l'organisation et à sa capacité à recueillir des d'informations à travers tout le territoire américain, est certainement un des grands facteurs de réussite de l'entreprise. L'importance des rapports cliniques est telle qu'il en arrive à valider les résultats de la standardisation animale par leur conformité aux résultats cliniques[19].

Les cliniciens qui s'occupent de diabète s'adaptent rapidement à la situation nouvelle créée par l'arrivée de l'insuline et mettent leur modèle d'étude et de compréhension de la maladie au service de la nouvelle thérapeutique. Il s'agit, on l'a vu, d'un modèle déjà très quantifié.

Les malades participent à la culture de la quantification développée par les médecins, en pesant les aliments qu'ils absorbent et en mesurant le sucre excrété dans leurs urines. Il ne faut pas oublier que les diabétiques, même avant l'insuline, n'étaient pas constamment à l'hôpital. On leur apprend donc à se surveiller et à se traiter seuls. Avec l'insuline, ils passent beaucoup plus de temps en dehors de l'hôpital et doivent donc impérativement se prendre en charge. De plus, ils apprennent vite à évaluer les effets positifs et négatifs de l'insuline. Parmi ces derniers, le plus redouté est l'hypoglycémie, crainte des patients autant que des médecins car elle peut provoquer une mort brutale à la suite de convulsions ou de coma. Les malades informent les médecins des symptômes qu'ils éprouvent après certaines injections. Patients et médecins apprennent ensemble à identifier les symptômes de l'hypoglycémie et à les situer sur une échelle de gravité assez bien codifiée. Sansum, un médecin de Californie, excellent informateur de Clowes, trace par exemple l'échelle suivante : "Pensée ralentie, extrême faiblesse, pouls et respiration accélérés, tremblement, sueurs, troubles visuels, perte de conscience, convulsions[20]."

On trouve dans le *Manuel* de Joslin une description des symptômes de l'hypoglycémie observés chez le lapin. Après une période préliminaire d'excitabilité, il observe un coma avec un rythme respiratoire très rapide et des pupilles dilatées. La moindre stimulation provoque des convulsions qui peuvent entraîner la mort en quelques minutes par insuffisance respiratoire. Il est difficile de savoir si cette description clinique a été utilisée par les physiologistes. Il se peut que ceux-ci aient pensé à l'utiliser afin de déterminer le meilleur moment pour mesurer la glycémie chez le lapin. Surtout, elle permet de comparer les symptômes chez l'animal, qui ne peut décrire ce qu'il ressent, et chez l'homme. La richesse de la clinique humaine est bien sûr sans équivalent et permet d'apprécier beaucoup plus finement le statut glucosé du patient. Certains patients savent évaluer assez précisément leur taux de glycémie dans les premiers stades de l'hypoglycémie. La mesure instantanée de la glycémie, possible depuis près de vingt ans, permet de le vérifier.

On peut donc dire que jusqu'à la fin de l'année 1924 au moins, la standardisation de l'insuline fut une entreprise difficile qui n'a pu être menée à bien que grâce à la circulation continue d'informations entre les patients, les cliniciens et les chercheurs de l'industrie. La participation des médecins à l'entreprise fut d'autant plus facile qu'ils avaient déjà œuvré à standardiser leurs pratiques. Dans cette configuration, les patients sont à la fois ceux qu'on soigne et la partie essentielle du dispositif qui permet de tester l'insuline.

LES ESSAIS CLINIQUES, HIER ET AUJOURD'HUI

Comment ont été organisés les essais cliniques de l'insuline en 1922? Il faut se garder ici de tout anachronisme en les évaluant à l'aune des essais cliniques randomisés (ECR) d'aujourd'hui. À l'époque, on évalue les effets étonnants de l'insuline par un ensemble de signes cliniques et biologiques. Le malade traité par le nouveau médicament retrouve rapidement des forces et de la vivacité et gagne du poids. Le sucre disparaît ou diminue fortement dans les urines et la glycémie, mesurée plus rarement en raison des difficultés techniques et de la longueur de cette mesure, diminue également pour se rapprocher de la normale. L'acétone disparaît des urines.

En raison des faibles quantités d'insuline produites au début par les laboratoires Lilly, le Comité de l'insuline de l'Université de Toronto décide de distribuer la précieuse hormone à un petit groupe de cliniciens choisis parmi l'élite des spécialistes du métabolisme et du diabète[21]. Les résultats de ces essais sont publiés en 1923 dans un numéro spécial du *Journal of Metabolic Research* (édité par Allen). On y trouve au moins deux caractéristiques communes : la description clinique abrégée des cas et des tables dites "statistiques" donnant pour chaque cas des résultats biologiques[22].

Bien que courte, la description de chaque cas inclut les données cliniques importantes pour chaque malade, la date d'apparition de la maladie, et des données quantifiées comme la perte de poids (un élément important pour évaluer la gravité de l'état du patient), le volume d'urines émises quotidiennement, les données biologiques et métaboliques avant et après le traitement par insuline. Le nombre de patients étudiés par chaque équipe varie, allant de 20 pour le plus petit groupe à 161 pour l'étude publiée par Allen, qui est fier d'avoir le plus grand nombre de patients traités. Son article occupe de ce fait 80 pages, contre une moyenne de 15 à 20 pour les autres[23].

Les signes cliniques importants sont présentés sur des tableaux qui comportent surtout les variables quantifiables, mais parfois aussi des données qualitatives (soif, douleur, faim, etc.). Ces tableaux sont soit individuels, retraçant l'évolution d'un cas sur plusieurs jours ou semaines, soit statistiques, regroupant les données du groupe de patients étudiés. Dans ce dernier cas, on trouve, le plus souvent en bas du tableau, une moyenne des valeurs trouvées pour l'ensemble des patients. De surcroît, dans la plupart des articles, des tableaux illustrent ces résultats par des courbes ou des colonnes. La mise en forme des données, que Bruno Latour considère comme caractéristique de la fabrication des faits scientifiques (nettoyage des données, transformation en graphiques divers incorporés dans le texte) est donc déjà un dispositif important des articles médicaux[24].

On peut constater, par ailleurs, que les auteurs sont soucieux de présenter des cas relativement homogènes puisque les malades qui sont atteints d'infections sévères, de coma ou de gangrène n'apparaissent pas dans les tableaux. En même temps, les malades testés présentent des diabètes nécessairement sévères, ne serait-ce qu'en raison des faibles quantités d'insuline disponibles en ces débuts de production industrielle. On réserve donc le précieux médicament pour ces patients. Les différents auteurs insistent dans leur discussion sur cette relative homogénéité des cas observés. Chez deux auteurs apparaît l'idée de sujets témoin. Allen, qui comme on l'a dit, n'était pas d'une nature confiante, fait surveiller étroitement ses patients, notamment leur régime alimentaire. Il affirme clairement que l'insuline ne peut être administrée qu'aux patients dignes de confiance[25]. Sa rigueur s'étend à la surveillance des protocoles : il est particulièrement attentif à ne pas laisser des facteurs mal contrôlés perturber les résultats et va jusqu'à faire pratiquer chez quelques patients des injections de sérum physiologique alternant avec les injections d'insuline pour éliminer l'influence éventuelle de facteurs psychologiques. Des jours sans insuline s'intercalent alors entre les jours de traitement. Dans l'article de Fletcher et Campbell, l'effet hypoglycémiant de l'insuline est testé sur des sujets contrôles : 15 des sujets testés par ce groupe sont diabétiques alors que 5 ne présentent pas de diabète. L'article ne précise pas si le consentement des sujets a été sollicité. On peut voir dans ces pratiques une première forme de sujet témoin et de médication placebo dans les essais cliniques. En revanche, on ne trouve dans aucun des articles de considérations sur la signification des moyennes présentées.

L'histoire de la thérapeutique dans le diabète sucré est une histoire complexe, marquée par l'apparition de nouvelles insulines, plus purifiées et de durée d'action variable, et par l'invention après 1950 des hypoglycémiants oraux, qui permet de séparer les diabètes sucrés en "insulino-dépendant" et "non insulino-dépendants". Cette histoire est aussi marquée par une longue controverse sur la nécessité d'associer ou non un régime alimentaire strict à l'insuline. Car si la nouvelle hormone est d'abord considérée comme une panacée, la découverte progressive des complications graves qui surviennent inéluctablement dans le diabète sucré, malgré le traitement par l'insuline, constitue un chapitre important de l'histoire de la maladie[26]. On peut distinguer deux phases d'inégale longueur dans l'histoire de la controverse sur les régimes. Durant la première phase, qui dure jusqu'à la fin des années 1970, les prises de position contrastées sur les régimes alimentaires se situent dans le prolongement des toutes premières discussions sur cette question, dès les années 1920. L'enjeu essentiel est celui de l'équilibre entre l'apport d'insuline et le régime alimentaire, et les arguments sont tirés de registres moraux (laisser plus ou moins d'autonomie au patient), cliniques (l'observation des complications et de leur lien éventuel avec les résultats biologiques des malades) ou expérimentaux (diabète provoqué chez des animaux de laboratoire). La seconde période débute vers 1980 et se caractérise par la prolifération des technologies destinées soit à aider les malades et les médecins à contenir la maladie, soit à obtenir des données comme les grands essais cliniques randomisés. La controverse sur les régimes en recouvre en fait une autre d'ordre pathogénique, sur le rôle de l'hyperglycémie dans la genèse des complications. C'est pourquoi cette controverse peut être désignée comme une "controverse glucose" de même que l'hypothèse qui fait l'objet de la controverse comme une "hypothèse glucose".

En 1993 paraissent les résultats de l'enquête du Diabetes Control and Complications Trial Research Group qui est acclamée comme ayant définitivement confirmé l'hypothèse glucose[27]. Il est intéressant de s'arrêter quelques instants sur cet essai car c'est l'un des "plus longs, des plus complets et des plus coûteux" jamais réalisés dans toute l'histoire de la médecine[28]. L'enquête, parrainée par le NIH, soutenue et sponsorisée par le National Institute of Diabetes and Digestive and Kidney Diseases (NIDDK), et préparée de 1982 à 1983, débute en 1984 pour se terminer en 1993. Elle porte sur 1 441 patients sélectionnés soigneusement à partir d'une première cohorte de 7 000. De multiples comités encadrent l'étude pour assurer son objectivité et la sécurité des malades. L'objectif de l'étude est à la fois de confirmer l'hypothèse glucose et de déterminer si un contrôle rigoureux de la glycémie permet de diminuer l'ampleur et la gravité des complications dans le diabète sucré. L'étude porte sur deux groupes de patients atteints de diabète sucré insulino-dépendant (ou diabète de type 1), dont le premier est composé de patients traités par une thérapie conventionnelle et le second par une thérapie intensive. La thérapie conventionnelle repose sur l'administration d'insuline une ou deux fois par jour alors que la thérapie intensive prévoit des doses plus faibles mais plus fréquentes d'insuline, notamment avant chaque repas, avec un contrôle plus strict de l'alimentation et de l'exercice physique. Le second groupe ne comporte que des patients dûment sélectionnés et motivés, décidés à accepter les contraintes de la thérapie intensive. La durée moyenne d'observation est de 3 à 9 ans, avec une moyenne de 6,5 ans. Les résultats montrent une baisse de l'hémoglobine glycosylée d'environ 2 % chez les patients traités de manière intensive par rapport à celle du groupe traité par des moyens conventionnels. C'est un résultat important si l'on considère que la valeur considérée comme satisfaisante pour l'hémoglobine glycosylée varie entre 6 et 8 %[29]. La complication à la fois la plus redoutée et la mieux étudiée, la rétinopathie, constitue la cible essentielle des recherches en la matière. L'enquête conclut que la thérapie intensive retarde de plusieurs années son apparition chez les patients non atteints de rétinopathie et ralentit clairement sa progression chez les patients déjà atteints. Les concepteurs et réalisateurs de cette étude affirment qu'elle met un terme à la "controverse glucose" et doit encourager une pratique diabétologique axée sur un contrôle rigoureux de la glycémie. Beaucoup de diabétologues affirment qu'il y aura désormais une ère post-DCCT, comme il y eut une ère post-insuline, puis une ère post-Hagedorn[30] et une ère post-hypoglycémiants oraux.

Cette reconstruction historique est l'œuvre des réalisateurs de l'essai. Une recherche un peu plus approfondie et l'interrogatoire de quelques diabétologues montrent que les choses ne sont pas aussi simples. En premier lieu, cette reconstruction efface les enquêtes qui dès la fin des années 1970 avaient été réalisées en Belgique et en France et qui semblaient déjà confirmer l'hypothèse glucose et encourager la pratique expérimentale de la thérapie intensive[31]. À partir des années 1980, de nouvelles enquêtes sont lancées, notamment en Grande-Bretagne et en Scandinavie, qui ouvrent la voie pour le futur DCCT Research Group. Il faut toutefois porter au crédit de ce dernier d'avoir mené l'enquête sur une durée nettement plus longue que les essais précédents, ce qui est évidemment important pour l'étude des complications tardives de la maladie.

Mais surtout, la reconstruction historique faite par le DCCT Research Group efface la primauté des pratiques sur la théorie. La thérapie intensive a non seulement précédé la confirmation définitive de l'hypothèse glucose par le DCCT Research Group, mais elle fait au premier chef partie des facteurs qui l'ont rendue possible, puisque cet essai comporte toute une partie expérimentale fondée sur l'utilisation de cette nouvelle forme de thérapie. Il a fallu faire preuve d'audace, anticiper sur la science et innover au niveau des pratiques pour lancer la thérapie intensive. Par ailleurs, une difficulté majeure n'est pas résolue par l'essai DCCT : il n'est pas possible de traduire facilement les résultats de l'enquête dans la pratique. La thérapie intensive nécessite des équipes multidisciplinaires, des patients motivés, des médecins formés à cette thérapie. Ces conditions sont difficiles à reproduire dans la pratique quotidienne, sans compter leur coût économique. En somme, on se trouve dans un cas de figure proche de celui qu'on rencontre souvent quand on analyse les apports de la biologie à la médecine clinique. Ces apports sont souvent limités par que le fait que les modèles expérimentaux sont assez loin des réalités cliniques.

Pour conclure sur le chapitre des essais cliniques, le rapprochement entre les essais de 1922 et les grands essais contemporains ne vise pas ici à faire apparaître les uns comme supérieurs aux autres, mais plutôt à poser une question, à partir d'un constat : même si l'insuline n'a jamais été le médicament miracle qu'on espérait, elle reste un des médicaments les plus actifs qui aient jamais été mis au point. En 2003, on peut affirmer qu'on n'a pas inventé de molécule aussi efficace depuis plus de trente ans. À l'inverse du dispositif d'évaluation des effets de l'insuline mis au point en 1922, simple mais fécond, l'organisation moderne des essais cliniques fait de plus en plus appel au gigantisme alors que les médicaments testés ne représentent souvent qu'un progrès minime par rapport à ceux qu'on utilisait avant eux. Très souvent, le résultat de ces essais est contesté ou remis en question, et ce, de plus en plus rapidement. On peut donc se demander s'il n'y a pas un lien entre les deux termes du constat : à médicament peu efficace, grands essais randomisés. Ce qui ne signifie pas que ces essais n'aient pas de valeur, mais plutôt qu'ils signent une certaine impuissance de notre médecine, méconnue du grand public, voire des spécialistes.

CONCLUSION

Sans permettre d'épuiser la question des différents usages de la quantification en médecine, l'exemple du diabète sucré permet d'en examiner un certain nombre, dans une maladie où la quantification a sans doute joué un rôle précoce en comparaison avec d'autres pathologies. À première vue, il n'y a pas grand-chose de commun entre les efforts pour définir une pathologie de façon quantitative, la gestion de l'incurable par une pratique quotidienne de la mesure, la standardisation d'un médicament et l'invention des essais cliniques randomisés. Mais il faut d'abord remarquer que cette disparité des pratiques médicales reflète le statut complexe d'une médecine occidentale qui s'est construite au carrefour de plusieurs sciences. S'il y a unité de la médecine, elle n'est sans doute pas à rechercher au niveau des savoirs qu'elle mobilise au lit du malade, mais plutôt dans sa finalité : restaurer une norme valorisée par les malades[32].

Certains historiens ont développé l'idée qu'il existait une "économie morale des sciences" qui se manifestait le plus clairement dans les processus de quantification[33]. Pour eux, mesurer de façon précise et exacte est un acte moral autant que scientifique. C'est doublement vrai pour la médecine clinique, qui fait intervenir, souvent de façon implicite, des valeurs morales dans ses pratiques autant que dans ses traités théoriques. Quand Claude Bernard cherche à éliminer les valeurs esthétiques ou morales de la médecine, celles-ci reviennent à son insu dans la terminologie, esthétique ou morale, qu'il utilise pour caractériser la santé (équilibre, harmonie). Quand les premiers diabé-tologues exhortent leurs patients à suivre une discipline marquée par la mesure, ils mènent de toute évidence un combat d'ordre moral, dans lequel les "mauvais" diabétiques sont stigmatisés. Quand la firme Lilly s'acharne à mettre en œuvre une standardisation rigoureuse de l'insuline, c'est pour répondre aux objectifs éthiques qu'elle s'est fixé, même si l'éthique devient en même temps un argument commercial. Les ECR peuvent être considérés comme la mise en œuvre d'une évaluation plus précise, plus fiable, plus objective et donc désintéressée des effets des médicaments. Mais la quantification a aussi ses excès.

Canguilhem a bien montré comment la conception purement quantitative de la maladie faisait bon marché de la subjectivité du malade et du qualitatif dans la définition des pathologies[34]. Le régime calculé à la calorie près qu'Allen administrait à ses patients a engendré des protestations violentes à son époque, chez les médecins autant que chez les patients. Les résultats quantitatifs qu'il obtenait étaient sans doute satisfaisants, mais ils ne s'accompagnaient d'aucune sensation de bien-être chez les malades ainsi traités. Quant aux ECR, ils ont aussi leurs détracteurs parmi les médecins qui les accusent d'effacer l'individualité de la maladie, ou parmi les sociologues des sciences qui affirment qu'aucun ECR ne peut être considéré comme un processus d'évaluation totalement objectif[35].

Dans un registre différent, Renée Fox a particulièrement examiné la question de l'incertitude en médecine. Parmi les différents facteurs qui expliquent cette incertitude, elle remarque que le développement de nouvelles techniques performantes, loin de faire disparaître l'incertitude médicale, souvent l'accentue. Elle souligne entre autres la tension accrue entre une médecine axée sur l'individu et celle qui s'intéresse au collectif, raisonne en termes de populations et construit ses connaissances à partir des résultats d'essais cliniques randomisés. À ce sujet, Fox fait remarquer que la médecine "fondée sur l'évidence" promue par des médecins de langue anglaise pourrait bien aboutir de façon paradoxale à aggraver ce qu'elle cherche à combattre.

Il n'est donc pas possible d'attribuer *a priori* une valeur positive, notamment sur le plan moral, à tous les processus de quantification en médecine. Il est intéressant à ce sujet d'observer que le terme de "rigueur" qui renvoie à la morale autant qu'à la scientificité, signifie aussi "dureté". Une thérapeutique rigoureuse peut aussi se révéler trop dure. De nos jours, malgré une confirmation de "l'hypothèse glucose" dans le diabète, plus personne n'oserait administrer les régimes de famine d'Allen. Le progrès ici est bien d'ordre moral.

NOTES

1 "Measurements of quantities of fats, carbohydrates and proteins consumed; the balance between the elements entering the organism and those leaving it through respiration and excretions; the relation between the material and energy exchanges of the body; and the effects upon all the relationships of differing conditions of nourishment, rest or exercise, age, health, and disease. By the twentieth century, the methods of measurement in this field were highly refined and there was a large body of accumulated knowledge." Frederic Lawrence Holmes, *Between Biology and Medicine : The Formation of Intermediary Metabolism, Four Lectures delivered at the International Summer School in History of Science* (Berkeley: Office for History of Science and Technology, University of California at Berkeley, 1992), 53–76. (Toutes les traductions en français de ce texte sont les miennes.)

2 Le quotient respiratoire est le rapport de la quantité de gaz carbonique expirée à la quantité d'oxygène inspirée, et donnait une indication de la quantité de glucides brûlée par l'organisme.

3 Le médecin et historien Chris Feudtner a particulièrement bien analysé cette quantification du statut métabolique des patients diabétiques dans le service de Joslin. Voir Christopher Feudtner, "Bittersweet : The Transformation of Diabetes into a Chronic Illness in Twentieth-Century America" (thèse de Ph. D., University of Pennsylvania, 1995), 231–2. Voir aussi *Bittersweet : Diabetes, Insulin, & the Transformation of Illness* (Chapel Hill : University of North Carolina Press, 2003).

4 C. Sinding, "Une molécule espion pour les diabétologues : L'Innovation médicale entre science et morale", *Sciences sociales et santé,* 18, 2000, 95–120.

5 F.M. Allen, *Studies Concerning Glycosuria and Diabetes* (Cambridge, Mass. : Harvard University Press, 1913).

6 F.M. Allen et J.W. Sherill, "Clinical Observations on Treatment and Progress in Diabetes", *Journal of Metabolic Research*, 1 (1922), 378–455.

7 C'est-à-dire, à l'époque, avant tout des théories nutritionelles et tirées des études des spécialistes du métabolisme intermédiaire. Sur l'histoire de la nutrition, voir Kenneth Carpenter, *Protein and Energy: A Study of Changing Ideas in Nutrition* (Cambridge : Cambridge University Press, 1994).

8 Elliot P. Joslin, *A Diabetic Manual for the Mutual Use of Doctor and Patient*, deuxième édition (Philadelphie : Lea & Febiger, 1919), 32. Cité par Feudtner, "Bittersweet", 314. L'insistance sur l'importance d'être intelligent pour un diabétique est une constante des écrits médicaux de l'époque.

9 Feudtner, "Bittersweet", 314.

10 "This is a disease which tests the character of the patient, and for success in withstanding it, in addition to wisdom he must possess honesty, self-control, and courage." Joslin, *A Diabetic Manual*, 17.

11 Michel Foucault, *Surveiller et Punir* (Paris : Gallimard, 1975).

12 Ilana Löwy, *Between Bench and Bedside: Science, Healing and Interleukin–2 in a Cancer Ward* (Cambridge : Harvard University Press, 1997).

13 F.G. Banting, C.H. Best, J.B. Collip, W.B. Campbell et A.A. Fletcher, "Pancreatic Extracts in the Treatment of Diabetus Mellitus: Preliminary Report", *The Canadian Medical Association Journal*, 2 (1922), 141–6, p. 141.

14 A.H. Lacey, "The Unit of Insulin", *Diabetes*, 16 (1967), 198–200.

15 M. Norton Wise, "Precision: Agent of Unity and Product of Agreement: Part iii – 'Today Precision Must Be Commonplace'", in Norton Wise (dir.), *The Value of Precision* (Princeton : Princeton University Press, 1995), 359.

16 John Patrick Swann, "Insulin: A Case Study in the Emergence of Collaborative Pharmacomedical Research", *Pharmacy in History*, 28 (1986), 3–13 et 65–74.

17 "The truth is I believe we shall have to rely almost entirely on tests carried out in the hospital on human cases."

18 "We are certainly not in a position to say that an absolutely reliable method of standardizing insulin is thus far available. We are still very dependent on large series of tests carried out in the co-operating clinics."

19 C. Sinding, "Making the Unit of Insulin: Standards, Clinical Work and Industry", *Bulletin of the History of Medicine*, 76 (2002), 231–70.

20 "Slow mentality, extreme weakness, rapid pulse and respiration, shaky feeling, sweating, visual disturbance, unconsciousness, convulsions." Sansum à Macleod, 16 janvier 1923, Insulin Committee Records, University of Toronto Archives, #82.0001, boîte 21.

21 Ce sont F.M. Allen et J.W. Sherill, du Physiatric Institute, Morristown,

N.J.; F.G. Banting, W.R. Campbell et A.A. Fletcher, au Toronto General Hospital, H.R. Geyelin et son groupe au Presbyterian Hospital, New-York; R. Fitz et son groupe au Peter Bent Brigham Hospital, Boston; E.P. Joslin et son groupe dans trois hôpitaux de Boston; R.M. Wilder et son groupe à la Mayo Clinic de Rochester, Minnesota; R.T. Woodyatt, au Sprague Memorial Institute et au Presbyterian Hospital de Chicago.

22 Il ne faut pas oublier que le terme de statistique, du latin "statisticus" (relatif à l'État), a d'abord désigné l'étude méthodique des faits sociaux par des procédés numériques simples (classements, dénombrements, inventaires chiffrés, recensements, tableaux).

23 F.M. Allen et J.W. Sherill, "Clinical Observations with Insulin. 1. The Use of Insulin in Diabetic Treatment", *Journal of Metabolic Research,* 2 (1922), 803–985.

24 Bruno Latour, *La Science en action* (Paris : La Découverte, 1989), 98–108.

25 "It is possible to adopt an inflexible attitude and declare that only the trustworthy patients deserve the benefits of insulin" (p. 961).

26 Voir Feudtner, "Bittersweet", 1995, et aussi, dans un registre différent, J.W. Presley, "A History of Diabetes Mellitus in the United States, 1880–1990" (thèse de Ph. D.), University of Texas at Austin, 1991) qui s'est intéressé à la persistance d'un taux de mortalité chez les diabétiques américains.

27 "The Diabetes Control and Complications Trial (DCCT): Design and Methodological Considerations for the Feasibility Phase", source? 35 (1986), 530–44.

28 S.V. Edelman, "Importance of Glucose Control", *Medical Clinics of North America,* (82) 1998, 665–87.

29 L'hémoglobine glycosylée est une fraction particulière de l'hémoglobine qui lie le glucose. Elle est présente chez tous les sujets, mais plus élevée chez les diabétiques; voir Sinding, "Une molécule espion".

30 Le Danois Hagedorn a inventé la première insuline à longue durée d'action. Voir Philip Felig, "Protamine Insulin: Hagedorn's Pioneering Contribution to Drug Delivery in the Management of Diabetes", *JAMA,* 251 (1984), 393–6.

31 D. Job, E. Eschwege, Guyot-Argenton J.P Aubry et G. Tchobrousky, "Effect of Multiple Daily Injections on the Course of Diabetic Retinopathy", *Diabetes,* 25 (1976), 463–9. J. Pirart, "Diabetes Mellitus and its Degenerative Complications: A Prospective Study of 4 400 Patients Observed Between 1947 and 1973", *Diabetes Care,* 15 (1978), 143–52.

32 Georges Canguilhem, *Le Normal et le pathologique* (1966, réedition, Paris : Presses universitaires de France, 1994).

33 Lorraine Daston, "The Moral Economy of Science", dans Arnold Thackray (dir.), *Constructing Knowledge in the History of Science* (Chicago : Osiris, University of Chicago Press, 1995), 10, 3–24; Robert E. Kohler, "Moral

Economy, Material Culture, and Community in *Drosophila* Genetics", dans Mario Biagioli (dir.), *The Science Studies Reader* (New York : Routledge, 1999).

34 Lawrence et Weisz ont fait le point sur la question du holisme en médecine dans leur ouvrage collectif *Greater Than the Parts: Holism in Biomedicine, 1925–1950* (New-York : Oxford University Press, 1998). Dans leur introduction, ils signalent notamment les usages éthiques que beaucoup de penseurs ont fait du holisme. Canguilhem, qui a défendu la portée éthique du vitalisme, peut incontestablement être compté au nombre de ces penseurs.

35 Voir par exemple E. Richards, "The Politics of Therapeutic Evaluation: The Vitamin C and Cancer Controversy," *Social Studies of Science*, 18 (1988), 653–701.

8

"Measures, Instruments, Methods, and Results": Jozefa Joteyko on Social Reforms and Physiological Measures

ILANA LÖWY

In August 1910, Jozefa Joteyko – a physiologist, a psychologist, a teacher of experimental psychology at the provincial *écoles normales* of Hainanut (Mons and Charleroi), and a pioneer and zealous advocate of pedology (the scientific study of childhood) – spoke to the Third International Congress for Family Education, held in Belgium. She called her talk "Measures, Instruments, Methods, Results."[1] The unification of measures and tests in pedology, Joteyko argued, is the precondition for the transformation of this domain into a scientific discipline.[2] She developed this idea in the opening speech of the First International Congress of Pedology, in Brussels, in 1911. Thanks to the unification of measures, methods, and terminology in pedology, she suggested, this science would make a great leap forward: "here, as elsewhere, the application of mathematical studies will be so very important. One can also understand why, even in pedagogic psychology, the precision of instruments plays such a crucial role."[3]

Joteyko, a Polish scientist active mainly in France and Belgium, was a highly prolific scientific worker. She was the author of many scientific publications in physiology and later in experimental psychology, won numerous scientific prizes, and was the first woman to teach (in a guest chair) at the Collège de France, a dedicated and enthusiastic teacher, an efficient organizer, and a successful scientific entrepreneur. Joteyko's career was, however, fraught with difficulties. She was unable to obtain a full-time university job, the enterprises that she founded were often short-lived, and her work and career are nearly totally forgotten. Joteyko sometimes receives mention in the context of the development of social sciences and pedagogy in Belgium, and her contribution to fatigue studies was discussed by Anson Rabinbach, who admired Joteyko's approach, and by François Vatin, who was much more critical.[4] This neglect is regrettable. Beyond its value to those concerned with women pioneers of science or central European scientific migration, Joteyko's career provides a telling illustration of intersections of the early-twentieth-century biological and medical sciences with economics, politics, and the social sciences. It also reveals the crucial role played by quantification in biology and medicine in a major social project – developed mainly in France and in Belgium – that aimed to promote the optimal development of human beings and the construction of a more rational and just society. Physiology writ large – that is, a scientific and quantitatively based study of all the functions of the human organism – was central to this project.[5] This paper looks in turn at Joteyko's life and career, her work on fatigue, her pedology and scientific measurement of children, and her efforts to transform physiology into a social science.

AN ATYPICAL CAREER

Jozefa Joteyko (1866–1928) belongs to the generation of central European women who in the late nineteenth century travelled "to the end of the earth" to acquire scientific and medical education.[6] She was born in Ukraine into a family of landowners (in the Eastern Territories of Poland most landowners were Polish, and most peasants, Ukrainian); her family moved to the Russian-governed duchy of Warsaw in 1873 to seek education for its children.[7] At that time governmental schools in Warsaw taught exclusively in Russian. The Joteykos, like many other wealthy households, organized private teaching for their children. After completing the equivalent of a high-school curriculum in Warsaw, Jozefa Joteyko persuaded her family to allow her to study abroad (again, a typical trajectory for a young Polish or Russian woman interested in science), and she studied natural sciences in Geneva (1886–88). In Geneva, she adopted a male look: simple dresses with a masculine cut, glasses, and short hair; she also ostensibly smoked cigarettes. In Geneva, she met Michalina Stefanowska, ten years older and a fellow Polish student, who became her friend, collaborator, and partner. Stefanowska, a former high-school teacher, opted for a career in biological research – a choice that may have influenced Joteyko.

The death of her father and the subsequent loss of a great part of the family's fortune obliged Joteyko, previously quite prosperous, to adopt a more modest way of life. In 1890 she moved with Stefanowska to Paris, where Stefanowska worked on a PhD in physiology and Joteyko studied medicine. Joteyko, however, became interested in physiology and prepared her MD thesis (1896) in Charles Richet's laboratory.[8] She remained in medicine and, after completing her studies in 1896, attempted to build a private practice in Paris. She later found that routine medical practice did not attract her. In the meantime Stefanowska obtained a temporary job at the Solvay Physiological Institute (before 1902, the Solvay Energy Laboratory) in Brussels. In 1898, Joteyko gave up her medical practice and obtained a similar job in Brussels.[9]

The Belgian industrialist, philanthropist, and social philosopher Ernest Solvay funded the Solvay Physiological Institute. He made a large fortune as a manufacturer of soda and used a substantial part of his income to finance scientific investigations, especially those destined to promote an optimal use of energy. An admirer of an "energetic" approach (promoted, by, among others, Wilhelm Oswald), he believed that the progress of humankind depended on a rational economy of energetic phenomena, including mental energies. Scientific research, he hoped, would devise means to optimize material and intellectual productivity. The Physiological Institute accordingly undertook research on physical and mental energies.[10] It provided excellent working conditions, but no permanent jobs. Simultaneously, Joteyko taught experimental psychology at the Psychology Laboratory of Brussels University (Laboratoire Kasimir), and she served as acting director from 1903 on. She became a protégée of Hector Denis, a professor of psychology at the Science Faculty of the University of Brussels, a prominent figure in Belgian academic life, and a friend as well as political ally of Solvay. (Solvay won election to the Belgian Senate, and Denis to the national assembly). Impressed by Joteyko's scientific skills and organizational abilities, Denis attempted to find her a full-time university job.[11]

At that time, Joteyko was ambitious, hard-working, gifted at synthesis and popularization (she wrote many monographs, mainly for medical students), and able at self-promotion.[12] Her *Titres et travaux* (curriculum vitae) of 1906 lists the 40-year-old's 106 publications and numerous honorary functions and scientific prizes.[13] Joteyko won the Desmett prize of the Royal Academy of Brussels in 1900 (with M. Radzikowski), the Dieudonnée Prize of the Royal Academy of Medicine of Belgium in 1901 (with M. Stefanowska), the Montyon

Prize in physiology of the Paris Academy of Sciences in 1901 (with M. Pachon), the Lallemand Prize of the Paris Academy (with M. Garnier), and again the Monyton Prize in 1903 (with M. Stefanowska and M. Radzikowski). She belonged to numerous learned societies, was president in 1904–5 of the Belgian Neurological Society, and headed the First Congress of the Belgian Society of Neurology and Psychiatry (Liège, 1905). Her *Titres et travaux* stressed her contribution to the mathematization of several domains of physiological investigation and her international reputation: "the holders of principal chairs of physiology, psychology, general pathology, psychiatry and pharmacology in Europe and in the United States include my works in their teachings."[14]

Until 1907, Joteyko wrote many of her scientific articles with Stefanowska, who was less ambitious than she. They were both feminists but held different views about the role of women. Joteyko fought for equality between the sexes and for allowing women to have a "man-style" career. She deplored the waste of human talent caused by the denial of educational and professional opportunities to gifted women, which condemned them to the domestic sphere and to routine tasks.[15] Stefanowska stressed the specificity – and, for her, natural superiority – of women. In her book on maternal love among animals, published in 1902, she argued that in the majority of higher animal species females are responsible for the well-being of offspring and thus for the species' survival. Thanks to the mechanisms of natural selection, females are therefore more resourceful, skilled, and brave than males of the same species – a rule that applies to humans as well.[16]

In 1906, Stefanowska decided to abandon scientific research and to return to Poland, where she became headmistress of a secondary school for girls. The two women's last collaborative effort was *Psychophysiology of Pain* (1909).[17] This mainly synthetic effort incorporated elements of Joteyko's and of Stefanowska's studies on pain (the asymmetry in distribution of cutaneous sensors for pain, the dissociation between tactile sensations and pain during anaesthesia, and relationships between pain and fatigue). In addition, one chapter discussed Joteyko's theory of "algogens" – the putative chemical mediators of pain. The book received a mixed reception. Some reviewers criticized its occasional repetitions, its abruptness on important points, and its lack of unified structure. Others saw it as a useful and accessible synthesis and praised the authors' innovative approach, which combined physiological, psychological, and moral issues.[18] Some saw a scientific study written by two women as a curiosity: "by itself, a female collaboration is sufficient to attract our attention; the fact that these two women are both physicians and both university professors makes it decidedly noteworthy, the more so because the book seems carefully written and well documented."[19]

In 1906 Hector Denis, unable to provide Joteyko with a permanent academic job, helped her to become a lecturer of experimental psychology at the *écoles normales* (teacher's training institutions) of the Belgian provinces of Hainanut (Mons and Charleroi). Before 1906 Joteyko had not been especially interested in education. She nevertheless rapidly became an enthusiastic advocate of applying the methods of experimental physiology to pedagogy and redirected her scientific and organizational efforts in this direction. The switch to pedagogy may have reflected genuine interest, an aspiration to change her research field after the break with Stefanowska, and a belief that a new domain could provide better career opportunities than physiology. Joteyko continued simultaneously to teach experimental physiology at the University of Brussels, to participate in physiologists' meetings, and to conduct physiological investigations. She worked with Varia Kipiani, a young Georgian who studied biology in Brussels. Joteyko shared with Kipiani militant vegetarian convictions and with her published a series of studies seeking to disprove that a vegetarian diet reduces strength, endurance, or the acuity of sensory perceptions.[20] However, from 1908 on, Joteyko worked mainly on the application of physiological measures to the study of children, and she became an enthusiastic adept and zealous promoter of the new science of pedology.

Joteyko employed her organizational skills to promote the institutionalization of pedology. She founded in 1908 a journal, *Revue psychologique*, specializing in childhood development, education, and the promotion of pedology. From 1909 on, she conducted an international summer course for teachers, The Pedology Seminar. She organized the first international congress of pedology in Brussels in 1911 (with 500 delegates from 20 countries). In 1912 she founded an independent institution, the International Faculty of Pedology.[21] She secured the patronage of important personalities, obtained financial support, and persuaded experts in psychology and pedagogy to teach in her faculty and to accept her students as visitors or trainees in their institutions. She also faced the animosity of her colleagues in Belgium. Raymond Buyse, later a professor at the School of Pedagogy of Louvain University, recalls that when Joteyko founded her faculty she was "a weak, solitary woman, and already a victim of the lowest kind of jealousy."[22] The faculty was a small private school, and approximately half of its students were Poles – undoubtedly a sign of Joteyko's imperfect integration within Belgian academe. Her students' recollections were, however, enthusiastic: they praised Joteyko as an inspiring and inventive teacher who provided them with unique, high-level training. Among these enthusiastic students was Maria Grzegorzewska, a young Pole who later became a devoted follower and then lifelong collaborator, companion, and friend.[23]

The First World War and German occupation of Belgium ended the faculty's activities and the publication of *Revue psychologique.* Joteyko and Grzegorzewska escaped to Paris, where Joteyko, unable to teach or to do research, turned to writing. She produced two books, one on fatigue and another on the scientific organization of labour. In 1916 she gave guest conferences at the Collège de France (in the Michonis chair), the first woman ever to teach there. Her inaugural lecture attracted a mixture of Polish expatriates and French feminists. While in Paris, Grzegorzewska specialized in the education of "abnormal children." With the proclamation of Poland's independence in 1918, Joteyko decided to return to her homeland, perhaps hoping for a university chair. This hope was thwarted. Being a woman was a major obstacle, and she had difficult relations with leading Polish psychologists. She viewed them as backward, poorly educated, and unscientific; they found her pretentious and aggressive and resented being lectured to by an outsider who had not shared the struggles and hardship of the years of foreign occupation.[24]

Grzegorzewska, who returned to Poland with Joteyko, became director of the new Institute for Special Pedagogy, which trained teachers to work with mentally handicapped children. Partly thanks to her intervention, Joteyko was named teacher of experimental psychology at the National Pedagogical Institute. She also taught experimental psychology at the University of Warsaw. She brought from Brussels instruments for physiological and anthropometric measurement and attempted to reproduce her laboratory teaching and research. In 1925, the Polish government decided, however, to close the institute and to create a (smaller) pedagogy department at the university. Joteyko lost her job and was unable to find another.

Thanks to Grzegorzewska's repeated interventions, she became honorary docent at the university's Medical School. She also taught summer courses for teachers and at the Institute for Special Pedagogy, served on several government commissions, and directed the Psychological Circle – a small, informal research group composed mainly of her ex-students at the Pedagogical Institute. In 1925, she founded a journal, the *Polish Archive of Psychology*, published by the Polish Association of Teachers of Elementary Schools.

Joteyko's life in Warsaw was described as Spartan: she lived in a small, sublet room on the sixth floor of an apartment building in a modest neighbourhood, ate sparingly, and limited her social life to contacts with a small circle of colleagues and friends. In the mid-1920s she developed a heart disease (perhaps linked to her excess weight; described as thin and agile as a young girl, she became a stately matron in her Brussels years). Her health deteriorated in 1927, and she died in 1928. Her friends noted that the Polish political and academic establishments responsible for the numerous disappointments in Joteyko's last years none the less organized a sumptuous official funeral for her.[25]

JOTEYKO ON FATIGUE: FROM PHYSIOLOGY OF THE MUSCLE TO DEBATES ON TAYLORISM

Joteyko prepared her MD thesis (1896) on muscular fatigue using Marey's myograph to study contractions of an isolated muscle from a frog's leg – a typical subject of research in Richet's laboratory. The modest scope of this thesis gives little indication of Joteyko's future scientific proclivities.[26] Between 1898 and 1906 she published extensively on two topics, pain and fatigue. Following Richet, she gathered both under the single heading "psychical defenses of the organism."[27] Her work on pain included quantitative studies of the distribution of pain receptors, conducted with Stefanowska, and attempts to prove a theory of "algogens" – supposed chemical transmitters of pain. Joteyko and Stefanowska measured pain with Chéron's algometer, which evaluated precisely the depth to which a needle penetrates the skin to induce minimal feeling of pain, and with a mechanical algesimeter, an instrument developed by Bjøernstroem to measure the thickness of a skin fold submitted to pressure. They insisted on the reproducibility and the precision of their measures, which precluded the interference of subjective elements. They concluded that women are more sensitive to pain than men (for them evidence of female superiority; "savages," they explained, are less sensitive to pain than civilized people) and that the distribution of pain sensors is not symmetrical: the left side of the body has as a rule more such sensors, in both right-handed and left-handed individuals. The two researchers investigated as well the relationship between the threshold of pain and fatigue.[28] Joteyko elaborated a theory of generation and transmission of painful impulses. Extending Frey's view that only specific sensors produce pain (which for her is not, as Richet and Wundt claimed, the expression of a general irritation of nerve endings), she proposed that specific chemical substances, the "algogens," mediate a feeling of pain. Measurements of the interval between painful stimulus and painful sensation, she argued, supported this chemical theory.[29]

Joteyko's physiological research on muscular fatigue led her to the application of physiological data to ergonomics and to pedagogy. She studied fatigue in animal models but simultaneously became interested in an "energetic" approach, strongly promoted by Solvay. The work of Angelo Mosso, inventor of the ergograph and author of the first major work on human fatigue (*La Fatica*, 1891), inspired her studies.[30] Joteyko investigated (with Stefanowska) muscular fatigue in laboratory animals as well as the relationships between mental or psychological exhaustion and muscular fatigue in humans.[31] She then devised a method for the quantitative measurement of mental (or intellectual) fatigue. Her conclusion was that such relationships are neither linear nor simple.[32] She employed research methods first elaborated by Mosse, and her investigations helped establish the new science of ergography, named after the principal instrument used in these studies.

Joteyko collaborated with Charles Henry, a physiologist, a psychologist, and the founder of scientific psychophysiologal aesthetics (he tried to elaborate a mathematical system for measuring aesthetic experiences), who worked at the Solvay Sociology Institute. Henry's goal was to harness the laboratory in the service of a social program. He aspired to introduce quantification, above all the "graphic method" developed by Jules Etienne Marey, into previously inaccessible domains, ranging from aesthetics and the study of art to investigation of intellectual effort.[33] Henry also studied quantification in medicine and saw the medical uses of instruments, such as the sphygmograph, as foreshadowing automatization and mechanization of complex events.[34] Influenced by Solvay's "energetism," he hoped to extend biological research methods to the social sciences. "It will be extremely interesting," he proposed, "to compare statistical graphs that describe the development of various social phenomena with analogous biological curves. This may be a way to determine the nature of perturbations of individual reactions by the so called social states, and to start a new discipline: social energetics."[35]

Henry's fascination with quantification echoed Joteyko's preoccupations.[36] Their joint attempt to develop a mathematical model of physical and intellectual fatigue – the "fatigue graphs" – was part of an effort to measure precisely human sensation and activities.[37] Joteyko complained about the insufficient mathematical training of biologists when mathematics was becoming indispensable for their research: "mathematical methods allow us not only to express in the form of general laws phenomena that have already been thoroughly studied, they can be utilized as a distinct method of research in physiology [to study new phenomena]."[38] Joteyko followed intensely the practical applications of fatigue studies. Her first major publication on that topic was her 1904 book on the role of fatigue in military training. Excessive fatigue, she proposed, is counter-productive and decreases the efficacy of training. Moreover, individuals who undergo military training reach a plateau after which their results do not improve with additional exercise. Joteyko maintained therefore that relatively short training of soldiers, six months at most, can produce excellent results. Her book, openly inspired by the pacifist theses of Jean de Bloch, contained a thinly veiled critique of the military. The preface was by her former teacher Charles Richet, known for his pacifist ideas.[39]

Joteyko also studied fatigue among industrial workers. She participated in 1905 in a study (co-ordinated by Emile Waxweiler, of the Institute of Sociology) on "workers' aptitude for mechanical work," conducted at the Mélotte Factory in Rémicourt – an agro-alimentary enterprise that employed workers who had migrated from the countryside and trained them in modern industrial methods. This investigation applied new methods such as photography and cinematography to analysing workers' tasks.[40] Joteyko strongly supported scientific studies of labour. She believed that governments should establish physiology laboratories to measure workers' fatigue under natural conditions. Such measures, she argued, are a precondition for a rational, science-based use of the labour force.[41] Yet she stressed that fatigue was not a simple physiological condition, but is the combined result of metabolic changes in muscles and of more complex neurological and psychological phenomena. Thus workers suffer at the end of the day from nervous fatigue and exhaustion, manifested by their increased sensibility to pain.[42] In a 1903 report from the psychophysiology laboratory of the University of Brussels, she emphasized that social problems relate closely to psychological ones and that the only way to study them seriously is through the methods of physiological psychology.[43]

Joteyko adopted the point of view of French and Belgian social reformers, gathered around the Musée Social and the *Revue de l'économie politique*, who believed that science-based solutions and appropriate education of workers would advance the interests of the popular classes and would help end sterile class antagonisms.[44] She associated with well-known Polish socialists, such as Edward Abramowski and Stanislaw Posner (Abramowski regularly published articles in *Revue psychologique*) and maintained contacts with French socialists as well. In 1907 she taught at the Worker's University (of socialist inspiration) in the Saint Gilles suburb of Paris, and during the First World War she and Grzegorzewska spent their summers in St Georges de Dionne in a socialist-inspired workers' cooperative.[45] She took her students at the International Faculty of Pedology to visit Belgian factories and mines in order to show them the advantages of efficient organization of labour and of applying scientific methods to improve workers' lives.[46] She saw in technical education for workers' children, which was being promoted in Belgium, an effective way to elevate workers' aspirations and to enrich their lives while maintaining their pride in their occupation. An appropriate education, she argued, can help young people to find jobs that correspond to their abilities and aspirations and can revalorize industrial labour. It can also reduce the number of sterile and useless labour conflicts: workers who understand how industry works will be less likely to raise unreasonable demands. [47]

In the first part of *La science du travail et son organisation* (1917), called "The Human Motor" (a title borrowed from Jules Amar's 1914 book), Joteyko argued that salaries should provide just compensation for workers' physical effort.[48] Pay should be therefore grounded in "energetic" laws. Employers should therefore provide a steep increase in pay for long hours and for work that produced fatigue, as well as equal pay for equal effort. During the war, Joteyko stressed, female factory workers successfully occupied male jobs but often received less than previous male incumbents. Such a disparity had no justification: people who furnish the same amount of work should receive the same salary.[49] Joteyko took her previous observation that an arithmetic rise of productivity entails a geometrical rise of fatigue as a starting point for advocating a shorter work week: at some point fatigue increases so sharply that workers are unable to regain their ability to work well even after a rest period, and overall productivity decreases. Shortening working hours often increases productivity and thus promotes the interests of both workers and employers. Joteyko nevertheless opposed trade unions' demand to establish a uniform legal length of work week. The optimal number of working hours in every profession and occupation, she argued, was a matter for scientific research to determine.[50]

La science de travail et son organisation (1917) and *La fatigue* (1920) also contributed to a debate on the introduction of Taylorism into France. French physiologists had divided on this issue. Some, such as Henry le Chatelier, enthusiastically supported Taylor's approach; others, such as Jean Maurice Lahy and Armand Imbert, strongly criticized it.[51] Joteyko admired the efficacy of Taylor's method and agreed with le Chatelier that it could raise productivity without increasing fatigue.[52] She believed that precise scientific measures of labour would serve workers' interests. She did not oppose the use of chronometers and did not view measurements of time to accomplish a given task as degrading to workers.[53] Yet she criticized Taylor's exclusive focus on productivity and his neglect of psychological and individual factors. Taylorism, she explained, pretends to be a scientific method, but in fact it is not based on truly scientific studies of fatigue. The system aims to increase productivity, not to manage personnel well, and may therefore easily lead to excesses, to exhaustion, and to ruthless exploitation of workers (especially when these are powerless and unable to negotiate their work conditions).[54] One need not, Joteyko concluded, accept Taylorism as an indivisible entity. It is possible to select some of its elements and to reject others. Nevertheless, "Taylorism, completed and revised, linked with recent findings in psychology and energetics, will become accepted only when it wins the agreement of worker's organizations such as trade unions and cooperatives."[55] Joteyko's 1921 monograph *Productivity and the Length of Labour Time* dwells on the importance of the "psychological factor," which regulates the way the "human motor" works. A truly scientific organization of industrial labour is thus antithetical to an excessive standardization of tasks and to the treatment of workers merely as part of the industrial machine; it takes into account individual differences in aptitude and aspirations.[56] Experimental psychology, Joteyko concluded, may be an efficient tool for increasing productivity while making industrial labour less oppressive. It will allow the economy to enlarge its domain and to become individual without ceasing to be social.[57]

Attempts to promote the "Taylorization" of housework illustrate, Joteyko argued, the intrinsic limitations of a purely mechanical attitude to organization of labour. In principle a scientific organization of activities such as cleaning, shopping, cooking, and dishwashing can be useful. However, enthusiastic advocates of Taylorism at home produced a purely utilitarian view of domestic labour that assumed that women will be happy to specialize as domestic workers and will take pride in efficient execution of domestic tasks. Such specialization will, however, become too absorbing for women and confine them exclusively to their familial milieu: "such a trend contrasts with the evolution of the family in modern societies in which women are encouraged to leave the family home, and where multiple functions which previously belonged exclusively to the domestic sphere became collectivized and socialized." But, she noted, attempts to rationalize domestic tasks such as cooking and cleaning may be helpful for organizations that transcend the family – for example, workers' co-operatives.[58]

Joteyko was sympathetic to workers' aspirations. Her attitude to scientific management revolved around contradictory images of industrial labour. She oscillated between an idealized view of factory work, presented as a worthy accomplishment of human potential, and a realistic view, which recognized the unavoidable drudgery and hardship of such work. She viewed workers alternately as craftspeople (hence the demand for more initiative and creativity) and as people condemned to repetitive and wearing tasks (hence the demand for free time to regenerate physical strength and for general education to incubate interests outside the work sphere). She sincerely admired the working class yet felt a strong elitism, grounded in a belief in "elites of the spirit." This tension shaped her efforts to construct a quantitative science of education.

MEASURING CHILDREN: THE RESEARCH PROGRAM OF PEDOLOGY AND ITS TRANSFORMATIONS

Before she accepted (in 1906) a lectureship in experimental psychology at the two *écoles normales* (teacher training schools) of the Belgian province of Hainanut, Joteyko had little interest in pedagogy. She grasped quickly the opportunities offered by her new job. Identifying enthusiastically with the newly created domain of "pedology," she endeavoured to redirect her previous interest in experimental physiology to the study of childhood.[59] The term pedology was first employed by an American researcher, O. Chrisman, in his thesis at the University of Jena in 1896. Chrisman wrote about "poeidology"; Emile Blum popularized this term in an article published in *Année psychologique* in 1899 and transformed it into "pedology." Blum advocated the development of a general science of childhood, which would take into account all aspects of development and growth and have a strong practical orientation. "Pedology" had numerous meanings, but proponents stressed physiological studies and exact measurements. Its essence was "an experimental study, investigation of fact, either induced or observed, but in both cases fully controlled. It is thus a true Science."[60] Its opponents identified pedology – or at least some of its variants – with excesses of scientism. Albert Binet criticized its excessive distance from a daily pedagogical practice: "pedology seems to be an exquisitely precise machine, a mysterious, brand new locomotive that, at a first sight, commands admiration, but the various elements are not well connected one to the other, and the machine has one major defect: it does not work."[61]

Joteyko adopted Blum's definition of pedology as a domain that includes theoretical and practical components. Pedology, she proposed, has in some ways a narrower field of application than psychology or physiology because it deals only with children. Yet it has a broader scope because it studies all aspects of the development of human beings. It has to combine methods borrowed from several sciences, while also developing its own method.[62]

Joteyko aspired to becoming a leader of the new discipline, and Brussels was an excellent place to develop it. The Institute of Sociology, founded by Solvay, promoted scientific studies of childhood and created in 1910 a Group for the Study of the Sociology of the Child. Ovide Decroly (1871–1932), a neurologist, psychiatrist, and pioneer in the development of special pedagogy for abnormal children, in 1906 founded (together with Emile Waxweiler) the Belgian Society for Pedotechnics.[63] Joteyko was a founding member of both groups and collaborated with Decroly, Waxwiller, and their colleagues in the collective effort to develop an objective "science of childhood." She argued that only a precise, experimental approach leads to the understanding of the intellectual and moral nature of children.[64]

Joteyko insisted on the importance of the pedology laboratory. Such a facility should include instruments for anthropomorphic measures (Broca's compass, cephalometer, pelvimeter), for the graphic method (chronograph, kymograph, polygraph), for studies of respiration and circulation (Marey's pneumograph, plethysmograph, sphyngomyograph, Verdin's spirometer), for studies of movements (dynamometer, ergograph, Marey's myograph), and for studies of skin sensations (Cheron's algesimeter, esthesiometer, Richardson's pulverisator), as well as material to test acoustic, gustative, olfactory, and visual sensations.[65] The new science of pedology, she explained, will complete the task of eugenics: while eugenics promotes "wellborn children," pedology promotes "well-educated" ones.[66] Joteyko's interest in eugenics probably had its source in her early work at the Solvay Institute. There she collaborated in studies – such as the research, co-ordinated by Emile Waxweiler, on "the influence of urban life on degeneration in children" – that stressed heredity. However, the Belgian variant of eugenics, like the French one, was a "soft," neo-Lamarckian one, that focused on interactions between heredity and environment.[67] Scientific studies, grounded in precise measurements, should allow the evaluation of each child's potential, and subsequently the development of health and education strategies aimed at optimizing that potential. In the long term, such studies will also improve the human race. Children will develop better muscles and better brains, and these modifications, fixed in their organism, will shape future generations.

A fully equipped pedology laboratory such as the one that Joteyko installed in the *écoles normales* of Mons and Charleroi was both a teaching and a research tool. Simplified versions, she argued, should routinely be used to follow up every school-age child. Schools should keep medico-pedagogical files (*carnets scolaires*) of their pupils, including results of systematic anthropomorphic and physiological measures made in pedology labs.[68] Each file should contain observations concerning the child's heredity, health status, and progress at school. Teachers and physicians should be familiar with the principles of pedology and should know how to evaluate results of its investigations. Critical to this process was the institutionalizion of pedology and its transformation into a full-fledged academic subject.[69] Each university should thus have a pedology faculty, which would train experts and conduct independent research. Joteyko viewed the International Faculty of Pedology in Brussels as the model for such an institution.[70]

The faculty's curriculum lasted three years,[71] with the first two dedicated to preparation for a "licence" and the last year to autonomous research leading to a "doctorate." Lectures and laboratories usually took place in the afternoons, leaving mornings free for individual studies and excursions to educational and cultural institutions. These excursions, and the practical *stages* offered to students, were among the faculty's most characteristic features. The curriculum emphasized natural sciences: anthropometrics, biology, physiology (with a special course on the physiology of muscles and nerves). It reflected Joteyko's belief in grounding all the psychological disciplines in "psychophysics" and therefore in experimentation and quantitative measures.[72] Other subjects were more traditional: didactics, experimental pedagogy, experimental psychology, history of education, physical education, school hygiene, and sociology of children. The faculty had four laboratories – anthropometrics, chemistry, experimental psychology, and physiology – for teaching and for research. The results of studies conducted by the staff and students appeared in the *Revue psychologique.* Joteyko stressed the moral importance of experimentation and of acquiring habits of precision and objectivity.[73] She aspired to develop in her students the "scientific spirit of a humble submission to experimentally confirmed facts" and used to say that 12 years of work with frog's muscles taught her to slowly elaborate solid and well-grounded theories.[74]

After moving to Poland in 1919, Joteyko remained faithful to the experimental method. She attempted to ground her teaching at the National Pedagogical Institute in laboratory investigation and experimentation. She taught in parallel a course in "pedology" at the National Institute of the Deaf in Warsaw.[75] However, her shift from "pedology" to "experimental psychology" denoted a change in orientation and the weakening of links with physiology. Students in the psychology lab learned to use physiological instruments such as the cardiograph, kymograph, pneumograph, or sphyngomyograph, but the focus had altered to more specific psycho-physiological investigations, such as measuring rapidity of reactions to stimuli, spatial orientation, and manual dexterity. In addition, the students learned to employ psychological tests, such as the Binet-Simon tests, the Otis test, and the Stanford educational test. These tests occupied a growing role in Joteyko's effort to make pedagogy a quantitative science.[76]

In the 1920s, Joteyko, who had better relationships with government officials than with academe, became involved in debates on school reform.[77] She advocated a unified, obligatory schooling system until the age of 14, and then "scientific selection" of pupils, which would separate those going on to general high schools leading to university from those destined for professional high schools and vocational training. Another round of selection at the age of 18 would choose those apt to join the ranks of university students.[78] Joteyko proposed to introduce some flexibility into the testing process. Some children, she explained, develop more slowly than others and should have a second chance to enter a general high school; similarly some young adults find their way only later in life and should have access to university after passing appropriate examinations.[79] Nevertheless, scientific tests of aptitude should become the backbone of the educational system: "the best results and the best support for creative forces can be achieved only through an expert selection, a difficult and demanding task which will demand the 'psychologisation' of large domains of life."[80] Hence Joteyko's recommendation to open departments of experimental psychology in all universities and medical schools and to create a Central Psychological Institute, which would supervise psychological tests, centralize their results, and develop new tests, better adapted to Polish conditions.[81]

Joteyko believed strongly in education providing equal opportunity to each child, promoting development of all talents, and enriching the world of underprivileged children. She also praised manual labour, craftsmanship, and practice-oriented occupations. The aim of selection, she argued, was not to create a hierarchy among individuals. Professional and vocational education was not an inferior trajectory. Clerical, "white collar" jobs can be more monotonous and less creative that many manual occupations. She praised the vocational training in Belgium, which provided children who went to professional schools with elements of general culture and opened up "worker's universities," such as the one at Charleroi. The Belgian system, she argued, produced well-educated and open minded workers, proud of their achievements and able to adapt to new tasks.[82]

Yet Joteyko promoted a "soft" version of biological determinism. Tests and psychological investigations, she explained, help to discover the "natural talents" of each child, often masked by differences of social origin. A rational educational system will help each individual to find an occupation that corresponds to inborn aptitudes: "a place for every man and each man on his place."[83] A just and efficient system will thus promote a more rational distribution of workers and replace class-based elites with intellectual ones – that is, with people able to develop a high level of abstract thinking.[84] The aim of pedology and of experimental psychology, Joteyko proposed in 1908, is to put an end "to the mediocrity that strangles us, and according to which everybody is shaped in the same mould because everybody is educated in the same way."[85] The goal of psychological testing, she argues in one of her last articles, is "to provide a selection which we may call natural."[86] The current "laissez faire" approach, which selects children on the basis of their achievement in school, favours those from privileged background. Only a scientific selection "can attenuate anti-democratic, anti-national or anti-feminist pressures, because the decisive factor will not be the candidates' origins, nationality or sex, but their talents."[87] Many Polish teachers, struggling in the 1920s for the democratization of the school system, remained unconvinced by her passionate advocacy of the application of scientific methods to pedagogy. They resisted her promotion of science-based selection, thus increasing her feelings of intellectual isolation.[88]

PHYSIOLOGY AS AN APPLIED SOCIAL SCIENCE

The dominant feature of Joteyko's professional life was her aspiration to make scientific new domains of activity through codification, standardization, and precision. "Role hybridization" and opening up of new areas of activity are common professional strategies for outsiders.[89] This did not, however, work for Joteyko. One possible reason may be that she attempted to compete with men in a male-dominated arena, using what are normally considered masculine methods – graphs, mathematical forms, and precise measurement – and accusing her adversaries of being backward-looking and unscientific. Her style of scientific writing deliberately conveyed the impression that she was mastering complex and difficult domains, as did her occasionally aggressive way of calling attention to her achievements. Joteyko also employed other strategies. She secured the support of influential male mentors (Richet, Denis), cultivated strong friendships with female collaborators, and later in life developed protective, motherly relations with students and younger co-workers.[90] Some of Joteyko's difficulties were probably contingent, rooted partly in her character and abilities and partly in chance events, such as the the First World War, which destroyed her efforts to promote pedology teaching in Belgium. Nevertheless, her double marginality as a foreigner and as a woman undoubtedly restricted her chances of achieving full professional success.[91]

We may contrast Joteyko's difficulties with the success of the approach chosen by her student and friend Maria Grzegorzewska. Grzegorzewska is celebrated in Poland as the pioneer of "special education" of mentally handicapped children. She was successful where her teacher and mentor failed, due most probably to her cultivation of a "gender-appropriate" research style in a "gender-appropriate" domain. Grzegorzewska adhered at first to Joteyko's ideas about the importance of physiological studies in pedagogy and conducted such research, focused mainly on sensory perceptions of handicapped children. However, she viewed tests mainly as tools that facilitate classification, indicate possibilities of intervention, and measure progress; she came to stress subordination of empirical investigations to educational and moral goals.[92] Moreover, Grzegorzewska had chosen to specialize in the low-prestige field of special education. She did not attempt to compete with powerful men on their own turf; she took a job that nobody wanted.

In 1909 Joteyko published a small volume on muscular functions, destined mainly for students of science and medicine.[93] The book was part of the series *Encyclopédie scientifique,* directed by Dr Toulouse and dividing the sciences into philosophy of science, pure sciences, and applied sciences. The philosophy of science stood alone and had no subdivisions, perhaps because the authors assumed that there is one correct scientific method and only one way to think about science. The divisions between pure and applied sciences were often quite different from today's. Thus microbiology, pathology, and physiology, but also anthropology, ethnography, political economy, psychology, and sociology appeared under the heading "normative biological sciences." The "applied biological sciences" were applied psychology, applied sociology, biological industry, hygiene and public medicine, and pharmacology.

Although Joteyko published a volume in Toulouse's series (and later invited him to be a sponsor of her International Faculty of Pedology), she resisted his distinction between pure and applied sciences. It is impossible, she argued, to differentiate clearly the roles of the researcher and of the practitioner.[94] Her lifelong efforts to measure with precision different physiological parameters and to use these measures in practice-oriented fields, such as education or the organization of industrial labour, appear to be attempts to close the gap between "normative" and fundamental biological sciences and the domains of applied sociology and psychology, but also of political action. Charles Richet promoted a similar view of physiology. In his preface to Joteyko's study of military fatigue, he explained that, "under its modest appearance, this book has a considerable theoretical and practical importance. It is indeed one of the first times that sociological problems which play a role in present-day political life [*ceux qui relèvent de la politique vivante, actuelle*] were tackled from a physiological point of view."[95]

Social scientists frequently link normalization with the use of science to control human beings – a perspective identified with Michel Foucault. Foucault indeed pointed to the controlling potential of science. But he was aware of the hopes and aspirations that accompanied the rapid growth of scientific knowledge in the nineteenth century:

> Le XIXe siècle a été le siècle dans lequel on a inventé un certain nombre des choses très importants, que ce soit la microbiologie par exemple, ou l'elecromagnetisme, etc., c'est aussi le siècle dans lequel on a inventé les sciences humaines. Inventer les sciences humaines, c'est en apparence faire de l'homme l'objet d'un savoir possible. C'était de constituer l'homme comme un objet de la conaissance. Or, dans le même XIXe siecle on éspérait, on révait le grand mythe eschatologique suivant: faire en sorte que cette connaissance de l'homme soit telle que l'homme puisse être par elle libéré de ses alienations, liberé de toutes les déterminations dont il n'était pas maître, qu'il puisse, grâce a cette connaisance qu'il avait de lui même, redevenir ou devenir pour la première fois maître de lui-même. Autrement dit, on faissait de l'homme un objet de conaissance pour que l'homme puisse devenir sujet de sa propre liberté et de sa propre existence."[96]

Foucault's insight may aptly sum up Joteyko's dreams and aspirations. Joteyko shared the nineteenth-century project of harnessing science to the task of controlling and reshaping human fate, at both the individual and the collective levels. Far from being "unnatural," science, Joteyko proposed in 1920, can help us to recover our lost instincts. The recent recognition of the importance of physical activity for school children, or of the role of manual activities and drawing in education, was not the result of a spontaneous decision to "return to nature," but the consequence of scientific investigations that displayed the value of certain activities in children's development. The progress of science, Joteyko argued, promoted the rediscovery of natural instincts and impulses suppressed by modern civilization. Gustave Le Bon had proposed that education is the art "de faire passer le conscient dans l'inconscient," but, Joteyko suggested, the opposite statement is even truer: education is increasingly becoming the art of "faire passer l'inconscient dans le conscient."[97] The opposition between "scientific knowledge" and "intuition" or "instinct" is entirely artificial: far from distorting true human nature, science is a tool for enhancing it. "All the complicated psychological apparatus employed to test children, all the efforts of creative pedagogy, have only one goal: to provide the right conditions for a natural development of the child."[98]

The nineteenth century's "eschatological project," Foucault proposed, had radically subverted itself. The development of human sciences – and especially of psychology and of psychoanalysis – not only did not enhance human beings' ability to become subjects of their own consciousness (the "auto-theologization of man"), but had the opposite effect: it led to the dissolution of the very notion of human nature.[99] Joteyko acted on the opposite conviction. She postulated continuity between biological, psychological, and sociological studies, believed that methods developed in the natural sciences will play a key role in social sciences, economy, or education, and perceived the objectification of human bodies through quantitative physiological measures as a means of human self-perfection and emancipation. Indeed Joteyko was praised for being "a biotechnician who aspires to shape human life in the most rational way."[100] Some of her attempts to apply physiological measures to social uses may seem naïve or futile, and some may have suffered distortion from her wish to advance her professional aims and to find a stable place in academe.[101] At their best, nevertheless, these efforts represent a sincere aspiration to increase human freedom through the use of measures, instruments, and research methods borrowed from the natural sciences. They also illustrate the intrinsic tensions and ambivalence in any such enterprise. Early-twentieth-century physiology, like present-day genetics, was a contested field.

NOTES

1 I follow the Polish spelling of Joteyko's first and last names, which appear in the majority of her later publications. Earlier, she frequently adopted the spellings Iosepha or Josephine and Ioteyko. Titles of all publications in Polish appear in English.

2 The paper later appeared in *Revue psychologique* (Brussels), a trimestrial journal founded and directed by Joteyko. Jozefa Joteyko, "Mesurations, instruments, méthodes, résultats," *Revue psychologique* 3 (1910), 404–7.

3 Jozefa Joteyko, "Unification des termes, des mésures et des notations en Pédologie," *Actes du Premièr Congrès International de Pédologie* (11–18 Aug. 1911) (Brussels: Librarie Misch & Thron, 1912), 51–2.

4 Anson Rabinbach, *The Human Motor: Energy, Fatigue and the Origins of Modernity* (Berkeley: University of California Press, 1992); François Vatin, *Le travail, sciences sociales et société: Essai d'épistémologie et de sociologie du travail* (Brussels: Editions de l'Université de Bruxelles, 1999). Rabinbach and Vatin do not discuss other aspects of Joteyko's career or her unusual biography.

5 Robert M. Brain, *The Graphic Method: Inscription, Visualization and Measurement in Nineteenth Century Science and Culture* (forthcoming). Brain discusses the social and cultural ramifications of a movement inspired by the teaching of the French physiologist Jules Etienne Marey. I am grateful to Brain for making his unpublished manuscript available.

6 Thomas Neville Bonner, *To the Ends of the Earth: Women in Search of Education in Medicine* (Cambridge, Mass.: Harvard University Press, 1992).

7 Testimonies on Joteyko's life appear in a special commemorative issue of *Polskie Archiwum Psychologji* 2, nos. 2–4 (1929). See also Maria Grzegorzewska, Jozefa Joteyko, (in Polish), Leaflet published by the Committee for the Commemoration of Achievements of Jozefa Joteyko (Warsaw, 1928); Otton Lipkowki, *Jozefa Joteyko: Life and Work* (in Polish) (Warsaw: PAN, 1968). These mainly hagiographical works provide many interesting details on Joteyko's life and work.

8 Richet considered Joteyko one of his best students. Nevertheless, he makes a sharp distinction between his male, French, and usually upper-middle-class students, destined for "aggregation," who later became trusted colleagues, collaborators, and friends, and foreigners, occasionally female, who worked in his laboratory. Charles Richet, *Souvenirs d'un physiologiste* (Paris: J. Peyronnet & Cie, 1932).

9 Stefanowska specialized at first in histology. She investigated the "piriform appendices" dendritic nerve cells, which, she claimed, were true functional structures and not artifacts or pathological phenomena. See

M. Stefanowska, "Evolution des cellules nerveuses corticalles chez la souris," *Annales des sciences médicales et naturelles de Bruxelles* (1898); M. Stefanowska, "Les appendices terminaux des dendrites cérébraux: Leurs différents états physiologiques," *Archives des sciences physiques et naturelles* (Geneva) (1901). Reprints in Stefanowska's file, Library of Warsaw University.

10 On Solvay's "social energetics" and its role in the development of social sciences in Belgium, see Jean François Cromboy, *L'univers de la sociologie en Belgique de 1900 à 1940* (Brussels: Editions de l'Université Libre de Bruxelles, 1994).

11 On Joteyko's career in Belgium, see Kaat Wils, "Iozefa Ioteyko et la pédologie en Belgique," unpublished paper delivered at the meeting "Construire les sciences de l'homme: quelle rôle pour les femmes ?" Paris, 13–15 June 2001.

12 Her publication list includes 267 items. S. Sedlaczek and I. Skowronkowna, "Bibliography of the Works of Jozefa Joteyko," *Polskie Archiwum Psychologji* (1929), 173–86.

13 Iosepha Ioteyko, *Résumé des travaux scientifiques* (Gand: Volsksdrukkerie, 1906).

14 Ibid., 4.

15 For example, I. Ioteyko, "La coéducation dans l'enseignement supérieur," *Actes du Premier Congrès International de la Pédologie,* 416; Wils, "Iozefa Ioteyko et la pédologie en Belgique."

16 Michalina Stefanowska, *Motherly Love in the Animal Kingdom* (in Polish) (Warsaw: J. Sikorski, 1902). We can contrast Stefanowska's argument with the one of sociobiologists who link male domination with freedom from the burden of pregnancy and from caring for offspring.

17 Iosepha Ioteyko and Michalina Stefanowska, *Psychophysiologie de la douleur* (Paris: Alcan, 1909).

18 Ioteyko and Stefanowska, *Psycho-physiologie de la douleur,* review (anonymous) of the book in *Revue de l'Université de Bruxelles,* quoted by Wils, "Iosepha Ioteyko et la pédologie en Belgique," Stefanowska's file, Library of Warsaw University.

19 Remy de Gourmont, "La dépêche de Toulouse" (newspaper cutting, Joteyko's file, Library of Warsaw University, JF-UW, 9 Oct. 1908). The information provided by "La dépêche de Toulouse" was incorrect: Stefanowska had a doctorate in natural sciences, not in medicine; and neither author was a "university professor."

20 Vegetarians still quote these studies today as proof of the innocuousness of a vegetarian regime.

21 Joteyko's attempt to create an alternative institution outside academe that would apply a scientific approach to the solution of social problems recalls earlier efforts of Dick May (Jeanne Weill). May helped develop

the Musée Social and in 1899 founded and became the permanent secretary of an alternative teaching institution, the Ecole des hautes études sociales, that aspired to harness science to the solution of social goals. Christophe Prochasson, "Dick May et le social," in Colette Chambelland, ed., *Le musée social en son temps* (Paris: Presse de l'Ecole Normale Supérieure, 1998), 43–58.

22 Letter of Raymond Buyse to the Committee for the Commemoration of Achievements of Jozefa Joteyko, 102. See also Wils, "Iosepha Ioteyko et la pédologie en Belgique."

23 On Gregorzewska, see I. Jaroszewska, M. Falski, and R. Woroszynski, eds., *Maria Grzegorzewska* (in Polish) (Warsaw: Instutut Wydawniczy Nasza Ksiegarnia, 1969); Ewa Zabczynska, ed., *Maria Grzegorzewska: A Pedagogue in the Service of Mentally Handicapped Children* (in Polish) (Warsaw: Wydawnictwo Wyzszej Szkoly Pedagogiki Specjalnej, 1985).

24 Lipkowski, *Jozefa Joteyko, Life and Work*, 48. According to Lipkowski, the main opponents of a university appointment for Joteyko were Professors Wladyslaw Witbicki and Bohan Nawrocki.

25 "Memoirs: Collection of Short Testimonies on Joteyko" (in Polish), *Polskie Archiwum Psychologji*, 97–158.

26 Ioteyko, *La fatigue et la réspiration élémentaire du muscle* (MD thesis) (Paris: Ollier-Henri, 1896).

27 I. Ioteyko, "Les défenses psychiques: I. La douleur, II. La fatigue," *Revue psychologique* 3 (1910), 3–22, 147–55; Charles Richet, *La défense de l'organisme: cours de physiologie de la Faculté de Médecine de Paris*, reproduced in *Physiologie: travaux de laboratoire de M. Richet*, vol. III (Paris: Alcan, 1895), 458–573.

28 I. Ioteyko and M. Stefanowska, "Recherches algésymetriques," *Bulletin de l'Académie Royale de Belgique*, classe des sciences, 2 (1903), 199–282; I. Ioteyko and M. Stefanowska, "Asymétrie dolorifique," *Journal de Neurologie et de Psychiatrie* 8 (1903) (unpaginated reprint in Joteyko's file,) Cf. also I. Ioteyko "Mesure de la force musculaire, de la sensibilité tactile et de la sensibilité à la douleur de soixante dix élèves des écoles normales de Hainanut," *Revue psychologique* 1 (1908), 51–9.

29 I. Ioteyko, "Les substances algogènes," *Journal de neurologie*, Brussels (1905), reprinted, Bruxelles, L. Severeyns, JF-UW; I. Ioteyko, "Une théorie toxique de la douleur," *Revue Générale des Sciences Pures et Appliqués* 5 (1906), 240–3. Joteyko grounded her argument on the existence of specific "pain-inducing" chemical substances in observations of dissociation of thresholds of tactile and pain sensibility under the influence of analgesic substances and in the fact that pain can persist long after the disappearance of its immediate cause.

30 Rabinbach, *The Human Motor*, 133–6.

31 She draws on a tradition of studies of intellectual fatigue through the use of physiological measures – for example, A. Mosso, *La fatigue intellectuelle et physique* (Paris: Alcan, 1894); A. Binet and V. Henri, *La fatigue intellectuelle* (Paris: Librairie C. Reinvald, 1898).

32 I. Ioteyko, "À propos de la fatigue cérébrale," *Revue psychologique* 8 (1901), 577–82; I. Ioteyko, "La fatigue intellectuelle et sa mesure," *Conférence de Laboratoire Kasimir, Revue de l'Université de Bruxelles* (1903), reprinted, Bruxelles: A. Lefèvre, 1903 in JF-UW.

33 Brain, *The Graphic Method,* chap. 40.

34 Ibid.

35 Charles Henry, *Mémoire et habitude* (Paris : Hermann et Fils, 1911), 5.

36 Charles Henry, *Mesure des capacités intellectuelles et énergétiques* (Brussels: Institut Solvay, Travaux de l'Institut de Sociologie, 1906).

37 I. Ioteyko and Charles Henry, "Sur l'équation générale des courbes de fatigue," CR *Académie des sciences,* Paris (24 Aug. 1903). Ioteyko and Henry quote, as their model, Solvay's book, *Notes sur les formules d'introduction à l'énergétique physio-et psycho-sociologique* (Brussels 1902).

38 I. Ioteyko, "Les lois de l'ergographie: Etude physiologique et mathématique," *Bulletin de l'Académie Royale de Belgique* 5 (1904), 560.

39 I. Ioteyko, *Entraînement et fatigue de point de vue militaire* (Brussels: Misch & Thron, 1905), preface by Charles Richet. Richet published a book praising pacifism two years later. See Charles Richet, *Le passé de la guerre et l'avenir de la paix* (Paris: Ollendorf, 1907).

40 Crombois, *L'univers de la sociologie en Belgique de 1900 à 1940,* 60–2.

41 I. Ioteyko, "Sur la mésure de la fatigue professionnelle," *Proceedings of the XIIIth International Congress of Demography and Hygiene* (Brussels, 3–6 Sept. 1903) ; I. Ioteyko, *Enquête sur la fatigue des ouvriers à l'atelier Melotte* (Brussels : Publications de l'Institut de Sociologie de Bruxelles, 1906). For studies on the physiology of labour in Belgium, see Eric Geerkens, « La rationalisation dans l'industrie belge de l'entre-deux-guerres," (PhD thesis, Université de Liège, 2002), 21–6.

42 Ioteyko and Stefanowska, *Psycho-physiologie de la douleur,* 114. Such increased sensitivity to pain was observed in female factory workers.

43 I. Ioteyko, "Rapport quinquennal sur les travaux du laboratoire de psycho-physiologie de l'Université de Bruxelles" (1903), quoted by Ioteyko, "Discours d'ouverture," *Actes du Premier Congrès International de Pédologie,* 25.

44 Janet Horne, "Le libéralisme à l'épreuve de l'industrialisation: la réponse du musée social," in Chambelland, ed., *Le musée social en son temps,* 13–26.

45 "Memoirs on Joteyko," *Polskie Archiwum Psychologji* 2, nos. 2–4 (1929), 113, 143. Grzegorzenka has similar inclinations; as a young woman she

taught at the Adam Mickiewicz People's University in Krakow, which popularized science among workers. Zabczynska, ed., *Maria Grzegorzewska*, 23–32.

46 "Memoirs on Joteyko," 117.

47 Jozefa Joteyko, "Les méthodes belges d'enseignement technique," *Revue générale de sciences pures et appliquées*, Paris, 10 (1917), 307–11; Jozefa Joteyko, *La science du travail et son organisation* (Paris: Alcan, 1917), 198–243. Cf. also Omer Buyse, "Le problème psychophysiologique de l'apprentissage," *Revue psychologique* 3 (1910), 377–99.

48 Jules Amar, *Le moteur humain et l'organisation scientifique du travail* (Paris: Dunod et Pinat 1914). Amar's title echoed his published thesis, *Le rendement de la machine humaine* (Paris: Ballière, 1910), and the study of Jules Etienne Marey, *La machine humaine* (Paris: Alcan, 1891).

49 Joteyko, *La science du travail et son organisation*, 139–40. Joteyko repeatedly affirmed in her writings that women are more resilient than men and that, as every zoologist knows, females of animal species tend to be the "strong sex" and males the "beautiful" one.

50 Ibid., 35–8.

51 For debates on the introduction of Taylorism in France, see Georges Ribell, "Les débuts de l'ergonomie en France à la veille de la première guerre mondiale," *le Mouvement social* 113 (1980), 3–36 ; on the role of applied psychology in these debates, see Vatin, *Le travail, sciences sociales et société*, 65–85.

52 Henry Le Chatelier, "La science économique," preface to F.W. Taylor, *Principes de l'organisation scientifique des usines* (Paris: Dunod & Pinat, 1912).

53 Jean Maurice Lahy, *Le système de Taylor et la physiologie de travail professionnel* (Paris: Masson, 1916).

54 Joteyko, *La science du travail et son organisation*, 86–8, 98–104; Jozefa Joteyko, *La fatigue* (Paris: Flamarion, 1920), 260–1. Lahy, trained as a physiologist and as an experimental psychologist, similarly proposed from 1904 on that studies of the "human motor" should always include a psychological dimension. Ribell, "Les débuts de l'ergonomie en France à la veille de la première guerre mondiale," 20–1.

55 Joteyko, *La science du travail et son organisation*, 111.

56 J. Joteyko, "La productivité et la durée du travail," *Revue de l'Institut de Sociologie de l'Institut Solvay* 1 (1921), 1.

57 Ibid.

58 Christine Freriks, "La tenue scientifique de maison," *Revue de la métallurgie* (1915), discussed by Joteyko, "La science du travail et son organisation," 92–4.

59 Ioteyko affirms that already in 1903, in the "Rapport quinquennal sur les travaux du laboratoire de psycho-physiologie de l'Université de Brux-

elles," she had drawn attention to the fact that "recently the term 'pedology' was coined to describe the scientific studies of childhood." I. Ioteyko, "Discours d'ouverture," *Actes du Premier Congrès International de Pédologie*, 25.

60 M.C. Schuyten, *La pédologie: synthèse* (Gand: Maison d'Edition Vanderpoorten, 1911), 10. Shuyten, a professor of pedagogy in Antwerp, collaborated systematically with Joteyko's *Revue psychologique*, as did other Belgian advocates of pedology such as Omer Buyse and Olivier Decroly.

61 Albert Binet, *Les idées modernes sur les enfants* (Paris: Flammarion, 1910), 131. Binet believed nevertheless that new tools developed by pedology could become very useful when combined with a holistic and practice-oriented approach to education.

62 Joteyko, "Unification des termes, des mésures et des notations en pédologie."

63 Cromboy, *L'univers de la sociologie en Belgique de 1900 à 1940*, 63–8.

64 Quoted by Jan Mazurkiewicz, "On Psychological Activity of Josepha Joteyko," *Polskie Archiwum Psychologji* 2, nos. 2–4 (1929), 56.

65 Josepha Joteyko, "Rapport sur les laboratories de pédologie des écoles normales provinciales de Hainaut (Mons et Charleroi)," *Revue psychologique*, 1 (1908), 28–39.

66 Jozefa Joteyko, "Les buts et les tendences de la Faculté Internationale de Pédologie," speech at the ceremony of inauguration of the International Pedologic Faculty, Brussels, 5 Nov. 1912, JF-UW.

67 Crombois, *L'univers de la sociologie en Belgique, de 1900 à 1940*, 68–71.

68 The First International Congress of Pedology included an exhibition of scientific instruments intended for such laboratories. Paul Menzerath, "Exposition scientifique," *Actes du Premier Congrès International de Pédologie*, 472–82.

69 Josepha Joteyko, "L'enseignement de la pédologie aux instituteurs et aux médecins," *Actes du Premier Congrès International de la Pédologie*; "Rapport sur les laboratories de pédologie des écoles normales provinciales de Hainaut."

70 Joteyko, "Les buts et les tendences de la Faculté Internationale de Pédologie."

71 "Programme général de la Faculté Internationale de Pédologie de Bruxelles (Ecole Supérieure des Sciences Pédologiques et Psychologiques)," *Revue psychologique* (1912), 273–83; J. Joteyko, "Les buts et les tendences de la Faculté Internationale de Pédologie de Bruxelles," *Revue psychologique* (1913), 116–24.

72 Joteyko's teaching notes for a course of physiology at the International Faculty of Pedology (undated); Joteyko's teaching notes for a short course in "psychophysics," conducted in April 1912 in Poland. Museum

Marii Grzegorzewskiej, Academia Pedagogiki Specjalnej im. Marii Grzegorzewskiej, Warsaw. Gregorzewska kept Joteyko's papers and nearly all of them disappeared during the Warsaw insurrection of 1944; only a few survived among Grzegorzewska's papers.

73 H. Radlinska, "Jozefa Joteyko as a Pedagogue" (in Polish), *Polskie Archiwum Psychologji* 2, nos. 2–4 (1929), 75–87; Jozefa Brugger, "Notes on the Organization of International Pedological Faculty in Brussels" (in Polish), *Polskie Archiwum Psychologji* 2, nos. 2–4 (1929), 88–96.

74 Letter of Raymond Buyse to the Committee for the Commemoration of Achievements of Jozefa Joteyko, *Polskie Archiwum Psychologji* 2, nos. 2–4 (1929), 103.

75 J. Joteyko, "Plan of Teaching at the National Institute for the Deaf, 1919–1920," Joteyko papers, Museum of Maria Grzegorzewska, Warsaw.

76 J. Joteyko, "Psychological studies at the National Pedagogical Institute, Warsaw" (in Polish), *Rocznik Pedagogiczny* 2 (1924), 15–44.

77 At that time, the Polish Ministry of Education dealt also with religion, and its official name was Ministry of Religious Cults and National Education (WROP).

78 J. Joteyko, "The Fate of Our Youth and the Reform of the School System" (in Polish), *Polskie Archiwum Psychologji* 4 (1926–7).

79 Radlinska, "Jozefa Joteyko as a Pedagogue."

80 Joteyko, "The Fate of Our Youth and the Reform of the School System."

81 Joteyko, *Methods of Testing Mental Abilities and Their Scientific Value*, 41–2; Joteyko, "Unity of the School System from the Point of View of Psychology and of Societal Needs" (in Polish), *Polskie Archiwum Psychologji* 1 (1926); Joteyko, *The Level of Intelligence of Pupils of Junior High Schools: Experimental Studies* (in Polish) (Warsaw: Sklad Glowny Ksiaznicy Poskiej Towarzystwa Nauczycieli Szkol Wyzszych, 1922), 15–20.

82 Joteyko, *La science du travail et son organisation*, 198–243; Joteyko, "La productivité et la durée du travail."

83 Jozefa Joteyko, *Methods of Testing Mental Abilities and Their Scientific Value* (in Polish) (Warsaw: Ksiaznica Atlas, 1924). The expression "une place pour chaque homme et chaque homme à sa place" she borrowed from James Harteness, *Le facteur humain dans l'organisation du travail* (Paris: Dunod & Pinat, 1916).

84 Joteyko's perception of psychological tests as a way to rationalize the labour force resonates with the ideas of Omer Buyse. Buyse, "Le problème psychophysiologique de l'apprentissage."

85 I. Ioteyko, "Notre programme," *Revue psychologique* 1 (1908), 3.

86 J. Joteyko, "Unity of the School System from the Point of View of Psychology and of Societal Needs."

87 Joteyko, "The Fate of Our Youth and the Reform of the School System." Joteyko energetically fought discrimination against women or, in Poland, against national minorities (Ukrainians, Lithuanians, Jews). She might, however, have had a different opinion of non-European races. Her Belgian colleague Omer Buyse visited U.S. schools and described enthusiastically the development of special methods of education for "ethnically retarded" people – that is, blacks. Blacks, Buyse explained, are incapable of abstract thought. Hence the need to develop an innovative approach to their education that links learning to the accomplishment of concrete tasks. Omer Buyse, *Méthodes americaines d'éducation générale et technique* (Paris: H. Dunod, 1908). Joteyko's teacher Charles Richet combined a sincere aspiration to promote the education of children from the lower classes and of women, as well as criticism of discriminatory practices against Caucasians (including Arabs and Jews), with racist propaganda directed against "inferior races," above all the black race. Charles Richet, *La sélection humaine* (Paris: Alcan, 1919).

88 Radlinska, "Jozefa Joteyko as a Pedagogue."

89 Joseph Ben David, "Roles and Innovations in Medicine," *American Journal of Sociology* 65 (1960), 557–68.

90 Her Warsaw students even nicknamed her "Little Mother" ("Matusia"). Testimony of Władsław Filipczyk, *Polskie Archiwum Psychologji* 2, nos. 2–4 (1929), 146.

91 The exemplary scientific career of Joteyko's compatriot Maria Curie-Skłodowska (1867–1939) was initially facilitated by her close association with Pierre Curie, with whom she won her first Nobel Prize.

92 Zabczynska, ed., *Maria Grzegorzewska*, 17.

93 Jozefa Joteyko, *La fonction musculaire* (Paris: Octave Doin, 1909).

94 Joteyko, "Les buts et les tendences de la Faculté Internationale de Pédologie."

95 Charles Richet, "Preface" in Ioteyko, *Entraînement et fatigue au point de vue militaire.*

96 Michel Foucault, "Foucault répond à Sartre," in M. Foucault, *Dits et écrits*, vol. I (Paris: Gallimard, 1994), 663–4. I am indebted to Michael Hagner for this reference. Cf. Michael Hagner, "Science and Medicine," in David Cahan, ed., *From Natural Philosophy to the Sciences: Writing the History of Nineteenth-Century Science* (Chicago: University of Chicago Press, in press).

97 Jozefa Joteyko, "Role of Knowledge and Intuition in Education" (in Polish) *Przeglad Pedagogiczny* (Jan. 1920), 5–15. In 1913, Joteyko explained that education consists of both making the conscious unconscious and of making the unconscious conscious. The first principle describes the assimilation of knowledge, and the second the development of creativity. Joteyko, "Les buts et les tendances de la Faculté Internationale de Pédologie de Bruxelles."

98 Joteyko, "Unity of the School System from the Point of View of Psychology and of Societal Needs."

99 Foucault,"Foucault répond à Sartre," 664.

100 Stefan Baley, "On the Scientific Activity of Prof. Dr. J. Joteyko," *Polskie Archiwum Psychologji* 2, nos. 2–4 (1929), 46. Baley was a professor of pedagogy at Warsaw University.

101 Vatin presents such efforts as reflecting a doubtful scientific orthodoxy and poor method. He views Joteyko's career as a "pathetic failure" that stemmed directly from her naïve scientism. Vatin, *Le travail, sciences sociales et société*, 75.

9

The Production of Biomedical Measures: Three Platforms for Quantifying Cancer Pathology

PETER KEATING AND ALBERTO CAMBROSIO

In his analysis of medicine as an "evolving synthesis of applied sciences," Georges Canguilhem described three processes that have transformed medicine in the modern era. First, the signs produced through medical intervention have replaced the symptoms presented by patients; second, the emergence of laboratory medicine has displaced the anthropocentrism embodied in bedside medicine; and, third, political demands have resulted in the rise of epidemiology as a social and economic science. The last in turn has entailed a shift of emphasis from health to safety and increasing reliance of clinical and public health authorities on biological monitoring techniques.[1] The quantitative analysis of data partakes in all these processes. Quantification, however, first appeared in medicine in the guise of medical statistics rather than as laboratory measurements. Consequently, most contributions to this volume focus on medical statistics and epidemiological research. In contrast, our contribution investigates the function of measurement in a domain – cancer pathology – that is representative of the other forms of quantification that have so profoundly altered diagnostic and laboratory medicine since the Second World War.

In using the term "quantification" outside its most obvious domains of application – namely, epidemiology and medical statistics – we follow the terminology of actors and institutions in our field of investigation, including the International Society of Diagnostic Quantitative Pathology. While the practices that we examine perhaps merely relabel in numerical, more objective terms[2] results already obtainable through other means, we show that quantitative techniques in pathology and affiliated domains have established new spaces of representation, which in turn have defined new objects and practices.[3]

But what exactly do actors mean when they speak of quantification in relation to cancer pathology? The process described in the subtitle of our article – quantifying cancer pathology – includes two overlapping, yet analytically distinct phenomena – namely, the quantification *of* pathology and quantification *within* pathology.

The quantification *of* pathology refers to the project of turning pathology – i.e., an institutional and epistemic configuration grounded in the qualitative analysis of pathological lesions as distinct from normal biological processes – into a quantitative endeavour based on the reduction of pathological to biological phenomena or, at least, on the alignment of the normal and the pathological.[4] Some observers see the reduction of pathological phenomena to a quantitative continuation of the normal as an effort to objectify medical diagnosis and thus eliminate the more subjective, often visual elements from diagnostic routines.[5] Proponents of reduction maintain that translating pathological lesions into continuous, biological variables opens the door not only to quantification but also to automation. Initiatives aiming – explicitly or implicitly – at the quantification of pathology generally originate with practitioners whose institutional basis lies outside pathology.

Quantification *within* pathology refers to the attempt to add a quantitative dimension to the analysis of pathological lesions, as defined within pathology. In this case the epistemic and institutional frame of reference remains pathological, and quantification refers to measurements made on specimens that are already categorized as pathological. As an example of this second kind of quantification, consider the aforementioned International Society of Diagnostic Quantitative Pathology, established in 1994 as the direct successor to the Committee for Diagnostic Quantitative Pathology, known originally – about 1981 – as the Committee for Diagnostic Morphometry. The society supports activities connected to quantitative microscopy and associated fields, including DNA cytometry, morphometry, quantitative immunohistochemistry, and stereology – that is, technologies related to the development of computerized instrumentation.[6] Here quantification designates first and foremost measurement. The material to be measured consists of tissues, cells, and organic substances whose status clinical selection and examination have determined to be pathological.

Both forms of quantification presuppose an alignment of the pathological and the biological – a process that has acquired special meaning since the Second World War and the concomitant rise of biomedicine. To illustrate this historically novel event, we examine three types of quantification in and of pathology. Each refers to a specific "platform," targeting different objects and points of measurement.[7] As an example of what we mean by platform, and as a way of introducing our three case studies, consider the case of a patient whose clinical signs suggest a lymphoid tumour. The clinician at this point requests a biopsy. A pathologist examines the resulting tissue sample and, with the help of a microscope and histochemical dyes, investigates the architectural arrangement and the shape and size of the cells in the sample. This morphological analysis can lead directly to a final diagnosis. But even in this case, and more so with difficult specimens, morphological analysis is nowadays frequently supplemented by immunophenotypic analysis. This second process combines panels of standardized antibodies via the use of computerized, laser-based equipment to detect the presence or absence of distinctive cell-surface molecules indicative of the diagnostic subgroup of the disease. A more recent, third diagnostic step involves molecular genetics. In it, suspicious cells are examined for culpable DNA fragments and genes through techniques such as DNA microarrays, RT-PCR, and Southern Blot.

Each of these three stages in the diagnostic process harnesses a configuration of techniques, instruments, reagents, diagnostic and laboratory skills, organic entities (cell morphologies, cell markers, genes), spaces of representations, diagnostic, prognostic, and therapeutic indications, and related aetiologic accounts.

We can label each of these configurations a distinctive biomedical platform, so that it is possible to speak of a morphological platform (we look at the example, going back to the 1920s, of the Pap test), an immunophenotypic platform (example: leukemia from 1970 on), and a molecular genetic platform (example: DNA microarrays from the 1990s on). Although they emerged in historical succession, each new platform did not replace the previous platform(s). Rather, new platforms articulated and aligned themselves in complex ways with the pre-existing ones and thus integrated into an expanding set of clinical-biological strategies.

MORPHOLOGY

Morphological investigations under the microscope are prototypical examples of visual exercises whose competent performance requires pattern-recognition skills.[8] Morphology, so it seems, blossoms in a world dominated by tacit knowledge and subjective expertise. How under these conditions can it possibly be quantified? The road to quantification, in this case, is indeed problematic, and it runs through two related, but distinct fields. First, one has to modify the principles underlying the diagnostic activity: instead of *looking* at differences in the shape of cells, one *measures* some physical variable – for example, the quantity of light passing through a cell – that somehow correlates with its morphological structure. In order to do so, however, one has also to turn the pathological entity into a biological object. One must postulate that the quantity being measured varies across the entire spectrum of normal and cancer cells and thus collapses the epistemic, material, and institutional distinction that separates the investigation of the normal from the investigation of the pathological.

While several oncology subfields have attempted to quantify morphology, we illustrate our argument through an examination of a now-ubiquitous screening technology for cervical cancer, the Pap test.[9] That process combines two strategies of quantification: reducing a pathological singularity, in this case cervical cancer, to a biological continuum; and automating the visual skills of Pap technicians by replacing them with computer-based morphometric technologies.

The first strategy would appear to be an instance of the quantification *of* pathology, and a successful one; despite a controversial history, the Pap test is now widely used. While the test has indeed enjoyed a successful career, it has done so not because it has quantified pathological diagnosis but rather because it has produced a new kind of diagnostic activity – screening – that is decidedly not diagnostic and that has formed a bridge between biology and medicine.

First developed by George Papanicolaou in the 1920s, the test was not, as originally conceived, diagnostic in nature. It was a method of classifying cells taken from the cervix and examined under a microscope. Sometimes those cells were deemed perfectly normal, in which case the slides examined fell into class I. Sometimes they appeared to indicate cancer, and the slides fell into classes IV and V. Classes II and III lay somewhere in between. At no point in the procedure did one diagnose cancer. The classification thus represented a proto–"biology of cancer," with a visible continuum between normal and pathological cells.[10]

Papanicolaou encountered two obstacles to the acceptance of his test. First, many pathologists believed that a microscope showed nothing in particular to distinguish cancer cells from normal cells.[11] Second, pathologists marginalized his work by noting that he was neither a pathologist nor a clinician, but an anatomist. Unsurprisingly, most subsequent developments in this field took place outside departments of pathology and were widely promoted by non-pathologists.[12] Papanicolaou himself had foreseen the problem and had used the biological terminology of classes in order to avoid conflict with pathologists.

None the less, even though the technique was entirely dependent on traditional microscopic techniques of cell identification, it took a veritable campaign conducted by the American Cancer Society and the National Cancer Institute before the Pap smear and its interpretation finally entered clinical medicine in the United States and Europe in the postwar era.[13]

The continuum between the normal and the pathological created by Papanicolaou's classification raised the question: at what point did the biology of cervical cells slide into disease? In other words, although the test was "hailed as the ultimate tool in cancer detection and prevention,"[14] it was not always clear in the 1940s and 1950s how pathologists should read the findings of a positive Pap smear (i.e., the presence of cancerous cells). In particular, some pathologists doubted that cancerous changes detected on the outermost tissue of the cervix (the epithelium), and referred to as carcinoma *in situ*, would inevitably lead to a genuine or invasive cancer of the cervix. An early practitioner of the Pap smear, Dr Lewis Robbins, has recalled disputes of the 1940s: "The Pap smear isn't diagnosing cancer, it's diagnosing a precursor. Why do they call it cancer then? Because nobody would pay any attention if they called it dysplasia (abnormal tissue). If you call it carcinoma *in situ*, then they will examine it, do something with it. I remember a battle at Roswell Park in 1946, the pathologist was saying that the Pap smear is no good. One physician said carcinoma *in situ* is not cancer, but we have to call it cancer. The pathologist said we can't call it cancer if it doesn't metastasize or if it hasn't already metastasized. But we did."[15]

These problems persisted well into the 1950s. To answer these and other questions, such as the age at which women were most in danger of developing cervical cancer, the National Cancer Institute (NCI) undertook experimental mass-screening programs for cervical cancer beginning in the late 1940s.[16] By the late 1950s, NCI was funding six separate experimental screening projects.[17] Preliminary results showed that "vaginal cytology readily lends itself to use as a mass screening device."[18] As defined in the 1950s: "Screening tests sort out apparently well persons who have a disease from those who probably do not. A screening test is not intended to be diagnostic."[19] As we noted at the beginning of this section, we have here the emergence of a new kind of activity. Rather than reducing pathology to a biological, and thus potentially quantitative, endeavour, it produced a new interface between biology and medicine. In other words, the Pap test uses biological techniques in and around pathology prior to or following diagnosis. It is an example of the search for biological markers to be used for prognosis and the monitoring of therapy or for pre-diagnostic screening. Based on biological techniques, these approaches all lend themselves to quantification in ways that traditional pathological techniques do not.

Prostate cancer has raised similar issues with respect to biological markers as substitutes for pathological criteria in diagnosis and prognosis. The discovery of the prostate specific antigen (PSA), which is present in both normal and pathological prostate cells, raised considerable hopes in the early 1990s about an efficient method to diagnose and predict prostate cancer. By the late 1990s, however, most organizations of screening experts had refused to recommend PSA screening[20] despite repeated claims that higher-than-normal serum PSA levels correlated well with the development of the cancer.

Three major problems had confounded clinical use of this biochemical variable. First, not all individuals who had elevated levels of PSA had prostate cancer. As PSA levels are a continuous biological variable, categorization of individual specimens assumed cut-off points that were invariably imperfect. For example, if the normal range is set at less than 4.0 ng/mL, then, as it turns out, abnormal levels between 4.0 and 10 ng/mL are positive for prostate cancer approximately 25 per cent of the time. In other words, an abnormal PSA reading is not diagnostic for prostate cancer.

Second, while PSA readings may be prognostic – the higher the reading, the greater the chance that the individual harbours prostate cancer – the use of PSA in treatment, as opposed to diagnosis and screening, has its own problems. In particular, whereas almost 98 per cent of patients with metastasized (and therefore inoperable) prostate cancer have PSA levels in excess of 40 ng/mL, some patients with local (and therefore operable) cancers express the same excessive levels. The problem has thus become how to correlate PSA levels with more specific pathological signs in order to articulate staging criteria with PSA levels.[21] Third, because of the nature of prostate cancer and its large number of relatively benign cases, prognosis is ultimately of greater importance than diagnosis. The NCI Progress Review Group convened in 1998 to study prostate cancer recommended: "NCI should place major emphasis on the development, validation and application of biologic markers or determinants that can provide reliable prognostic information."[22] It concluded: "The ultimate strategy for defeating prostate cancer calls for developing ways to distinguish the harmless (indolent) cancers from the potentially lethal and developing effective ways to prevent or treat the potentially lethal cancers."[23]

PSA levels in prostate cancer are, by definition, a quantitative biological variable. But in what sense is the Pap test a quantitative tool? First, the Pap test and biochemical measurements share the idea of a gradual transition from the normal to the pathological. In the Pap test, this is expressed by a continuum of cell classes. There is, however, a more evident sense in which the test relates to quantification – namely, through the attempt to automate the test by substituting various forms of measurement for visual inspection. Precisely because the test displays a continuous biological variable, much time and money have been devoted to its quantification.

Efforts reached a high point in the early 1970s with NCI's inauguration of its Cytology Automation Program.[24] Designed to fund applied research destined to automate the Pap test, and run by a Committee on Cytology Automation, the program received funds from the recently announced War on Cancer.[25] Although the program's money went as often to "pure technology" and "general biomedical applications" as to "clinical applications,"[26] the resulting instruments were intended to become devices for the automatic detection of cervical cancer cells.[27]

This did not happen. In 1978, reorganizations within NCI reduced the Committee on Cytology Automation to a purely advisory capacity.[28] Two years later, NCI abolished the committee, and the program ended, somewhat acrimoniously, having failed to achieve its objectives.[29] Why did NCI think that it could automate a medical activity – namely the diagnosis of cervical cancer – by funding instrument development? As we see below, various rationales have underlain cervical-cytology instrument development since the 1950s.

NCI announced its original intentions to produce an automated cytology instrument with a 1955 press release headlined: "Can a machine distinguish between cancer and normal cells? The Government and the American Cancer Society are betting $100,000 that it can."[30] That same year, Airborne Instruments Limited of Long Island, New York, received a grant to develop what came to be known as the Cytoanalyzer. Moving back and forth over a microscope slide, the device measured the area and density of cells on the slide by transforming the variation in light passing through the sample on the slide into an electric current. Researchers could then run the current through a computer supplied with rules to distinguish a normal from an abnormal current.[31]

Between 1955 and 1961, Airborne Instruments produced a number of instruments field-tested by NCI and outside collaborators. In 1961, they reported a trial showing no false negatives and a mere 15 per cent of false positives – "a very effective screening level." It would be, however, the last time that anybody achieved a false negative rate of 0 per cent – today considered next to impossible. The Cytoanalyzer subsequently disappeared.[32] Reviewing the situation in 1965, the director of NCI's Diagnostics Research Division concluded that, even though the device "performed its purpose well," its "biological programming" did not work.[33]

Rather than abandoning the whole project, NCI turned to its chief contractor for yet another device, with greater computing capacity. Developed in the period 1961–63, CYDAC grew directly out of the Cytoanalyzer program, but differed in one major respect. Rather than scanning hundreds of cells looking for normal and abnormal cells, it scanned hundreds of cells and reconstituted a digitized image of a normal cell. In developing CYDAC, NCI had in effect abandoned clinical medicine and devices for the wider field of biological instrumentation, automating the pathological by digitizing the normal. Indeed, the instrument was to digitize microscope images of cells and thus transform a classification of normal cells based on morphological appearances into one based on measures of those same images. Yet CYDAC measured the same variable as the Cytoanalyzer – namely, cells' ability to absorb different amounts of light. CYDAC, however, had its field-test in chromosome analysis, where it lost out to immunocytochemical analytical techniques.

Even with this shift within the NCI program, the idea that a machine could automate the Pap test did not go away. In 1963, L.A. Kamentsky, an IBM engineer, and Myron Melamed, a pathologist at New York's most prominent cancer research facility, the Sloan-Kettering Memorial Hospital, began research in the automation of the Pap test. Their collaboration would last for more than a decade.[34] In the absence of a specific pathological criterion distinguishing cancer cells from normal cells, the two men needed a biological variable. Kamentsky developed a spectrophotometer that exploited the ability of the cell's nucleus and its constituent nucleic acids to absorb light at a specific wavelength. Measurements of the amount of ultraviolet light absorbed by cells in the apparatus showed that some cancer cells absorbed more light than normal cells.[35]

However, by the time Kamentsky had perfected his instrument, the field had changed considerably. No longer the strict purview of NCI and the American Cancer Society, the Pap test had become a relatively common procedure, and over 120 government-supported schools of cytotechnology had produced an abundance of cytotechnologists.[36] Moreover, since 1966, the Pap test had been a reimbursable procedure under Social Security only if performed by a pathologist or by an individual certified by George Wied's American Society of Cytology at the University of Chicago – a form of unofficial quality control for the Pap test. If the Society did not like the device, then it would not fly.

In the late 1960s, Wied announced the (unofficial) rules of the game for automation of the Pap test – in effect 0 per cent false negatives, or 100 per cent success in cancer detection. The machine could not miss any cancer cells, even though cytotechnicians and pathologists sometimes did. There was a Catch-22: the machine had to perform as well as pathologists, but if it did, then it was equivalent to a device that intentionally produced misdiagnoses and was hence subject to civil litigation. The only way out of the paradox was to make the machine judgment-proof through the reduction of the false negatives to zero. Moreover, according to Wied, the use of cellular criteria such as the absorption of light was no substitute for what cytopathologists really do. In reality, cytopathologists never evaluated single cells. Rather, they looked at "cell patterns" and "associations of cells." Consequently "[a]ny method that removes cells from their 'pattern' tends to decrease diagnostic accuracy."[37]

The ideal machine became one that replaced human judgment. On these grounds, Kamentsky's spectrophotometer failed. Yet the initial confusion now dissipated: there would be no machine to replace human judgment. This did not, of course, preclude automation if the machines could be infallible. Rather than automating morphology, Kamentsky was redefining the biologically normal cell on the basis of new instruments.

Kamentsky and Melamed articulated this movement from the automation of clinical tasks to biological automation in the late 1960s. Presenting their machine in a special issue of the IEEE journal published in 1969,[38] they pointed out that, despite the origin of the demand, an automated instrument did not primarily identify pathological cells: it identified "specimens that are entirely normal." They drew this lesson explicitly from the attempt to automate the Pap test. After the initial identification of abnormal cells, it would be possible to think of "separating, concentrating or marking abnormal cells in a specimen."[39] The project to automate the Pap test had again produced an apparatus that measured and identified, on the basis of that measurement, different biological entities without actually diagnosing anything. In a sense, it was adequate to the task, as the Pap test did not actually diagnose anything either.

As American initiatives in Pap test automation wound down, interest in Europe and Japan heated up. Between 1975 and 1981, the Europeans developed eleven Pap automation systems,[40] and between 1983 and 1987 four of these went into limited clinical trials funded by the European Community as part of a larger program entitled Concerted Action Automated Analytical Cytology (CAAAC). Despite these initiatives, in their final report to the European Community, the researchers admitted that "the early hopes and expectations of the CAAAC have not been fulfilled."[41] Yet work continues, as many people believe that the reasons for the commercial "failure" of the devices were more economic than technical.[42] In particular, enthusiasts suggest that the fragmented European market, composed of many small test laboratories, could not shoulder the high cost of the systems.

As for the U.S. market, centralized into seven "Pap test mills" handling tens of thousands of tests a year, the International Academy of Cytology had erected a formidable barrier to entry by insisting on 0 per cent false negatives,[43] based partly on the assumption that this was potentially the accuracy of human analysts and thus the only level of acceptable risk from the actuarial and litigation point of view. A series of articles critical of the "Pap mills" and exposing their elevated levels of false negatives appeared in the *Wall Street Journal* in 1987 and laid that myth to rest, thus rekindling interest in automation in the United States.[44]

In 1992, a review of cytopathology automation noted a sea change since 1987:[45] several commercial systems had appeared and produced preliminary positive results. Subsequent events have done nothing to bolster enthusiasm. By 1998 none of the systems mentioned in the 1992 review had found broad clinical use.[46] A report in 2000 from a French medical-technology assessment team, citing similar findings from an Australian study of 1998 and a New Zealand study from 2000, concluded that the automated systems were inferior to manual techniques.[47]

We have suggested that the ambiguous relationship between medical devices and biological instrumentation has beset the history of attempts to automate the Pap test. As we saw above, the project has been a relative failure, even though it produced biological instrumentation in more than one instance. The persistent ambiguity and the failure can be partly understood within the larger framework of the relations between the normal and the pathological and, in particular, between the quantitative measurement of the normal and the qualitative definition of the pathological.

There is an institutional coda to our story. We pointed out that screening, as embodied in the Pap test, functions as a bridge between pathology and biology. We also noted in the introduction that there is an International Society of Diagnostic Quantitative Pathology (ISDQP), whose activities correspond to what we have defined as quantification within pathology. (ISDQP) has its mirror image in the European Association for Analytical Cellular Pathology (ESACP), set up in 1986 as successor to the aforementioned CAAAC program. Both ISDQP and ESACP focus on computer-based methods for cell measurements. Yet, despite its name, and as opposed to ISDQP, ESACP also draws members from within biology. As the newsletters of both societies noted:

> For many years, there have been two societies in the field of Quantitative Pathology that have their main activities in Europe: the [ESACP] and the [ISDQP]. The ISDQP originates from a Working Group of the European Society of Pathology, and has traditionally been a society of pathologists, mainly concentrating on applications of analytical techniques. The ESACP, on the other hand, has had a bigger input from biologists focusing on research. Both Societies have realized that over the last few years, the Societies have grown to share similar objectives and goals and that there is a great deal of overlap between the two groups ... The officers of the two Societies have therefore had several talks to discuss possible further collaborations ... We believe that this collaboration will be fruitful to both Societies.[48]

If we take the ESACP as an instance of the quantification of pathology and the ISDQP as quantification within pathology, the distinction between these two strategies of quantification seems to be disappearing. However, the main motive for the closer collaboration, or even possible merger, is failure to attract members. Their activities have remained marginal to the pathology profession.

This does not mean that attempts to quantify pathological practices have reached a dead end. Rather, they have moved on from morphology to the development of novel quantitative platforms such as immunophenotyping and molecular genetics, which replace the visual inspection of cells with the measurement of biomedical entities – cell markers and genes – that are present in both normal and pathological specimens.

IMMUNOPHENOTYPING

"Immunophenotyping" (IPT) refers to the investigation of distinctive markers or antigens on the surface of cells using antibodies that selectively bind to these substances. Fluorescent dyes conjugated to the antibodies enable researchers to visualize the bound antibodies with sophisticated equipment to do the visualizing and counting. In the simplest case, the equipment may consist of a fluorescence microscope, but in most cases it involves a computerized apparatus able to count thousands of fluorescent cells per second.

IPT, however, began in leukemia research in the 1970s as a quest for unique cell-surface markers that were, in other words, pathognomonic (distinctive diagnostic signs) for cancer cells.[49] Soon IPT gave rise to a new etiological account of leukemia: cancer cells were not mature, degenerated cells but normal cells with arrested development. The markers detected by IPT are thus "normal" markers of cells frozen at a given developmental stage. One speaks no longer of leukemia-specific markers but of leukemia-associated markers. In other words, through the alignment of biological and pathological variables it became possible to speak, in a strong sense, of a *biology* of leukemia.[50]

The detection of cell markers became in principle a quantitative issue, insofar as one had to examine many cells and detect the presence of "normal" markers in "abnormal" quantities or on an "abnormal" number of cells. Moreover automatic methods measured fluorescence intensities above a certain threshold and analysed (and displayed) the resulting measurements with the help of statistical algorithms. While IPT resorts to advanced measurement tools, its results are only partly quantitative: the tools presuppose a qualitative distinction between normal and abnormal cells that is essential for setting up and calibrating the instrument as well as for interpreting the resulting data. Thus while the initial horizon was the quantification *of* pathology, this process led to semi-quantitative measurements of normal entities that stand in complex relation to pathological entities.

IPT developed in a distinctive institutional environment. In the 1970s a number of cancer research institutions around the world made large investments in cancer immunology and immunobiology. Michael Stoker initiated one such enterprise when he became the scientific director of Britain's Imperial Cancer Research Fund (ICRF). Stoker defined his investment as strategic research – i.e., research that "might have a bearing on cancer but which is just as likely to lead to benefits in other fields," such as biology. Unsurprisingly, he believed that "medicine, as we all know, is one of the branches of biology" and that, even though the recent revolution in biology had had little impact on medicine, its consequences would begin to affect the clinic: "just you wait!"[51]

One of Stoker's key investments centred on a project set up by a biologist, Melvin Greaves, to characterize acute leukemias according to a new biological classification of immune cells into B and T cells. The system rested largely on the proteins on the cell surfaces – the "cell surface markers." Greaves's research bore fruit in the mid-1970s: he had characterized a number of disease entities according to their cell surface antigens. Normally these antigens appeared in hematopoiesis, when normal blood and immune cells develop from an original stem cell. The cell surface markers signalled stages in this process of development and differentiation. As we saw above, Greaves and others in the field projected a novel relationship between the normal and the pathological: malignant leukemia cells expressed the markers of their stage of differentiation, prior to transformation into and subsequent expansion as a malignant clone.

A propos the continuous relationship of the normal to the pathological, "lineage fidelity" maintained that malignant cells could further differentiate and mature within a given cell lineage. There could be no "de-differentiation," or reversion to a "foetal phenotype," as pathologists had claimed. Rather, the leukemia cells remained "'frozen' in a particular cell lineage compartment but ha[d] an essentially normal cell surface phenotype."[52] Lineage fidelity – the consistent correspondence between normal and leukemia phenotypes – suggested that "no qualitatively unique and consistent leukaemia 'markers' may exist or be required."[53] And, since the cell surface remained essentially unchanged during the malignant process, one need not look for mutant genes that transformed the molecular architecture and gave rise to "foreignness." "Rather, it [was] suggested that subtle alterations uncoupling the controls that integrate[d] proliferation and differentiation [were] all that [was] required."[54]

That leukemia cells retained the immunophenotypic properties of normal cells did not earn universal acceptance. One of the foremost American experts in leukemia therapy, Donald Pinkel, a clinical researcher at St Jude's Hospital in Memphis, Tennessee, observed: "Leukemia cell phenotypes are disorderly and asynchronous, not just arrested in maturation. At no stage of normal B-lymphocytic differentiation can one find cells that look like those of B-cell leukemia." Thus "we cannot extrapolate from leukemia to normal hematopoietic differentiation. Attempts to draw conclusions about normal lymphocyte differentiation by study of leukemia cell populations can yield erroneous results. On the other hand, leukemia cells can be good sources of antigens and genes involved in growth and differentiation. Leukemias are useful tools for study of hematopoietic differentiation but not models."[55]

Undeterred, Greaves and co-workers insisted that they had "not seen a single T plus B phenotype cell in something like 2000 cases of lymphoid leukemia examined over 7 years." It was "remarkable that such a high proportion of leukemias [had] a phenotype consistent with normal gene expression and that 'mixed' or 'illegitimate' phenotypes occur[ed] so infrequently."[56] Yet reports of empirical results pointing to lineage "infidelity" or "promiscuity" demanded a reply. Greaves's team, on the point of biological victory over pathologists, did so by raising doubts about the competence of the researchers reporting incidents of infidelity and asked whether the results corresponded to an "identity crisis for cells, ... antibodies, or investigators."[57]

Two points are crucial here. First, although Greaves suggested that pathology was nothing more than biology – or, at least, supervenient on biology – and that knowledge of the normal translated directly into and was in some sense superior to knowledge of the pathological, because more fundamental, he was unable to dispense entirely with the pathological. Indeed, while the different types of malignancy aligned with different stages of normal blood-cell development, there was a pathological event – "uncoupling" – at the basis of the malignant process.

Second, even though the relationship between biology and pathology appeared to be a one-way street, subsequent events have redressed the balance in the other direction. Cases of lineage infidelity have accumulated: acute mixed-lineage leukemia (AMLL) would have been impossible, or at least unlikely, according to Greaves's position during the 1980s. Moreover, since the appearance of the initial mixed-lineage reports, the MLL gene has been isolated and related to chromosomal translocations associated with acute human leukemia.[58] In other words, mutation, not uncoupling, lay behind the "foreignness" that Greaves had sought to deny. Rather than normal development serving as the sole source of illumination of normal and pathological hematopoietic processes, the pathological situation becomes a tool for investigating normal processes. Researchers in pathology are now in a position to ask: "What can we learn from leukemia as for the process of lineage commitment in hematopoiesis?"[59]

Beneath the polemics, a process of exchange created new biological *and* pathological knowledge – in short, new biomedical knowledge. If one wished to describe this episode in terms that captures at least some of the complexities – most of which we have glossed over here – one would have to begin by describing the history of those cell surface "markers" that allowed immunobiologists to enter into communication with the pathologists in the first place. One would then outline how these entities came to occupy a space of representation that lies between the normal and the pathological without reducing one to the other. We could then start understanding the interactions between fundamental and clinical research in terms other than subordination or application. For our present purpose, the computerized equipment for performing IPT measurements has become ubiquitous in pathology (or, at least, hematopathology) laboratories. What at first seemed a bold attempt to quantify pathology has turned into a reasonably successful quantification within an altered pathology, still within the specialty's institutional boundaries.

MOLECULAR GENETICS

Proponents of the IPT platform have sometimes described it as an example of "molecular morphology," thus creating a metaphorical bridge between the traditional morphological techniques used by pathologists and the new molecular approaches championed by biomedical scientists.[60] A similar rhetorical strategy is apparent in molecular genetics – for instance, in the name of a recent initiative, the Cancer Genome Anatomy Project (CGAP).[61] Established in 1996, CGAP aims to redefine anatomical pathology at the level of the molecular changes that occur as a normal cell becomes a cancer cell.

Molecular genetics is thus the most recent platform (started in the 1990s) designed to quantify biological entities in the service of pathology. Given the field's recent and impressive techno-scientific and industrial growth, the existence of several variants comes as no surprise. We focus on the most recent – DNA microarrays (also called biochips), whose market is growing at a spectacular rate.[62] Microarrays allow for the simultaneous inspection of the activity of hundreds or thousands of genes, as opposed to the single genes and mutations addressed by previous molecular-genetic techniques. While molecular genetics may have shifted measurement to the level of genes, the process seems one of realignment rather than of reduction.

How does a DNA microarray experiment work?[63] A microarray consists of a small, solid surface (a glass or, more rarely, nylon slide of a few square centimetres), with individual DNA samples (up to thousands of them) arranged in a grid.[64] In a typical run, a technician investigates the differential expression of genes between, for example, a breast cancer specimen and a normal tissue specimen. The genetic material extracted from the two specimens is labelled with different fluorescent dyes (for example, green and red) and incubated with the microarray. Genes that are expressed (i.e., show some activity) in the sample tissues hybridize with their counterpart fixed to the microarray, and the result becomes visible as a fluorescent spot at a specific grid location. Thus "the fluorescent signal at the spot in the array representing each individual gene provides a quantitative readout of the level of expression of that gene in the sample. This simple procedure offers a systematic way to monitor expression of tens of thousands of genes simultaneously, in thousands of samples per year."[65] Reading the results of a microarray run, however, requires more than visual inspection. Rather, a scanner must first perform fluorescence measurements, which undergo further treatment by computer algorithms. The algorithms may take into account fluorescence thresholds, execute statistical tests, and correct for all sorts of sources of "noise" (irregular spots, dust, and so on). The resulting values are then translated into colour-coded diagrams and, most important, rearranged through the use of statistical clustering algorithms, to allow for meaningful inspection and witnessing by researchers.[66]

Despite the problems and debates about "proper" performance, a microarray quantitatively describes the level or intensity of gene expression as tracked through the measurement of fluorescence intensities. In addition to establishing the presence of a (qualitative) gene mutation that produces altered gene products, one can follow the abnormally high or low level of expression of a set of genes characterizing the pathological behaviour of a cancer cell. Do we not have here a tool for the quantification of diagnosis? We would certainly seem to have the beginnings of the automation of cancer diagnosis. As described by Todd Golub of Harvard Medical School: "The idea here was that you put a sample on a microarray, you press a button, and out comes the answer. It's this tumor or that tumor."[67] The routine clinical use of microarray techniques depends on finding solutions to a number of problems.

First, how much independent and novel information concerning diagnosis, classification, and prognosis can the technique provide? Todd Golub, Eric Lander, and their colleagues at the MIT Center for Genome Research knew that microarrays needed independent status in order to obtain clinical success. Among the earliest and most often-cited entrants into the diagnostic field, they invented a technique "that automatically discovered the distinction between acute myeloid leukemia and acute lymphoblastic leukemia without previous knowledge of these classes" and claimed that it could provide "a general strategy for discovering and predicting cancer classes for other types of cancer, independent of previous biological knowledge."[68] In a subsequent special editorial for the *New England Journal of Medicine* – "Genome-Wide Views of Cancer" – Golub concluded that previous taxonomies were dispensable and clinical practice would have to adjust.[69]

Echoing Golub, a review in the *Journal of Clinical Pathology* warned pathologists that if they did not embrace the technology, they might have to leave the field: "If pathologists neglect the potential of these processes at an early stage, it is not unthinkable that in the future their task will be limited to judging whether or not a sample contains material for microarray analysis or whether a tumor's histology is compatible with the more precise diagnosis made by geneticists or chemists, or just handing over samples to specialists from other disciplines after dissection. Even worse, such samples may be taken from the specimen before they are sent to the pathology department."[70]

Similarly, the *Journal of Pathology* tells its readers: "As pathologists in the future, none of us will be able to avoid DNA microarrays and there may come a time when tumor RNA is routinely run on arrays to give an accurate read-out of the patient's prognosis, and even a prescription for treatment!"[71]

It would certainly seem as if we have finally found the quantification of pathology. Yet, although the previous quotes paint pathologists as passive receptacles for new technologies in the basic sciences, biomedicine entails considerably more interaction and offers a number of options and strategies to pathologists and clinicians. Pathologists have appropriated the microarray technologies for their own purposes. Guido Sauter and his colleagues at the Basel Institute of Pathology, in collaboration with the NIH Human Genome Research Institute, have developed a tissue microarray that inverts the principle of the DNA microarray. Rather than following thousands of genes through a single tissue specimen, they have organized thousands of specimens on a single slide in order to follow a single gene product.[72] In the *Journal of Molecular Diagnostics*, Peter Lichter pointed out: "Although they stress the point that their study was accomplished within 2 weeks, this number does not account for the previous efforts to carefully analyze archived material for the generation of the arrays."[73] These specific arrays presupposed the activities of pathologists who classify and preserve pathological material.

To what extent do microarrays apply biology to pathology – or quantify previously unquantifiable lesions? To answer this question we must ask whether microarrays provide a simple, independent measurement of the intensity of gene expression in a given (normal or pathological) cell. The answer is no: the biology has been articulated with the pathology to produce a mixed measure.

Let us take, for instance, the highly cited microarray profile of two different lymphoma populations published in 2000 as a result of a collaborative project between Stanford University and NCI.[74] The authors claimed to have shown that a formerly single disease entity corresponded, when examined with microarray technology, to two molecularly distinct diseases. Molecular genetics, they argued, thus succeeded in a domain where morphology "largely failed owing to diagnostic discrepancies arising from inter- and intra-observer irreproducibility."[75] The visual demonstration consisted in the display of the colour patterns produced by the differential expression of hundreds of genes sorted according to three colour-coded categories of intensity: high (red), medium (black), and low (green).

These distinctive colour patterns – once again, the result of various statistical manipulations – constituted the characteristic *signature* of distinct pathological entities.[76] Two things are worthy of note here. First, the researchers had characterized the starting material – the tissue samples from which the genetic material was extracted – as normal or pathological according to morphological and IPT criteria. Second, and most important, they ultimately translated the pathological events into a qualitative pathological sign – a "signature" – rather than into a quantitative expression of biological data.

Thus, as in the case of IPT, we witness the alignment of the normal and the pathological, rather than the reduction of the latter to the former through quantification. Microarray experiments literally juxtapose the gene expression patterns characterizing normal and pathological material within a single, digitally produced representation. For instance, Staudt's group at the NCI assembled the results from 202 array experiments into a single map, where the gene expression of lymphoid malignancies sat side-by-side with the gene expression of normal immune responses.[77] The databases of gene expression obtained though the study of normal immune response thus help in the analysis of a pathological situation such as immune-cell cancers.[78] In a move reminiscent of the aetiological accounts provided by IPT, understanding the pathological mechanisms involves relating the malignant process to the normal stages of development and the physiology of immune cells. But, as with IPT, the pathological mechanisms maintain a distinct identity: while based on quantification, they do not reduce the pathological to a quantitative expression of the normal.

The issues so far discussed transcend mere epistemic considerations; they relate directly to and resonate with the material and social organization of biomedical work. In practice, the use of microarray technology or, more generally, of molecular-genetics techniques has added a further level to morphological and immunophenotypic diagnostic categories.[79] This does not mean that there are no surprises or that levels of alignment automatically fulfil expectations.[80] How will the quantification and its supporting technology fare in routine immunopathological applications?

Microarrays can align with work already under way. Researchers in Finland, for example, have applied them to investigate patients first classified according to traditional clinical, morphological, cytogenetic, immunophenotypic, and staging techniques. Their microarray did not monitor thousands of genes. A Becton-Dickinson subsidiary, Clontech, simplified and focused the process by producing "application-targeted arrays" that selected genes that reflected the specific functions and disorders of the cells in question. Thus, using the Atlas of Human Hematology Array[81] (containing 440 genes), the investigators isolated a cluster of up-regulated genes of known normal and pathological function.[82]

Indeed, some commentators have suggested that the use of thousands of genes to differentiate within cancer classes constitutes overkill. The theory of oncogenes says that, at best, several hundred genes mutate in most cancers.[83] Molecular profiling is thus more of the same; just as immunophenotyping articulated with histology, so too will molecular profiling ultimately have to address its relation to morphology. A keynote speaker at the inaugural meeting of the Association for Molecular Pathology, held at a gathering of the United States and Canadian Academy of Pathology, suggested: "In a sense, pathologists already use gene expression studies diagnostically on a daily basis in the form of immunohistochemistry. Expression profiling provides a supraexponential increase to the amount of gene expression data available on a given tumor, but lacks the topographical information of immunohistochemistry."[84]

The talk's *plus ça change* attitude, however, belied its more serious purpose: a call to arms for pathologists. Unlike immunohistochemistry or even cytogenetics, "expression profiling may require less prior expert histopathological 'triage' than any prior ancillary technique."[85] Given these conditions, will expression profiling evolve into another "ancillary" technique or become an alternative to expert surgical pathology? "The extent of involvement of the pathology community in the further development of microarray-based expression profiling as a diagnostic test may determine the nature of its ultimate relationship to conventional tissue-based diagnoses."[86]

Here is one form of involvement. Spurred by the work done in Staudt's laboratory, a French group of haematopathologists took up the challenge of producing a study "to aid in the transition of microarray technology into routine use."[87] They sought correlations between microarrays and existing immunohistochemistry techniques. They concluded: "in the future, pathologists might be able to analyse by [immunohistochemistry] potential markers of interest previously identified by array technology."[88]

Closer to the clinical world, a review in the *Journal of the American Medical Association* enumerated "possible pitfalls that may undermine the authority of the microarray platform."[89] The problems – sample selection, comparability, archiving, and clinical and biological significance – all revolved around regulation and articulation of microarrays with existing techniques for determining gene function, such as RT-PCR and knock-out mice. While none of the pitfalls seemed fatal, their solution is part of the deployment of microarrays as a functioning biomedical platform, not an external problem. They are inherent to the management of microarrays.[90]

A recent review in *Nature Genetics Reviews* also warns clinical readers of problems attendant on alignment of microarrays with existing routines in pathology. Gene expression studies require intact genetic material. Freezing tissue may preserve genetic material but compromises morphology. Formalin fixation also degrades genetic material to an unknown extent. Procedures such as those that use alcohol may be safe. But even here one must, for example, process the material with considerable dispatch: "investigators face an uphill battle in convincing surgeons and practicing pathologists to process the tissue obtained at surgery rapidly to preserve all the macromolecules of interest."[91]

Pathological expertise and mobilization of the underlying routines are essential to isolating the initial pathological material. Biopsy specimens are three-dimensional structures with a variety of cell populations. Explicit comparison between normal and pathological cells depends on a prior visual inspection of the biopsy material in order to separate the two types. None the less, some pathologists fear losing time during biopsy to placate microarray enthusiasts less than losing control over the resulting specimens and the downstream information.

Promoters of the microarray platform for routine clinical use know that these work-arounds and problems may block its adoption. Addressing a clinical audience, Golub admitted that microarrays are "often viewed as screens to identify markers for traditional diagnostics, such as immunohistochemistry, for routine clinical use" and that "the feasibility of routine clinical use of microarrays ... has yet to be established."[92] On the pathologists' side, a symposium held by the Royal College of Pathologists in 2000 on the molecular genetics of solid tumours agreed that, "aside from the use of gene rearrangement studies in hematological malignancies, genetic information has thus far offered little in the way of disease diagnosis and patient management."[93] The gathering set up a committee to develop a framework for introduction of molecular diagnosis into routine practice, for "there is a risk that technology will be used simply because it is available."[94]

CONCLUSION

We began by noting that this essay stood apart from most of the other contributions in this book. Rather than focusing on explicitly quantitative specialties – such as medical statistics and epidemiology – we have explored the processes through which a largely qualitative, visual practice – cancer pathology – has recently acquired a quantitative dimension. While discussions of medical statistics and epidemiology often raise questions concerning the historical and epistemological role that these specialties have played within medicine, nobody doubts the centrality of pathology to the practice of medicine. We further examined the role and meaning of quantification in the field of pathology by separating two analytically distinct strategies. One aims at turning cancer pathology itself into a quantitative endeavour, thus transforming simultaneously the epistemic, institutional, and material configuration of the specialty. The second, more mundane strategy involves injecting selected quantitative techniques and tools into the specialty.

Perhaps these strategies are only analytically separable; if we conceive of any given specialty as a network of tools, notions, skills, practices, and so on, then the distinction appears mere artifice. We do agree that, beyond the continued existence of the pathology label, the cancer pathology of the year 2000 is quite different from that of the 1950s. Also, our distinction between quantification *of* and *within* pathology refers to polar ideal types rather than to actual configurations of action. We none the less maintain that this distinction is quite useful for relating quantification in/of laboratory medicine to the larger post-1945 transformation of medical activities and, in particular, to the rise of biomedicine. For, despite short-term disturbances – debates and controversies that characterize the daily surface of medical activities – the last decades have seen a fundamental realignment of the relations between biological and clinical activities, or, in more conceptual terms, between the normal and the pathological. As we have tried to show, however, realignment does not mean reduction. Measurement of biopathological variables has certainly allowed researchers to pursue quantification in and of pathology. But the case studies in this essay show that, despite rhetoric and appearances, quantification proceeds just in and around pathology – none of our examples offers an instance of the quantification of pathology.

By resorting to the surface/depth metaphor and by contrasting short- with medium-term events, we obviously invite questions about the level at which our analysis operates. We have investigated the activities of human actors by citing excerpts from their pronouncements. We have also evoked the role of institutions and other social organizations. But, most important, we have structured our case studies around three platforms – morphology, immunophenotyping, and molecular genetics – that consist of many interconnected components, human skills being only one of them. This approach has allowed us to move seamlessly from laboratory techniques to institutional matters, from human skills to aetiological accounts and instrumental standards.

Quantification, when analysed as part and parcel of a set of practices in a given field, cannot be reduced to professional strategies or treated as a purely epistemic issue. It participates in all the above.

ACKNOWLEDGMENTS

Research for this paper was made possible by grants from the Social Science and Humanities Research Council of Canada (SSHRC) and Quebec's Fonds de Recherche sur la Société et la Culture (FQRSC). We would like to thank Gérard Jorland, Annick Opinel, George Weisz, and the Mérieux Foundation for inviting us to the October 2002 Conference on Quantification in the Medical and Health Sciences, where we presented the initial version of this article. We would also like to thank André Ponton, head of the Chip MicroArray Expression Laboratory at the Montreal Genome Centre, for introducing us to the technical subtleties of DNA chips.

NOTES

1 Georges Canguilhem, "Le statut épistémologique de la médecine," *History and Philosophy of the Life Sciences* 10 Suppl. (1988), 15–29. For a partial translation, see François Delaporte, ed., *A Vital Rationalist: Selected Writings from Georges Canguilhem* (New York: Zone Books, 1994), 141–6 and 152–7.

2 Theodore M. Porter, "Objectivity as Standardization: The Rhetoric of Impersonality in Measurement, Statistics, and Cost–Benefit Analysis," *Annals of Scholarship* 9 (1992), 19–59.

3 For a detailed discussion of the notion of spaces of representation, see Hans-Jörg Rheinberger, *Toward a History of Epistemic Things: Synthesizing Proteins in the Test Tube* (Stanford, Calif.: Stanford University Press, 1997).

4 Georges Canguilhem, *The Normal and the Pathological* (New York: Zone Books, 1989).

5 The objectification of pathology does not necessarily require quantification. Telepathology is an example of an attempt to overcome diagnostic subjectivity by making patient specimens available for collegial inspection.

6 Y.U. Collan and G.M. Mariuzzi, "Organized Quantitative Pathology: Short Review of the Activities of the Committee for Diagnostic Quantitative Pathology from 1981 to the Foundation of the International Society of Diagnostic Quantitative Pathology in 1994," *Pathologica* 87 (1995), 318–25. G.M. Mariuzzi and Y.U. Collan, "Some Reflections on the History and Presence of Quantitative Pathology," *Pathologica* 87 (1995), 215–20.

7 Peter Keating and Alberto Cambrosio, *Biomedical Platforms: Realigning the Normal and the Pathological in Late-Twentieth-Century Medicine* (Cambridge, Mass.: MIT Press, 2003).

8 For a detailed analysis of the learning of visual skills in a haematopathology laboratory, see Paul Atkinson, *Medical Talk and Medical Work* (London: Sage, 1995), especially chap. 4.

9 The history of the Pap smear has recently attracted the attention of several authors. See, for example, Monica J. Casper and Adele E. Clarke, "Making the Pap Smear into the 'Right Tool' for the Job: Cervical Cancer Screening in the USA, circa 1940–95," *Social Studies of Science* 28 (1998), 255–90; Adele E. Clarke and Monica J. Casper, "From Simple Technology to Complex Arena: Classification of Pap Smears, 1917–90," *Medical Anthropology Quarterly* 10 (1996), 601–23; Vicky Singleton and Mike Michael, "Actor-Networks and Ambivalence: General Practitioners in the UK Cervical Screening Programme," *Social Studies of Science* 23 (1993), 227–64; Patricia A. Kaufert, "Screening the Body: The Pap Smear and the Mammogram," in Margaret Lock, Allan Young, and Alberto Cambrosio, eds., *Living and Working with the New Medical Technologies: Intersections of Inquiry* (Cambridge: Cambridge University Press, 2000), 165–83; Eftychia Vayena, "Cancer Detectors: An International History of the Pap Test and Cervical Cancer Screening, 1928–1970," PhD thesis, University of Minnesota, 1999. Our purpose here is not to provide an alternative account of that complex process, but to focus on a single element: quantification and its relation to the normal–pathological dichotomy.

10 When the Bethesda system supplanted the Papanicolaou classification in 1988, among the four reasons cited for abandoning the classification was: "The Papanicolaou classes have no equivalent in diagnostic histopathologic terminology." While it never did have an equivalent, there was always hope that it would. V. Schneider, "The Bethesda System: The European Perspective," in Peter Pfitzer and Ekkehard Grundmann, eds., *Recent Results in Cancer Research 113: Current Status of Diagnostic Cytology* (Berlin: Springer-Verlag, 1993), 113–5.

11 Heinz Grunze and Arthur I. Spriggs, *History of Clinical Cytology: A Selection of Documents* (Darmstadt: E. Giebeler, 1980), 89–90.

12 Ibid., 89.

13 Casper and Clarke, "Making the Pap Smear," 261–2.

14 Leopold G. Koss, "The Papanicolaou Test for Cervical Cancer Detection: A Triumph and a Tragedy," *Journal of the American Medical Association,* 261 (1989), 737.

15 Quoted in Walter S. Ross, *Crusade: The Official History of the American Cancer Society* (New York: Arbor House, 1987), 87.

16 Memorandum to Director (7 July 1958), National Cancer Institute Archives, National Institutes of Health, Bethesda, Md. (NCI Archives).

17 By 1958, in the course of these research projects, over 300,000 of a projected 1.3 million slides had been examined. In 1961, 30 of every 100 women reported having had at least one Pap test. By 1966, a survey of women showed that this number had risen to 67 of every 100 (or at least 43 million tests). A survey of pathologists (all the members of the College of American Pathologists) carried out by the Cancer Control Program the same year estimated the number of women tested at 15.7 million. In any event, millions of tests were being done, which meant that thousands of cytotechnicians had to be trained. As of 1971, there were 110 approved schools of cytotechnology. See Carl Baker (Director of the National Cancer Institute), "Memorandum for the Assistant Secretary for Health and Scientific Affairs, July 9, 1971," NCI Archives.

18 John Roderick Heller, "Evaluation of the Validity of Uterine Cytology," speech to the International Cancer Cytology Congress, Chicago, 8 Oct. 1956, NCI Archives, AR-5610–003862.

19 Commission on Chronic Illness, *Chronic Illness in the United States*, vol. 1 (Cambridge, Mass.: Harvard University Press, 1956). More generally, see J.M.G. Wilson and G. Jungner, *Principles and Practice of Screening for Disease* (Geneva: World Health Organization 1968).

20 Richard Klausner, *The Nation's Investment in Cancer Research: A Budget Proposal for Fiscal Year 1999* (Bethesda, Md.: National Cancer Institute), 30.

21 P. May, R. Hartung, and J. Breul, "The Ability of the American Joint Committee on Cancer Staging System to Predict Progression-Free Survival after Radical Prostactectomy," *BJU International* 88 (2001), 702–7.

22 Don Tindall and Peter Scardino (Chairs), Progress Review Group, *Final Report, Defeating Prostate Cancer: Crucial Directions for Research* (Aug. 1998), 4. www.prg.nci.nih.gov/prostate/finalreport

23 Ibid., 15.

24 On the program, see Chester J. Herman and Bill Bunnag, "Goals of the Cytology Automation Program of the National Cancer Institute," *Journal of Histochemistry and Cytochemistry* 24 (1976), 2–5.

25 On the political framework of cancer research in the United States, see Mark E. Rushefsky, *Making Cancer Policy* (Albany: State University of New York Press, 1986).

26 "Committee on Cytology Automation," Annual Report, 15 Aug. 1981, Federal Records Center, Washington, DC, RG-443-97-0019, 3–4.

27 Cytology Automation Contract Program: Annual Report Summary, July 1, 1973 to June 30, 1974, NCI Annual Report, 1974, vol. II, S-1.

28 "Minutes of the Committee on Cytology Automation," 29 June 1978 (NCI Archives), 2.

29 Even though the Cytology Automation Program shut down in 1980, funding for a number of these grants continued under the new Cancer Diagnosis Research Program. At the final meeting of the Cytology

Automation Committee, longtime chair Chester Herman claimed that the reasons for closure boiled down to a mere question of macroeconomics: the political commitment to national screening programs had evaporated with the advent of the economic downturn. Department of Health and Human Services, Committee on Cytology Automation: Annual Report, 15 Aug. 1981, 3.

30 Press Release, National Cancer Institute, 20 Jan. 1955 (NCI Archives), AR-5501–003191.

31 W.E. Tolles, "The Cytoanalyzer: An Example of Physics in Medical Research," *Transactions of the New York Academy of Sciences* 17 (1954), 251.

32 In 1962–3, however, Sandritter and his colleagues in Germany developed a hand-operated cytophotometer explicitly modelled on the Cytoanalyzer. Following a field trial with approximately 9 per cent false positives, they recommended that "an automatic prescreening with a cytophotometer is advisable." W. Sandritter, Bertha L. Lobel, and G. Kiefer, "Photometric Cytodiagnosis of Vaginal Smears," *Journal of the National Cancer Institute* 32 (1964), 1221.

33 Elie M. Nadel, "Computer Analysis of Cytophotometric Fields by CYDAC and Its Historical Evolution from the Cytoanalyzer," *Acta Cytologica* 9 (1965), 203.

34 Louis A. Kamentsky, Herbert Derman, and Myron R. Melamed, "Ultraviolet Absorption in Epidermoid Cancer Cells," *Science* 142 (1964), 1580–83; Louis A. Kamentsky, Myron R. Melamed, and Herbert Derman, "Spectrophotometer: New Instrument for Ultrarapid Cell Analysis," *Science* 150 (1965), 630–1.

35 Kamentsky, Derman, and Melamed, "Ultraviolet Absorption." Citing this paper in 1969, Melamed and Kamentsky summarized its conclusions as follows: "It has been shown that at least some of the cancer cells from epidermoid carcinomas of the human uterine cervix are relatively rich in nucleic acids." Myron R. Melamed and Louis A. Kamentsky, "An Assessment of the Potential Role of Automatic Devices in Cytology Screening," *Obstetrical and Gynecological Survey* 24 (1969), 921.

36 See George L. Wied, "History of Clinical Cytology and Outlook for the Future," in George L. Wied, Catherine M. Keebler, Leopold G. Koss, Stanley F. Patten, and Dorothy L. Rosenthal, eds., *Compendium on Diagnostic Cytology*, 7th ed. (Chicago: Tutorials of Cytology, 1992), 2.

37 George L. Wied, "Automated Cell Screening: A Practical Reality or a Daydream?" in David Maclean and Demetrius Evans, eds., *Cytology Automation, Proceedings of the Second Tenovus Symposium, Cardiff, 24–25 October, 1968* (Edinburgh: E. & S. Livingstone, 1970), 45.

38 Louis A. Kamentsky and Myron R. Melamed, "Instrumentation for Automated Examinations of Cellular Specimens," *Proceedings of the Institute of*

Electrical and Electronic Engineers (Special Issue on Technology and Health Services) 57 (1969), 2007–16.

39 Ibid., 2007.

40 For a description and review, see Hugo Banda-Gamboa, Ian Ricketts, Alistair Cairns, Kudair Hussein, James H. Tucker, and Nasseem Hussain, "Automation in Cervical Cytology: An Overview," *Analytical Cellular Pathology* 4 (1992), 25–48.

41 Ibid., 34.

42 See, for example, J. Tucker and B. Stenkvist, "Whatever Happened to Cervical Cytology Automation?" *Analytical Cellular Pathology* 2 (1990), 259–66.

43 International Academy of Cytology, "Specifications for Automated Cytodiagnostic Systems Proposed by the International Academy of Cytology," *Analytical and Quantitative Cytology* 6 (1984), 146. Although this de facto standard was announced in 1986, cytopathologists had promoted and tacitly accepted it for a number of years.

44 See Walt Bogdanich, "Lax Laboratories," *Wall Street Journal*, 2 Nov. 1987, 1, and "False Negative," *Wall Street Journal*, 2 Feb. 1987, 1. Bogdanich received a Pulitzer Prize for these reports.

45 James Linder, "Automation in Cytopathology," *American Journal of Clinical Pathology* 98 Suppl. 1 (1992), S47–S51.

46 Dawn H. Grohs, "Impact of Automated Technology on the Cervical Cytologic Smear: A Comparison of Cost," *Acta Cytologica* 42 (1998), 165–70.

47 Sandrine Baffert, Stéphane Jouveshomme, Emmanuel Charpentier, A. Souag, D. Tiah, M.-C. Vacher-Lavenu, and E. Fery-Lemonnier, "Évaluation médicale et économique d'un système d'analyse des frottis cervico-utérines (FCU) assistée par ordinateur," poster presented at the 2nd French Health Economists Conference, Paris, 1–2 Feb. 2001.

48 Gerrit Meijer and Peter Hamilton, "Cooperation between the ISDQP and the ESACP," *Diagnostic Quantitative Pathology Newsletter* 31 (Aug. 2000), 4.

49 A detailed account of this and related developments appears in Keating and Cambrosio, *Biomedical Platforms*, especially chaps. 4 and 5.

50 Melvyn F. Greaves, *Biology of Acute Lymphoblastic Leukaemia* (London: Leukemia Research Fund, 1981); Jacques J.M. Van Dongen and Henk J. Adriaansen, "Immunobiology of Leukemia," in Edward S. Henderson, T. Andrew Lister, and Mel F. Greaves, eds., *Leukemia*, 6th ed. (Philadelphia: Saunders, 1996), 83–130.

51 Michael Stoker, "New Medicine and New Biology," *British Medical Journal* 281 (1980), 1678–82.

52 George Janossy, M.M. Roberts, D. Capellaro, Melvyn F. Greaves, and G.E. Francis, "Use of the Fluorescence Activated Cell Sorter in Human Leukaemia," in W. Knapp, K. Holubar, and G. Wick, eds., *Immunofluores-*

cence and Related Staining Techniques (Amsterdam: Elsevier/North-Holland Biomedical Press, 1978), 111.

53 Melvyn F. Greaves, "'Target' Cells, Cellular Phenotypes, and Lineage Fidelity in Human Leukaemia," *Journal of Cellular Physiology* Suppl. 1 (1982), 113.

54 Melvyn F. Greaves, Domenico Delia, Jean Robinson, Robert Sutherland, and Roland Newman, "Exploitation of Monoclonal Antibodies: A 'Who's Who' of Haematopoietic Malignancy," *Blood Cells* 7 (1981), 273.

55 Donald Pinkel, "Curing Children of Leukemia," *Cancer* 59 (1987), 1683.

56 Greaves et al., "Exploitation of Monoclonal Antibodies," 272.

57 Melvyn F. Greaves, L.C. Chan, A.J. Furley, S.M. Watt, and H.V. Molgaard, "Lineage Promiscuity in Hemopoietic Differentiation and Leukemia," *Blood* 67 (1986), 2–4.

58 Paul M. Ayton and Micheal L. Cleary, "Molecular Mechanisms of Leukemogenesis Mediated by MLL Fusion Proteins," *Oncogene* 20 (2001), 5695–707.

59 C.A. Schmidt and G.K. Przybylski, "What Can We Learn from Leukemia as for the Process of Lineage Commitment in Hematopoiesis?" *International Reviews of Immunology* 20 (2001), 107–15.

60 Günter Valet, "Analytical Cellular Pathology and Biology: Presence and Future," *Analytical Cellular Pathology* 18 (1999), 3.

61 See www.cgap.nci.nih.gov

62 Aileen Constans, "The State of the Microarray," *Scientist* 17 (2003), 34.

63 There are many useful introductions to microarrays, some of which are available on the world wide web. A very simple, popularized introduction is available on the "Educational Resources" and "Slide Tour" links of the CGAP Project; see www.cgap.nci.nih.gov For a professional introduction see, for instance, www.Gene-Chips.com, where, in addition to an overview of the basics of the technology and a bibliography, one can find an extensive list of microarray academic and industrial sites. *Nature Genetics* published two special issues – in 1999 (vol. 21, Jan. Suppl.) and 2002 (vol. 32, Dec. Suppl.) – with several reviews on biochips.

64 There are, in fact, two main variants or formats of microarrays. In the first case, a robot deposits DNA spots onto a coated glass slide; this approach allows for the use of two different fluorescent colours (and thus the simultaneous analysis of, for example, a control and a diseased tissue sample) on the same microarray. In the second kind, developed and sold by Affymetrix under the trademark GeneChip, photolithographic methods synthesize hundreds of thousands of oligonucleotides on a small glass surface. For a description and comparison of these two formats, see, for example, David Gerhold, Thomas Rushmore, and C. Thomas Caskey, "DNA Chips: Promising Toys Have Become Powerful Tools," *Trends in Biochemical Sciences* 24 (1999), 168–73. For an illustrated

description of microarray equipment, see Vivian G. Cheung, Michael Morley, Francisco Aguilar, Aldo Massimi, Raju Kucherlapaty, and Geoffrey Childs, "Making and Reading Microarrays," *Nature Genetics* 21 Suppl. (Jan. 1999), 15–19. For simplicity's sake, and because most of the important early contributions in pathology used the "spot" microarray format, we confine our discussion to examples concerning this format.

65 Howard Hughes Medical Institute website; Description of Patrick Brown's research concerning microarrays: www.hhmi.org/research/investigators/brown.html

66 All these manipulations raise, of course, several problems concerning the regulation of the production and reporting of microarray data. See, for example, Aileen Constans, "Challenges and Concerns with Microarrays," *Scientist* 17 (2003), 35–6.

67 Douglas Steinberg, "DNA Chips Enlist in War on Cancer," *Scientist* 14 (2000), 1. T.R. Golub, D.K. Slonim, P. Tamayo, C. Huard, M. Gaasenbeek, J.P. Mesirov, H. Coller, M.L. Loh, J.R. Downing, M.A. Caligiuri, C.D. Bloomfield, and E.S. Lander, "Molecular Classification of Cancer: Class Discovery and Class Prediction by Gene Expression Monitoring," *Science* 286 (1999), 531–7.

68 Ibid., 531.

69 T.R. Golub, "Genome-Wide Views of Cancer," *New England Journal of Medicine* 344 (2001), 601–2.

70 A.M. Snijders, G.A. Meijer, R.H. Brakenhoff, A.J.C. van den Brule, and P.J. van Diest, "Microarray Techniques in Pathology: Tool or Toy?" *Journal of Clinical Pathology: Molecular Pathology* 53 (2000), 293.

71 Nicola J. Maughan, Fraser A. Lewis, and Victoria Smith, "An Introduction to Microarrays," *Journal of Pathology* 195 (2001), 6.

72 Jan Richter, Urs Wagner, Juha Kononen, André Fijan, James Bruderer, Ulrico Schmid, Daniel Ackermann, Robert Maurer, Göran Alund, Hartmut Knönagel, Marcus Rist, Kim Wilber, Manuel Anabitarte, Franz Hering, Thomas Hardmeier, Andreas Schönenberger, Renata Flury, Peter Jäger, Jean Luc Fehr, Peter Schraml, Holger Moch, Michael J. Mihatsch, Thomas Gasser, Olli P. Kallioniemi, and Guido Sauter, "High-Throughput Tissue Microarray Analysis of Cyclin E Gene Amplification and Overexpression in Urinary Bladder Cancer," *American Journal of Pathology* 157 (2000), 787–94. See also Juha Kononen, Lukas Bubendorf, Anne Kallioniemi, Maarit Bärlund, Peter Schrami, Stephen Leighton, Joachim Torhorst, Michael J. Mihatsch, Guido Sauter, and Olli-P. Kallioniemi, "Tissue Microarrays for High-Throughput Molecular Profiling of Tumor Specimens," *Nature Medicine* 4 (1998), 8447; Joachim Torhorst, Christoph Bucher, Juha Kononen, Philippe Haas, Markus Zuber, Ossi R. Köchli, Frank Mross, Holger Dieterich, Holger Moch, Michael Mihatsch,

Olli-P. Kallioniemi, and Guido Sauter, "Tissue Microarrays for Rapid Linking of Molecular Changes to Clinical Endpoints," *American Journal of Pathology* 159 (2001), 2249–56.

73 Peter Lichter, "New Tools in Molecular Pathology," *Journal of Molecular Diagnostics* 2 (2000), 172.

74 Ash A. Alizadeh, Michael B. Eisen, R. Eric Davies, Chi Ma, Izidore S. Lossos, Andreas Rosenwald, Jennifer C. Boldrick, Hajeer Sabet, Truc Tran, Xin Yu, John I. Powell, Liming Yang, Gerald E. Marti, Troy Moore, James Hudson Jr., Lisheng Lu, David B. Lewis, Robert Tibshirani, Gavin Sherlock, Wing C. Chan, Timothy C. Greiner, Dennis D. Weisenburger, James O. Armitage, Roger Warnke, Ronald Levy, Wyndham Wilson, Michael R. Grever, John C. Byrd, David Botstein, Patrick O. Brown, and Louis M. Staudt, "Distinct Types of Diffuse Large B-Cell Lymphoma Identified by Gene Expression Profiling," *Nature* 403 (2000), 503–11.

75 Ibid., 503.

76 A.L. Shaffer, Andreas Rosenwald, Elaine M. Hurt, Jena M. Giltnane, Lloyd T. Lam, Oxana K. Pickeral, and Louis M. Staudt, "Signatures of the Immune Response," *Immunity* 15 (2001), 384.

77 Louis M. Staudt, "Gene Expression Physiology and Pathophysiology of the Immune System," *Trends in Immunology* 22 (2001), 37.

78 Louis M. Staudt and Patrick O. Brown, "Genomic Views of the Immune System," *Annual Review of Immunology* 18 (2000), 829–59.

79 Ibid., 845.

80 Golub et al., "Molecular Classification of Cancer," 533.

81 An extended product description appears in "Atlas™ Neurobiology and Hematology/Immunology Arrays," *Clontechniques* 13 (Oct. 1998); online edition available at www.clontech.com/archive

82 Y. Aalto, W. El-Rifai, L. Vilpo, B. Nagy, M. Vihinen, J. Vilpo, and S. Knuutila, "Distinct Gene Expression Profiling in Chronic Lymphocytic Leukemia with 11q23 Deletion," *Leukemia* 15 (2001), 1721–28.

83 Richard Wooster, "Cancer Classification with DNA Microarrays: Is Less More?" *Trends in Genetics* 16 (2000), 328.

84 Marc Ladanyi, Wing C. Chan, Timothy J. Triche, and William L. Gerald, "Expression Profiling of Human Tumors: The End of Surgical Pathology?" *Journal of Molecular Diagnostics* 3 (2001), 92.

85 Ibid.

86 Ibid., 93.

87 J.P. Dales, J. Plumas, F. Palmerini, E. Devilard, T. Defrance, A. Lajmanovich, V. Pradel, F. Birg, and L. Xerri, "Correlation between Apoptosis Microarray Gene Expression Profiling and Histopathological Lymph Node Lesions," *Journal of Clinical Pathology: Molecular Pathology* 54 (2001), 17.

88 Ibid., 23.

89 Hadley C. King and Animesh Sinha, "Gene Expression Profile Analysis by DNA Microarrays: Promises and Pitfalls," *Journal of the American Medical Association* 286 (2001), 2280.

90 See, for example, Mei-Ling Ting Lee, Frank C. Kuo, G.A. Whitmore, and Jeffrey Sklar, "Importance of Replication in Microarray Gene Expression Studies: Statistical Methods and Evidence from Repetitive CDNA Hybridization," *Proceedings of the National Academy of Sciences of the USA* 97 (2000), 9834–9; see also M.J. Becich, "Information Management: Moving from Test Results to Clinical Information," *Clinical Leadership and Management Review* 14 (2000), 296–300.

91 Lance Liotta and Emanuel Petricoin, "Molecular Profiling of Human Cancer," *Nature Genetics Reviews* 1 (2000), 49.

92 Sridhar Ramaswamy and Todd R. Golub, "DNA Microarays in Clinical Oncology," *Journal of Clinical Oncology* 20 (2002), 1941.

93 I.P.M. Tomlinson and M. Ilyas, "Molecular Pathology of Solid Tumors: Some Practical Suggestions for Translating Research into Clinical Practice," *Journal of Clinical Pathology: Molecular Pathology* 54 (2001), 202.

94 Ibid.

PART THREE

Statistics and the Underdetermination of Theories

10

La sous-détermination des théories médicales par les statistiques : Le cas Semmelweis

GÉRARD JORLAND

L'historiographie du débat académique de 1836 sur la méthode numérique en médecine conclut à un refus des statistiques médicales qui se serait maintenu pendant plus d'un siècle. George Weisz a mis en pièces ce consensus et montré que des arguments statistiques n'ont jamais cessé d'être échangés dans les controverses académiques – concernant les techniques chirurgicales beaucoup plus que les traitements de médecine interne, pour lesquels on ne disposait pas toujours d'un indice de létalité[1].

Mais l'ambition du docteur Louis excédait largement la seule utilisation des nombres en thérapeutique. Il voulait constituer une *médecine statistique* au sens où l'on parle aujourd'hui de mécanique statistique, en l'occurrence une anatomo-pathologie statistique faisant fonds de l'observation clinique en série rendue possible par la nouvelle médecine hospitalo-universitaire — et la controverse académique de 1836 portait bien sur ce programme de recherche.

Toutefois, George Weisz a fort bien souligné que les arguments statistiques n'ont été concluants dans aucune des discussions académiques qu'il a présentées. Dans la première, sur le traitement de la pleurésie purulente en 1836, Louis est intervenu avec une statistique de 150 cas. Il était en dispute continue avec Bouillaud, qui l'a une fois de plus contré avec sa propre statistique. S'ensuivit une discussion sur la validité de tous ces chiffres que George Weisz conclut en ces termes : "Cette question finit par s'éteindre tandis que d'autres prenaient sa place[2]."

La seconde controverse – trachéotomie *vs* tubage dans l'opération du croup – opposa Trousseau à Eugène Bouchut, lequel n'était pas membre de l'Académie mais dont la position était défendue par un membre éminent, Malgaigne. Des chiffres furent produits de part et d'autre "mais dans ce cas," commente George Weisz, "le débat académique ne semble pas avoir été à l'origine d'un changement de conception [...] Il a plutôt fait émerger un consensus sur l'efficacité de la trachéotomie[3]." De même, dans les discussions sur l'excision chirurgicale des tumeurs cancéreuses et la ponction des kystes ovariens, respectivement en 1854–1855 et en 1856–1857, "les nombres échangés ne pouvaient pas conduire à un accord [...] parce que la mort ou la survie étaient rarement en jeu[4]."

Dans la controverse sur le traitement du rhumatisme aigu par la saignée en 1853–1854, où Bouillaud produisit une statistique de 600 observations et Piorry, qui le soutenait, de 58, "personne," remarque George Weisz, "ne fit grand cas de leurs chiffres. Ceux de Bouillaud en particulier semblent avoir été rapidement mis à l'écart[5]." Et plus loin : "Bouillaud [...] ne cessa de citer des statistiques de toutes sortes, de même que Piorry. Toutefois, ces statistiques n'étaient pas convaincantes pour les autres académiciens si bien que les décisions furent prises sur d'autres bases[6]."

La critique par Malgaigne des chiffres qu'avança Trousseau en faveur de la trachéotomie fait comprendre pourquoi ces arguments statistiques ne parvinrent pas à convaincre. D'abord, il y a comme toujours une critique des données : Malgaigne souligne de petites incohérences dans les chiffres avancés et de petites différences entre ces chiffres et ses propres relevés dans les registres d'hôpitaux. En outre, il ne peut pas s'expliquer comment un taux de mortalité d'environ 100 % avant 1848 a pu autant diminuer depuis.

Ensuite, une réinterprétation des chiffres, rectifiés ou non, est proposée. Malgaigne objecte ainsi que les trachéotomies pratiquées dans le privé ont un taux notoirement élevé de mortalité, et il cite un sondage informel des principaux praticiens parisiens, dont certains académiciens, qui donne 312 morts sur 346 opérations — beaucoup plus qu'aux Enfants malades, le plus insalubre des hôpitaux parisiens. Or, les statistiques des opérations à l'hôpital sont toujours plus défavorables que celles à domicile, les patients étant dans ce dernier cas plus riches, mieux nourris, mieux soignés et moins exposés à l'insalubrité et à l'infection des établissements publics. Malgaigne propose une nouvelle interprétation des chiffres : les statistiques ne sont si favorables à la trachéotomie que du fait que des internes inexpérimentés opèrent prématurément, bien avant que les parents ne les y eussent autorisés à domicile.

Les statistiques sont en effet toujours susceptibles d'une multiplicité d'élaborations et d'interprétations. En d'autres termes, et c'est l'objet de cette étude, il y a une sous-détermination des théories, en l'occurrence médicales, par les statistiques, comme il y en a une par l'expérience. Je voudrais le montrer en prenant un autre exemple de discussion à l'Académie de médecine, exemple que n'a pas retenu George Weisz bien qu'il soit de la même époque, la décennie 1850. Cette controverse a porté, à la fin de l'hiver et au printemps 1858, sur le traitement de la fièvre puerpérale. Mais au lieu de concerner des statistiques thérapeutiques qui auraient départagé des traitements différents d'une même maladie, elle tourna autour de statistiques étiologiques, puisque les résultats du traitement proposé avaient pour objet de valider l'étiologie supposée de la maladie. Ces statistiques étaient donc de même nature que celles de l'école numérique du docteur Louis. Nous verrons que, dans ce cas, pas plus que dans ceux présentés par George Weisz, les arguments numériques n'ont été concluants. Les statistiques furent en effet l'objet de contestations et d'interprétations divergentes, mais aussi rationnelles ou vraisemblables les unes que les autres. La controverse a encore un double intérêt historique. D'une part, c'est la première maladie nosocomiale attestée; d'autre part, c'est le tribut payé par les femmes à la médecine hospitalo-universitaire.

PRÉSENTATION DE LA THÉORIE STATISTIQUE DE SEMMELWEIS À PARIS ET EDIMBOURGH

La fièvre puerpérale, une septicémie des femmes en couches dans la plupart des cas mortelle, est considérée à l'époque comme l'une des plus graves maladies. Guérard, qui a lancé la discussion académique, juge qu'elle "mérite d'être classée en tête des fléaux les plus dévastateurs[7]." Depaul, qui a ouvert la discussion, parle "d'une maladie qui, à toutes les époques, a été considérée comme l'une des plus graves [...] une maladie dont les ravages sont plus considérables que ceux de la fièvre typhoïde, du typhus et même du choléra[8]." Cruveilhier s'écrie : "Les statistiques des maisons d'accouchement seraient bien plus exactes si, au lieu de répartir les morts sur toutes les femmes reçues dans l'année, on relevait le chiffre de la mortalité par épidémie : ce chiffre serait effrayant[9]!"

On observe une augmentation considérable des décès par fièvre puerpérale au cours du temps. Guérard cite ces chiffres : dans une maternité anglaise, de 1789 à 1798, pour 100 à 300 accouchements par an, il y eut 1 décès sur 288 accouchements, de juillet 1812 à août 1815 il n'y en eut pas un seul sur 1 059 accouchements, mais de 1829 à 1838, il y eut 1 décès sur 39,3 accouchements. Dans une autre maternité de

Londres, de 1827 à 1846, pour 500 à 600 accouchements annuels, il y eut 1 décès sur 84,3 accouchements, en 1847, 1 sur 79, et en 1848, 1 sur 20,2[10].

L'étiologie de la fièvre puerpérale est connue depuis plusieurs années. En effet, un ancien chef de clinique de la Maternité de Vienne, le docteur Franz Hecktor Arneth, est venu présenter, dans les mêmes termes, les résultats des recherches statistiques de Semmelweis, à l'Académie de médecine en hiver 1851 puis à la Société médico-chirurgicale d'Édimbourg au printemps de la même année[11].

La disposition même de la Maternité de Vienne constitue une expérience toute faite. Par conséquent, décrire l'observation statistique de Semmelweis revient à raconter l'histoire de cette maternité. Elle a été fondée le 16 août 1784. En 1823, les dissections de cadavres y sont introduites à fin d'enseignement. Dans cet intervalle de 39 ans, sur 71 395 accouchements, il y a eu 897 décès, soit 1,25 %.

En 1833, une deuxième clinique d'accouchement a été ouverte, contiguë à la première. Pendant les dix ans précédant cette ouverture, sur 28 429 accouchements, on a compté 1 509 décès, soit 5,3 %.

Le premier tableau présenté par Arneth à Paris et à Édimbourg est relatif à la période qui a suivi cette ouverture. Il s'écarte du tableau XXII de Semmelweis[12]. Là où celui-ci compare les données relatives à chacune de ces cliniques pendant cette période, Arneth compare les données de l'ensemble de la maternité à celles de la seconde clinique. Et alors que le tableau de Semmelweis couvre la période 1833–1844, le sien ne s'étend que de 1834 à 1839. Enfin, tandis que celui-là donne les chiffres et les pourcentages, celui-ci ne reproduit que des pourcentages, légèrement différents d'ailleurs. Pour la commodité de l'exposé, je présente un tableau qui suit Semmelweis pour la période mais Arneth pour les termes de la comparaison (Tableau 1). Dans un cas comme dans l'autre, les chiffres montrent que le taux de létalité est à peu près le même dans la première et dans la seconde clinique ou dans l'ensemble de la maternité et la seconde clinique. Ainsi, pour la période 1833–1840, dans la première clinique ont eu lieu 23 066 accouchements dont 1 505 mortels contre 13 095 et 731 respectivement dans la seconde, soit un taux de létalité de 6,52 % contre 5,58 %. La conclusion qu'ils en tirent, c'est que la fièvre puerpérale n'est pas endémique, elle ne tient pas aux caractéristiques (orientation, aération, disposition, etc.) de chacune des cliniques.

Par décret impérial d'octobre 1840, les étudiants en médecine sont affectés à la première clinique et les élèves sages-femmes à la seconde. Arneth présente un second tableau des taux de létalité dans chacune des cliniques de 1839 à 1846 (Tableau 2). C'est le même que le tableau I de Semmelweis qui donne en plus les nombres d'accouche-

Tableau 1 Létalité comparée des deux cliniques avant la réforme de 1840

Années	*Mortes dans toute la maternité (%)*	*Mortes dans la seconde clinique (%)*
1833[1]	5,01	2,26
1834	8,06	8,60
1835	5,33	4,99[2]
1836	7,61	7,84[3]
1837	8,24[4]	6,95[5]
1838	3,75	4,94
1839[1]	5,05	4,52[6]
1840[1]	6,49	2,65[7]

Source : Semmelweis et Arneth.

1. D'après Semmelweis, tableau XXII.
2. Arneth donne 4,98.
3. Arneth ne donne qu'une décimale.
4. Arneth donne 8,28.
5. Arneth ne donne qu'une décimale; Semmelweis donne 6,99.
6. Semmelweis donne 4,05. Dans le tableau suivant, Arneth donne 4,6.
7. Semmelweis donne 2,06. Dans le tableau suivant, Arneth donne 2,6.

ments et de morts chaque année. Au total, de 1841 à 1846, 20 042 femmes ont accouché dans la première clinique et 1 989 sont mortes, tandis que 17 791 ont accouché dans la seconde clinique et 696 sont mortes, ce qui donne des taux de létalité de 9,92 % et 3,91 % respectivement.

Il apparaît déjà clairement que la ségrégation des étudiants en médecine et des élèves sages-femmes introduit une différence significative dans les taux de létalité respectifs des cliniques. Semmelweis en conclut que la fièvre puerpérale n'est pas épidémique.

Semmelweis est médecin assistant à la première clinique, celle réservée aux étudiants en médecine, du 27 février 1846 au 20 octobre 1846 puis de nouveau du 20 mars 1847 au 20 mars 1849. Cherchant systématiquement la cause des différences de létalité qu'il ne trouve ni dans les saisons ni dans l'encombrement, il l'identifie dans cette circonstance que les étudiants en médecine pratiquent des dissections en amphithéâtre ou y collaborent, ce que les élèves sages-femmes ne font pas. Arneth présente cette découverte en termes identiques à Paris et à Édimbourg.

Tandis que les élèves sages-femmes n'assistaient pas aux autopsies et que même les chefs de cette clinique ne venaient que rarement dans les salles de dissection où ils n'avaient pas de leçons à donner, les élèves de la première clinique étaient des médecins qui, se préparant à leurs examens, se vouaient tout spécialement à la pratique des accouchements et en même temps à des

Tableau 2 Létalité comparée des deux cliniques après la réforme de 1840

Années	*Clinique des étudiants en médecine (%)*	*Clinique des élèves sages-femmes (%)*
1841	7,8[1]	3,5
1842	15,7[2]	7,5
1843	8,9	6,1[3]
1844	8,2	2,3
1845	6,9[4]	2,03
1846	11,4	2,7

Source : Semmelweis et Arneth.
1. Semmelweis et Arneth donnent 7,7.
2. Semmelweis et Arneth donnent 15,8.
3. Semmelweis et Arneth donnent 5,9.
4. Semmelweis et Arneth donnent 6,8.

travaux anatomo-pathologiques; ou c'étaient des docteurs étrangers qui s'empressaient de suivre les leçons d'anatomie pathologique données par le savant professeur Rokintansky [que Rudolf Vichow aurait surnommé "le Linné de l'anatomie pathologique"].

Tous se livraient avec ardeur aux travaux anatomiques; ils ne se bornaient pas à faire de temps en temps une autopsie, mais chaque jour ils assistaient tous à huit ou dix opérations de ce genre, dont les sujets étaient fournis par le grand hôpital, dont la Maternité ne fait qu'une partie. Les dissections dont je viens de parler étaient très souvent faites par eux-mêmes, ou bien on se rendait à des leçons d'anatomie pathologique où toutes les pièces pathologiques de chaque jour, même du canal intestinal, étaient examinées et passaient de main en main. En outre, le chef de clinique d'accouchements donnait, presque sans relâche, un cours où l'on exerçait sur le cadavre des opérations obstétricales. Après de si longues opérations sur des cadavres, les élèves n'allaient que trop souvent, immédiatement, continuer la pratique d'accouchements à la Maternité. Ces divers travaux étant étrangers à la clinique des sages-femmes, M. Semmelweis soupçonna qu'en eux résidait la cause de la grande différence observée dans la mortalité de ces deux services. Cet observateur judicieux crut voir la source trop fréquente et funeste des maladies puerpérales dans l'inoculation des atomes cadavériques aux parties génitales, et il conçut l'espoir de réussir, en prenant des précautions nécessaires, à combattre victorieusement ces influences délétères et à réduire la mortalité qui décimait cette clinique[13].

Pour éliminer ces "atomes cadavériques", Semmelweis s'en remet à leur trace, c'est-à-dire à leur odeur, comme il est de mise depuis Lavoisier. Ayant constaté que le chlorure de chaux fait disparaître cette odeur, il présume que ce désinfectant, universel depuis Guyton

Tableau 3 Létalité dans la première clinique

Mois	*Accouchements*	*Décès*	*%*
1847			
Juin	268	6	2,23[1]
Juillet	250	3	1,20
Août	264	5	1,89
Septembre	262	12	4,58[2]
Octobre	278	11	3,95
Novembre	246	11	4,47[3]
Décembre	273	8	2,93
1848			
Janvier	283	10	3,53
Février	291	2	0,68
Mars	276	0	0
Avril	305	2	0,65
Mai	313	3	0,95[4]
Juin	264	3	1,13
Juillet	269	1	0,37
Août	261	0	0
Septembre	312	3	0,96
Octobre	299	7	2,34
Novembre	310	9	2,90
Décembre	373	5	1,34
1849			
Janvier	403	9	2,23
Février	389	12	3,08
Mars	406	20	4,92

Sources : Semmelweis, 393 ; Tableau XVI, 394.

1. Semmelweis donne 2,38.
2. Semmelweis donne 5,23.
3. Semmelweis donne 4,97.
4. Semmelweis donne 0,99.

de Morveau, détruit ces “miasmes cadavériques”. Il fait arrêter en mai 1847 que personne n’entrera dans les salles d’accouchement sans s’être lavé les mains et brossé les ongles au chlorure de chaux. Et il en vérifie l’effet sur les statistiques de décès. Arneth n’en donne que les chiffres bruts. Je reproduis donc le tableau plus complet de Semmelweis (Tableau 3). Au total, de juin à décembre, il y a eu 1 841 accouchements dans la première clinique et 56 morts, soit un taux de létalité de 3,04 %. Et tandis qu’Arneth s’arrête là, Semmelweis donne les chiffres des mois suivants jusqu’à la fin de ses deux années d’assistanat. En 1848, sur 3 556 accouchements dans la première clinique, on a compté 45 morts, soit un taux de létalité de 1,27 %.

Fin mars 1849, son assistanat prend fin. Bien que ne croyant pas à sa théorie, son successeur maintient ses prescriptions, de même que le frère de ce dernier, qui lui succède à partir de 1853. Néanmoins, le taux de mortalité n'a plus cessé d'augmenter[14], d'ailleurs dans l'une et l'autre des deux cliniques. On peut penser que les prescriptions n'ont pas été appliquées avec suffisamment de rigueur.

Ce n'était pas la première fois que les corps médicaux britannique et français entendaient parler de la découverte de Semmelweis. Dès novembre 1848, le *Lancet* publiait la discussion qui avait suivi une communication d'un docteur Routh à l'Assemblée des médecins anglais, lequel avait fait un stage à la première clinique de Vienne en tant qu'étudiant et en était revenu convaincu par la théorie de Semmelweis. Cette communication avait été publiée dans les *Medico-Chirurgical Transactions.* En France, la *Revue médico-chirurgicale* avait rendu compte d'un article de Semmelweis lui-même[15], puis d'un article de F. Wieger[16], médecin à l'hôpital de Strasbourg, sur les moyens prophylactiques employés par celui-là contre l'apparition de la fièvre puerpérale. Le compte-rendu de cet article fut utilisé au cours de la discussion académique, de manière fautive d'ailleurs, par Depaul[17].

Les deux communications d'Arneth, celle d'Édimbourg comme celle de Paris, étaient elles-aussi connues puisqu'elles avaient été citées au cours de la discussion académique. Toutefois, une commission composée de Ricord, Danyau et Moreau avait été nommée pour rendre compte de celle de Paris[18]. S'est-elle jamais réunie? Arneth aurait écrit au président de cette commission pour en connaître le rapport — sa lettre serait restée sans réponse[19]. Néanmoins, Henri de Castelnau rendit compte de cette communication dans la *Gazette des hôpitaux civils et militaires* dès le lendemain en termes condescendants.

Nous voudrions pouvoir user généreusement, envers notre honorable confrère d'outre-Rhin, des devoirs de l'hospitalité; mais les droits de la science et de la vérité passent avant toute autre chose, et nous ne pouvons nous dispenser d'exprimer la surprise que nous ont causée les opinions de M. Arneth. Puisque son voyage et son séjour à Paris avaient pour but spécial l'étude de la fièvre puerpérale, comment a-t-il pu ignorer qu'à la Maternité et à la Clinique de la Faculté les femmes accouchées sont précisément dans les mêmes conditions que celles des deux cliniques de Vienne, et que, nonobstant, les épidémies de fièvre puerpérale ne sont ni moins fréquentes, ni moins meurtrières rue de la Bourbe que place de l'École de Médecine? Si M. Arneth n'a pas ignoré ce fait, comment a-t-il pu conserver la moindre foi dans l'opinion que lui a transmise son honorable maître et compatriote? Nous ne saurions nous l'expliquer.

La cause invoquée par M. Arneth étant démontrée imaginaire, il serait inutile d'insister sur les avantages du moyen propre à détruire cette cause. Nous devons ajouter cependant que le chlorure de chaux, auquel M. Arneth reconnaît la propriété de détruire toutes les molécules cadavériques qui peuvent rester adhérentes aux mains après une dissection, n'est rien moins que sûr dans son action; le contraire même est aujourd'hui beaucoup plus probable. Si c'est, en effet, par l'odeur qu'on peut reconnaître la présence sur les mains des molécules cadavériques, il est certain que le chlorure de chaux n'enlève point cette odeur. Comme il a lui-même une odeur aussi forte que désagréable, il parvient bien à masquer plus ou moins celle du cadavre, mais jamais à la détruire; ce n'est qu'au bout de plusieurs heures que celle-ci disparaît entièrement, et souvent elle persiste plus longtemps que celle du chlorure. En outre, les observations récentes et les expériences extrêmement intéressantes et encore en cours d'exécution de M. Renault, d'Alfort, prouvent que le chlorure de chaux n'a aucune des propriétés antiseptiques qu'on lui avait si gratuitement accordées. Le chlorure de chaux employé comme antiseptique n'est, le plus souvent, qu'une cause de plus ajoutée aux autres causes d'infection[20].

Ainsi, non seulement la cause serait imaginaire, mais le remède pire que le mal! Or, le premier argument est faux, le second controuvé. Le premier argument est faux car, certes, la Maternité ne compte que des élèves sages-femmes et la Clinique de la Faculté que des étudiants en médecine, mais on pratique des dissections de cadavres dans l'une comme dans l'autre institution[21]. Castelnau ne pouvait pas l'ignorer, par conséquent son argument est de mauvaise foi. Le second est controuvé : Le chlorure de chaux n'a jamais cessé d'être un désinfectant, notamment dans les salles d'hôpitaux après chaque épidémie de fièvre puerpérale quand on ne peut rien faire d'autre que de les vider et de les assainir[22].

C'est tout le contraire qui s'est produit à Édimbourg. La communication du Docteur Arneth a été suivie d'une discussion, elle-aussi commentée au cours du débat académique de Paris quelques années plus tard. Trois interventions ont eu lieu, dont l'une par le Docteur Simpson, le découvreur de l'anesthésie chirurgicale au chloroforme[23].

En premier lieu, ils défendent à cette occasion la thèse du caractère contagieux de la fièvre puerpérale. Leur argument est toujours statistique, ils énumèrent des séries de cas dont le caractère collectif établit la contagiosité de la maladie. Par exemple, en 1814–1815 à la Maternité d'Édimbourg, sur 9 malades, 8 sont mortes, et 3 cas se sont déclarés en ville mais chez une sage-femme employée à l'hôpital. Ou encore cette *observation* statistique — les statistiques étant au XIXe siècle avant tout une méthode d'observation — qui laisse voir qu'il ne s'agit ni d'une épidémie (une "influence morbifique présente dans l'air"), ni d'une endémie ("ou émanant de la localité"). Sur 400 femmes accouchées à domicile dans différents quartiers de Manchester en 1840 par différentes sages-femmes en relation avec la maternité, 16 sont mortes. Il ne peut donc s'agir d'une endémie puisque la maladie est apparue dans différents quartiers de la ville; ni d'une épidémie puisque peu de femmes au bout du compte ont été touchées. Or, toutes les malades ont été accouchées par la même sage-femme. Il s'agit donc bien d'une contagion par le personnel soignant.

En second lieu, ils montrent, à l'aide d'exemples, que le personnel soignant est l'agent de transmission. Ainsi, le cas, mentionné et moqué lors de la discussion académique parisienne, de ce médecin qui, après avoir accouché une femme atteinte de fièvre puerpérale, contamina toutes ses autres patientes, que ce soit à Londres parce qu'il portait toujours les mêmes vêtements, ou au cours d'un voyage transocéanique parce qu'il s'était servi de linge qui avait été en contact avec ces vêtements dans ses malles. Ils font le rapprochement avec l'inoculation et la vaccination, où là aussi un médecin transmet une maladie, qu'il n'a pas mais qu'il transporte, à un malade, évidemment sous une forme atténuée dont celui-ci se remettra et qui le protégera sans qu'on sache très bien alors pourquoi, mais à laquelle il succombera parfois.

Ils établissent ensuite une corrélation avec d'autres maladies, comme les érysipèles, une observation nosologique proprement britannique et pertinente puisqu'il s'agit de la même cause, le streptocoque qui produit dans le premier cas une infection dermique. Ou comme la fièvre chirurgicale, le chirurgien jouant le même rôle que l'accoucheur : "les chirurgiens comme les accoucheurs sont occasionnellement les malheureux *media* de l'inoculation de matière morbide à leurs patients[24]." Simpson avait consacré un article à ce sujet dans le tome précédent de la même revue, lequel sera commenté lors de la discussion à l'Académie de médecine, et d'ailleurs approuvé, curieusement. Nous y reviendrons.

Et s'ils sont d'accord avec Semmelweis sur ses moyens prophylactiques, dont la simplicité même fait merveille, s'ils admettent comme lui que l'odeur trahit la présence d'une substance "morbifique", ils s'en séparent sur sa nature. Alors que Semmelweis adhère encore à la théorie de la putréfaction héritée de la révolution chimique de la fin du siècle précédent, eux pensent déjà en termes de "virus" ou de "sécrétion inflammatoire". Par exemple, à partir de l'expérience cruciale suivante.

Le docteur M. accouche une patiente un soir à minuit, une seconde le lendemain dans la matinée et une troisième le surlendemain dans l'après-midi, après que le bébé de la première fut mort mais avant de pratiquer l'autopsie pour déterminer la cause de sa mort. Cette autopsie ayant révélé une infection purulente de la plèvre, il change de vêtements et se lave soigneusement les mains au chlorure de chaux. Quatre jours après son accouchement, la première patiente présente des symptômes de fièvre puerpérale, le lendemain c'est au tour de la seconde et de la troisième, et toutes les trois en meurent. Dans ce cas, la cause de la contagion n'est pas l'autopsie du bébé mort-né, puisque les patientes ont toutes été accouchées auparavant et qu'aucune n'a été auscultée sans que les précautions hygiéniques de rigueur n'aient été prises. C'est la première patiente, la mère du bébé mort-né, qui devait porter la "matière morbide" avant de la communiquer au docteur M., qui a transmis la maladie aux deux autres patientes, et après qu'elle l'eut transmise elle-même à son propre fœtus.

Simpson conclut que si la mortalité est beaucoup plus élevée dans les maternités continentales que dans les îles britanniques, ce n'est pas à cause d'une quelconque supériorité obstétricale, mais d'une *croyance*, d'une croyance au caractère contagieux de la fièvre puerpérale ici et d'un défaut de cette même croyance (*the want of that belief*) là. Et il précise que si les médecins continentaux ne partagent pas cette croyance, c'est parce qu'ils n'imaginent pas qu'une contagion puisse être indirecte. Pour eux, toute contagion est par définition directe, de malade à malade; or ce n'est manifestement pas le cas dans la fièvre puerpérale. Ainsi Semmelweis lui même ne croit-il pas au caractère contagieux de la maladie pour cette raison précise[25]. "Combien de vies maternelles auraient pu être sauvées!" s'écrie-t-il.

On le voit donc, les médecins d'Édimbourg ont pris au sérieux la découverte de Semmelweis, ils ont discuté son explication, mais leurs désaccords théoriques ne les ont pas conduits à remettre en question la découverte elle-même, les faits que l'assistant de la maternité de Vienne avait mis en évidence.

DISCUSSION DE LA THÉORIE STATISTIQUE DE SEMMELWEIS LORS DU DÉBAT ACADÉMIQUE

Non seulement l'étiologie de la fièvre puerpérale était-elle bien identifiée, mais encore était-elle bien connue, notamment des discutants de l'Académie de médecine. Aussi bien Semmelweis que Simpson furent cités, le premier à six reprises, le second à cinq reprises. En quels termes?

Dans tous les cas, Semmelweis est cité de manière négative[26]. Au mieux, son étiologie soulève des réserves, au pire, elle est ouvertement rejetée; quant à sa prophylaxie, si elle laisse incrédule, elle est néanmoins préconisée, souvent de manière impérative. Par exemple, Depaul avoue être ébranlé par l'étiologie de Semmelweis et convaincu par sa prophylaxie "surtout en temps d'épidémie", tandis que Danyau, qui appartient à la même école dite "de la Maternité", entreprend de la discréditer :

Pourtant, les contradicteurs ne manquèrent pas à Semmelweis, et, parmi eux, les accoucheurs les plus distingués de son pays, Kiwisch, Scanzoni, Seyfert, Lumpe, etc.; il fut démontré qu'à Vienne, même antérieurement aux précautions recommandées par Semmelweis, la première clinique avait eu des époques de très faible mortalité; que la plus grande mortalité habituelle de la première clinique tenait à d'autres causes que celles qu'il avait signalées; que la seconde avait eu aussi ses moments de forte mortalité, et qu'il en était de même de la division des femmes payantes qui n'admet point d'élèves de l'un ni de l'autre sexe; d'un autre côté, qu'à Vienne aussi et ailleurs, ces lavages à l'eau chlorurée n'avaient pas empêché le développement de graves épidémies, que les résultats obtenus d'abord par Semmelweis à Vienne ne l'avaient point été à Prague, à Würzburg ou ailleurs, que des épidémies avaient eu lieu dans les endroits où les précautions prescrites étaient très rigoureusement suivies, et qu'elles avaient quelquefois cessé alors qu'on s'en était relâché ou qu'on les avait abandonnées tout à fait, bien que les travaux anatomiques, les autopsies, les exercices sur les cadavres continuassent[27].

Autrement dit, les chiffres sont critiqués avant d'être interprétés autrement : on retrouve les deux éléments de la sous-détermination des théories par les statistiques. Et pourtant, Danyau conclut que "nul, d'après les faits maintenant connus, ne pourrait, sans se rendre coupable d'une extrême imprudence et même d'un crime, passer de l'examen d'une femme morte de fièvre puerpérale à la chambre d'une femme en travail ou récemment accouchée". Et, de plus, il préconise lui aussi "d'employer largement les désinfectants dans les cas surtout où ses doigts auraient été en contact avec des sécrétions morbides". Que dit d'autre Semmelweis?

En revanche, l'identification par Simpson des fièvres chirurgicale et puerpérale retient l'attention, notamment de Dubois, le patron de l'obstétrique française à l'époque, qui l'introduit dans la discussion[28] (Tableau 4) – peut-être parce qu'il s'agit de statistiques anatomopathologique comparatives qui jouissent encore de l'autorité du docteur Louis pour cette génération.

Par ailleurs, certains des discutants font état d'expériences du même ordre dans leurs propres pratiques[29]. Danyau les résume en des termes que n'aurait certainement pas désapprouvés Semmelweis :

Dans tous les faits que je viens de citer, il y a une distinction à faire : dans beaucoup de ces cas, l'accoucheur venait de pratiquer une autopsie; ses mains et

Tableau 4 Fièvre chirurgicale et fièvre puerpérale

	Chevers 134 décès de fièvre chirurgicale	*Dugès 341 décès de fièvre puerpérale*	*Tonnelé 222 décès de fièvre puerpérale*
Péritonite	52 (0,39)	266 (0,78)	193 (0,87)
Métrite ou pus dans les veines		200 (0,58)	
Ovarite		48 (0,14)	
Métrite et ovarite			197 (0,89)
Pus dans les veines			112 (0,50)
Pneumonie	47 (0,35)		21 (0,09)
Pleurésie	35 (0,26)	40 (0,12)	43·(0,19)
Méningite	27 (0,20)		
Péricardite	14 (0,10)	6 (0,02)	1 (0,004)
Entérite	9 (0,07)	4 (0,01)	6 (0,03)
Cérébrite	9 (0,07)		
Cystite	8 (0,06)		
Artérite et aortite	4 (0,03)		
Bronchite, laryngite et diphtérie	4 (0,03)		
Phlébite	3 (0,02)		
Pus dans les muscles et les articulations	3 (0,02)	8 (0,02)	
Pus dans le foie, le pancréas, les muscles			19 (0,08)
Pus dans les articulations			10 (0,04)
Inflammation de la tunique vaginale	1 (0,007)		
Arachnoïdite		1 (0,003)	

Source : Simpson et Dubois. J'ai introduit les pourcentages.

ses vêtements étaient encore imprégnés d'émanations putrides, si même il ne portait aux doigts dans quelque repli épidermique quelque matière délétère. Aux cas de ce genre, dans lesquels la transmission ne paraît pas douteuse, et que M. Depaul nous a fait connaître, je pourrais ajouter celui d'une jeune femme auprès de laquelle je fus, il y a quelques années, appelé en consultation par un interne qui l'avait accouchée immédiatement après avoir ouvert le cadavre d'une femme morte de fièvre puerpérale. Sa cliente était atteinte de la même maladie et ne tarda pas à succomber[30].

Seul Dubois pousse l'obstination jusqu'à mettre en doute l'expérience de ses propres confrères. Il témoigne qu'il a lui-même assisté à de nombreuses autopsies, certes sans y prendre une part manuelle, puis est allé accoucher ses clientes sans prendre d'autre précaution que de changer de vêtements, or rien de fâcheux ne leur est arrivé[31].

Bref, les théories étiologiques et prophylactiques de Semmelweis et de Simpson sont parfaitement connues et, malgré les observations ou les expériences vécues, elles ne rencontrent, au mieux, que l'incrédulité. Pourquoi? Parce que ses raisons sont seulement statistiques. On le voit parfaitement dans les chiffres que donne Depaul à l'ouverture de la discussion et qui ne cesseront plus d'être commentés, constituant en quelque sorte la trame statistique des échanges.

LES STATISTIQUES DANS LA CONTROVERSE ACADÉMIQUE

Depaul présente les chiffres des accouchements et des décès de 1852 à 1856 à la Maternité de Paris, à la Clinique de la Faculté de Paris, à l'Hôtel-Dieu, à l'Hôpital Saint-Antoine et à l'Hôpital Saint-Louis, enfin à l'Hôpital Lariboisière qui venait d'être ouvert, et donc entre 1854 et 1856 seulement[32]. Comme il n'a pas le loisir de comparer, comme Semmelweis, des accouchements par des médecins à d'autres par des sages-femmes, il compare les accouchements hospitaliers aux accouchements en ville. Il présente ses chiffres par mois, toujours avec l'idée d'une corrélation entre les épidémies et les saisons. Je n'ai retenu que ceux de la Maternité et de la Clinique de la Faculté et les moyennes annuelles de tous les autres (Tableau 5).

Ces chiffres appellent plusieurs remarques que ne fait pas toujours Depaul. D'abord, le fait que Lariboisière, le plus moderne des établissements d'accouchement, construit conformément aux prescriptions de l'Académie des sciences à la fin de l'Ancien Régime, a le taux de létalité le plus élevé : Depaul ne fait que le constater sans chercher à l'expliquer. Symétriquement, on trouve le taux relativement très faible pour toutes les années et en moyenne de Saint-Louis. Là, Depaul avance trois explications possibles : "le nombre peu considérable des accouchements", mais ils restent plus nombreux qu'à Lariboisière et à Saint-Antoine; l'exposition est-ouest du service, conformément à l'aérisme dominant; et le faible encombrement – deux salles de huit lits chacune et huit chambres d'un lit. Dans une intervention ultérieure, il revient sur ce cas pour affirmer "qu'il s'est glissé quelque erreur dans ce relevé, qui n'a tenu compte, probablement, que des morts inscrites sous le nom de 'fièvre puerpérale', tandis que beaucoup, déclarées sous les noms de 'péritonite' ou de 'métro-péritonite puerpérales', n'y sont pas mentionnées, quoiqu'elles eussent eu très certainement pour cause la même maladie[33]." Autrement dit, lorsque les chiffres ne conviennent pas, au lieu de chercher à les comprendre, on en change. Or, il se trouve qu'à Saint-Louis, Malgaigne avait interdit de toucher les parturientes[34]. Mais celui-ci n'a pas participé à cette discussion académique.

Tableau 5 État comparatif des accouchements et des décès

	1852		*1853*		*1854*		*1855*		*1856*	
	Accouchements-	*Décès*	*Accouchements-*	*Décès*	*Accouchements*	*Décès*	*Accouchements*	*Décès*	*Accouchements*	*Décès*
					Maternité de Paris					
Janvier	296	»	230	»	260	»	334	»	291	1
Février	289	4	299	8	302	»	265	1	271	3
Mars	311	5	339	19	236	»	235	»	351	20
Avril	263	»	314	18	303	»	257	»	317	30
Mai	239	1	225	7	305	»	259	1	15	»
Juin	205	3	165	1	239	»	206	»	55	5
Juillet	236	1	193	1	262	1	241	4	184	2
Août	196	1	208	7	239	»	255	5	205	13
Septembre	211	9	177	1	236	»	31	1	213	13
Octobre	200	19	226	7	252	»	84	»	119	7
Novembre	217	3	216	»	289	»	102	»	185	4
Décembre	197	»	257	3	262	»	195	»	272	99
Totaux	2860	46	2849	72	3185	1	2464	12	2478.1	
Moyennes	1/62		1/39		1/3185		1/205		1/25	

Total des accouchements 13 836. Décès connus, 230
Proportion, 1/60 environ

Source : Depaul.

	1852		*1853*		*1854*		*1855*		*1856*	
	Accouchements-	*Décès*	*Accouchements-*	*Décès*	*Accouchements*	*Décès*	*Accouchements*	*Décès*	*Accouchements*	*Décès*
					Clinique de la Faculté					
Janvier	98	»	123	7	104	2	116	»	108	2
Février	103	»	52	5	95	1	89	1	81	1
Mars	117	2	2	»	97	3	116	4	79	»
Avril	92	1	»	»	93	1	104	4	107	7
Mai	117	3	76	1	81	»	99	2	66	5
Juin	76	»	96	2	54	6	88	2	9	»
Juillet	96	1	71	2	76	»	91	1	»	»
Août	104	1	93	4	58	1	85	1	65	12
Septembre	108	5	91	3	70	»	138	1	36	»
Octobre	105	1	87	»	90	2	123	1	»	»
Novembre	108	»	87	8	89	4	116	3	38	»
Décembre	109	8	69	»	96	2	101	6	41	32
Totaux	1233	22	847	32	1003	22	1266	26	630.5	
Moyennes	1/56		1/26		1/45		1/48		1/19	

Total des accouchements 4 979. Décès connus, 134
Proportion, 1/37

Source : Depaul.

Tableau 5 (*continué*)

Taux de létalité puerpérale dans les hôpitaux de Paris

	1852	*1853*	*1854*	*1855*	*1856*	*Moyenne*
Maternité	1/62	1/39	1/3 185	1/205	1/25	230/13 836 ou 1/60
Clinique	1/56	1/26	1/45	1/48	1/19	134/4 979 ou 1/37
Hôtel-Dieu	1/62	1/31	1/55	1/76	1/22	170/6 506 ou 1/38
Saint-Antoine	1/21	1/23	1/36	1/43	1/76	30/1 216 ou 1/40
Saint-Louis	1/660	1/346	0	1/152	1/813	9/3 748 ou 1/416
Lariboisière			1/24	1/22	1/26	56/1 382 ou 1/24

Source : Depaul; d'après Depaul.

Depaul a donc comparé ces chiffres à ceux, donnés par Tarnier dans sa thèse, des décès *post partum* en ville, dans le 12e arrondissement de Paris sur une seule année, 1856 : 14 décès pour 3 222 accouchements soit 1 sur 322, 17 fois moins qu'à la Faculté ou à la Maternité[35]. On remarquera que ces chiffres sont néanmoins supérieurs à la mortalité de Saint-Louis. On aurait pu s'attendre, en toute rigueur, à une recherche sur la salubrité exceptionnelle de cet hôpital : il n'en est rien. Toute la discussion tourne autour de la différence entre la létalité hospitalière et à domicile.

Depaul tire argument de ces chiffres pour réclamer la suppression des cliniques d'accouchement et leur remplacement par un service de secours à domicile, les accouchements en ville étant incomparablement plus sûrs. Cette position est soutenue par Cruveilhier, qui y ajoute l'ouverture de petits hospices hors de Paris où chaque accouchée aurait sa chambre[36].

On voit comment les statistiques induisent cette conclusion : alors que Semmelweis avait pu isoler statistiquement la cause des épidémies de fièvre puerpérale grâce à la disposition des lieux, l'existence de deux cliniques l'une pour médecins l'autre pour sages-femmes, qui constituait un véritable dispositif expérimental, Depaul ne le pouvait pas. Il ne pouvait que faire la différence entre la pratique hospitalière et la pratique de ville et donc conclure à la suppression de la première, là où Semmelweis le pouvait à la suppression des germes morbides transportés par les médecins accoucheurs à la suite de leurs travaux anatomo-pathologiques et inoculés aux parturientes. Autrement dit, les statistiques induisent des conclusions et c'est en raison de ces conclusions qu'on est conduit à les accepter ou à les réfuter. C'est ce qui s'est passé au cours de la discussion académique.

La discussion de cette statistique a suivi les deux moments de la sous-détermination que j'ai distingués : d'abord la critique des données, ensuite leur réinterprétation.

La critique des données s'est faite elle-même en deux temps : d'abord la critique de leur constitution, puis celle de leur pertinence. En ce qui concerne leur constitution, Tarnier avait établi la statistique du 12e arrondissement en relevant sur les registres d'état civil les noms des enfants nés à domicile et celui des femmes décédées. Le nom des enfants nés à domicile indiquait à la fois celui d'une femme accouchée à domicile et son domicile. Par conséquent, en rapprochant ces deux listes, il obtint le nombre des accouchées à domicile et celui des décédées à domicile des suites de leur accouchement.

Dubois objecta qu'il faudrait que toutes les femmes accouchées à domicile dans le 12e arrondissement et dont l'accouchement avait été fatal eussent succombé dans ce même arrondissement. Or certaines avaient pu être transportées dans un hôpital extérieur au 12e arrondissement de sorte que leur décès aurait été déclaré dans l'arrondissement de cet hôpital. Danyau en apporta un témoignage : l'une de ses anciennes élèves sages-femmes à la Maternité lui avait appris qu'au début de 1854 une épidémie de fièvre puerpérale avait précisément frappé cet arrondissement et qu'elle même avait eu 20 malades sur 35 accouchées. Or, sur les 14 décès parmi ces 20 malades, 8 appartenaient au 12e arrondissement et 6 aux localités voisines (la Glacière, la barrière de Fontainebleau, la Gare d'Ivry). Le nomadisme de la classe ouvrière et l'instabilité de ses unions en fournissaient l'explication[37].

Non seulement les décès d'un arrondissement ne sont pas forcément des malades de cet arrondissement, mais en outre tous les décès puerpéraux d'un arrondissement ne sont pas forcément comptabilisés comme tels. En effet, le secret médical empêcherait que les déclarations des causes de décès fussent sincères. Comme preuve qu'il en était bien ainsi, Dubois invoqua son expérience personnelle : la moyenne des décès dans sa propre clientèle privée était moins favorable que celle du 12e arrondissement selon Tarnier.

Danyau fit une autre objection, c'est que les résultats dépendent crucialement de la période d'observation. Les relevés faits par Tarnier à sa demande dans les registres d'état civil du 12e arrondissement indiquaient 20 mortes de fièvre puerpérales pour 1 205 accouchées pendant les quatre premiers mois de 1854, soit 1 décès sur 60 accouchées, ce qui était bien moins favorable aux accouchements en ville.

Quant à la critique de la pertinence de ces chiffres, Dubois et Danyau citèrent l'un et l'autre des cas où l'épidémie s'était propagée de la ville vers les hôpitaux et non l'inverse, voire même n'était apparue qu'en ville, comme par exemple à Brackel en 1852. Dans cette “petite ville de 3 000 habitants, l’une des plus salubres de toute la Westphalie”, en l’espace de 4 mois, sur 28 accouchées, 13 eurent la fièvre puerpérale et 12 succombèrent, seuls 2 nouveaux-nés des 13 malades survivant[38]. Et pour ruiner toute idée de létalité supérieure en ville qu’à l’hôpital, Dubois en vint à mettre en doute le caractère contagieux de la fièvre puerpérale et à relancer le débat, à ce propos, entre infectionnistes et contagionnistes.

Dubois et Danyau admettaient néanmoins que la létalité puerpérale était plus élevée dans les maternités qu’en ville. Ce qu’ils voulaient établir par leur critique des statistiques, c’était simplement que la mortalité par fièvre puerpérale en ville était bien supérieure à la statistique de Tarnier, de sorte que le problème n’aurait pas été résolu par la suppression des maternités. Et pour simplement réduire la mortalité de celles-ci au chiffre de la mortalité en ville, il suffisait d’une réforme consistant à “transporter dans les maisons d’accouchement les conditions relativement favorables de salubrité qu’on trouve dans la pratique privée[39].”

La critique de la pertinence des chiffres conduit ainsi à leur réinterprétation : loin de prouver qu’il faut fermer les maternités et développer la pratique de ville, ils soulignent l’urgence d’y introduire les conditions de salubrité des soins à domicile.

La véritable raison de l’opposition de Dubois et Danyau se trouve ailleurs : “les hôpitaux et cliniques d’accouchement ne sont pas seulement des établissements d’assistance publique, ce sont encore des écoles où se forment annuellement un grand nombre d’élèves[40].” La suppression des maternités mettrait fin à l’enseignement pratique. On retrouve ici ce trait caractéristique de la médecine française : la connaissance passe avant les soins.

Depaul a facilement répondu à la critique de la statistique de Tarnier que, tout compte fait des inévitables erreurs de relevé, la différence restait “énorme”, tellement qu’on “ne comblera jamais la distance qui sépare une statistique qui donne 1 mort sur 19 et celle qui n’en donne que 1 sur 322[41].” Et il l’étaya sur une autre, citée par Velpeau, une statistique de Trébuchet, fonctionnaire de la Préfecture de Police et secrétaire du Conseil d’hygiène de Paris, qui donnait une mortalité de 4 parturientes sur 1 000 à Paris, soit 1 sur 250.[42]

Et contre la réinterprétation de ses chiffres, contre la proposition de créer de petits établissements ou d’imposer les conditions de salubrité les plus draconiennes aux maternités, il fit état de la mortalité à Lariboisière, la plus élevée des statistiques qu’il avait fournies alors que c’était la maternité la plus “moderne”. Et réciproquement, pour soutenir la faisabilité des secours à domicile, il cita l’exemple de la Société médicale d’accouchement fondée en 1837 par des médecins que la mortalité dans les maternités horrifiait : de 1837 à 1841, elle pratiqua 1 258 accouchements à domicile sans dommage alors qu'au même moment, en 1841, sur 623 accouchées à la Clinique, il y eut 22 décès (1 sur 28).

Or malgré l'évidence statistique, ce sont ces critiques qui l'ont emporté, en tout cas qui ont emporté la conviction de Guérard, lui qui avait introduit la discussion et qui fut chargé de la conclure : "J'avoue, pour ce qui me concerne, que l'argumentation de M. Dubois a bien ébranlé mes croyances sur ce point particulier de la discussion. Je ne suis plus guère disposé à admettre la transmission de la maladie par l'intermédiaire des personnes qui assistent l'accouchée[43]." Et c'est ainsi que Semmelweis a perdu la bataille de Paris, et avec lui les malheureuses femmes qui accouchaient dans les maternités. Il faudra attendre la fin du siècle et la découverte du streptocoque, c'est-à-dire du microbe responsable de ce qu'on savait être une septicémie, pour lui donner raison à titre posthume. Combien de femmes, combien de mères, ont-elles été sacrifiées sur l'autel du réalisme médical?

NOTES

1 George Weisz, *The Medical Mandarins: The French Academy of Medicine in the Nineteenth and Early Twentieth Centuries* (New York et Oxford : Oxford University Press, 1995), chap. 7.

2 *Ibid.*, 168

3 *Ibid.*, 172.

4 *Ibid.*, 173.

5 *Ibid.*, 175.

6 Ibid.

7 "Le traitement de la fièvre puerpérale", *Bulletin de l'Académie de médecine,* 23(1857–1858), Guérard 367.

8 *Ibid.*, Depaul, 389.

9 *Ibid.*, Cruveilhier, 518.

10 *Ibid.*, Guérard, 942–943.

11 Franz Hecktor Arneth, "Note sur le moyen proposé et employé par M. Semmelweis pour empêcher le développement des épidémies puerpérales dans l'Hospice de la maternité de Vienne", lue à l'Académie de médecine dans la séance du 7 janvier 1851, *Annales d'hygiène publique et de médecine légale,* première série, 45 (1851), 281–90; "Evidence of Puerperal Fever Depending upon the Contagious Inoculation of Morbid Matter", communication à la Edinburgh Medico-Chirurgical Society dans la séance du 16 avril 1851, *Monthly Journal of Medical Science,* 12 (1851), 505–11.

12 Ignaz Philipp Semmelweis, *Die Aetiologie, der Begriff, und die Prophylaxis des Kindbettfiebers* (Pest, Vienne et Leipzig : C.A. Hartleben, 1861) trad. angl. par Frank P. Murphy, *Medical Classics*, 4, n5 (janvier 1941), 349–478; 4, n6 (février 1941), 481–589; 4, n7 (mars 1941), 591–715; 4, n8 (avril 1941), 719–73; édition en fac-simile (Birmingham, Ala. : Gryphon, The Classics of Medicine Library, 1981). Je cite d'après cette édition facsimile qui suit en continu la pagination de la traduction anglaise. Le tableau XXII se trouve à la page 457.

13 F.H. Arneth, "Note", 283–4; cf. "Evidence", 507–8.

14 Semmelweis, *Die Aetiologie*, tableau XXIII.

15 "De l'étiologie de la fièvre puerpérale, par le docteur Semmelweis", *Revue médico-chirurgicale de Paris*, 3 (1848), 298–9.

16 "Des moyens prophylactiques mis en usage au grand hôpital de Vienne contre l'apparition de la fièvre puerpérale, par F. Wieger," *Revue médico-chirurgicale de Paris*, 6 (1849), 173–5. Wieger est cité par Semmelweis mais à propos d'une correspondance ultérieure (*Die Aetiologie*, 451).

17 "Le traitement de la fièvre puerpérale", *Bulletin de l'Académie de médecine*, 23 (1857–1858) : Depaul, 424. Il fait du médecin de Strasbourg "l'introducteur du moyen prophylactique de M. Semmelweis au grand hôpital de Vienne".

18 *Bulletin de l'Académie de médecine*, 16 (1850–1851), 290.

19 Semmelweis, *Die Aetiologie*, 702–703.

20 Henri de Castelnau, rubrique "Séances des Académies", *Gazette des Hôpitaux civils et militaires*, jeudi 9 janvier 1851, en première page.

21 "Des moyens prophylactiques mis en usage…, par F. Wieger", 175; Semmelweis, *Die Aetiologie*, 447–50. Cf. Paul Delaunay, *La Maternité de Paris*, (Paris : J. Roussel, 1909), 172.

22 "Le traitement de la fièvre puerpérale", Depaul, 424.

23 *Monthly Journal of Medical Science*, 12 (1851), 70–81.

24 *Ibid.*, 73.

25 Semmelweis, *Die Aetiologie*, 387, 462–3, et 567 où il prétend que Simpson aurait abandonné cette idée.

26 "Le traitement de la fièvre puerpérale", Guérard, 367 et 376, Depaul, 424, Dubois, 413–4 et 648, Danyau, 561–2, Velpeau, 751.

27 *Ibid.*, Danyau, 561–2. Semmelweis a répondu à tous ses détracteurs, y compris ceux-là nommément, cf. *Die Aetiologie*, 591–771 : à Friedrich Wilhelm Scanzoni, 591–660, Bernhard Seyfert, 676–81, Franz Ritter Kiwisch, 681–6, Lumpe, 692–701.

28 "Le traitement de la fièvre puerpérale", Velpeau, 751, Dubois, 506–9 et 643, Cruveilhier, 543, Danyau, 558. James Young Simpson, "Some Notes on the Analogy between Puerperal Fever and Surgical Fever", *The Monthly Journal of Medical Science*, 11 (1850), 414–29.

29 “Le traitement de la fièvre puerpérale”, Guérard, 376–7, Depaul, 404–5, Dubois, 520, Danyau, 559–60.
30 Les autres cas sont ceux de transmission par une sage-femme, qui n’a donc pas pratiqué d’autopsie, comme celle de Manchester citée par Simpson lors de la discussion d’Édimbourg.
31 “Le traitement de la fièvre puerpérale”, Dubois, 642. Il raille un certain nombre de témoignages *a contrario* dans la littérature médicale anglaise, “indignes de figurer dans une enquête sérieuse” (643), comme celui mentionné *supra* p. 214.
32 *Ibid.*, Depaul, 396–401.
33 *Ibid.*, Depaul, 837–838.
34 “Des moyens prophylactiques mis en usage…, par F. Wieger”, 175.
35 “Le traitement de la fièvre puerpérale”, Depaul, 398. Cf. Stéphane Tarnier, *Recherches sur l’état puerpéral et sur les maladies des femmes en couches* (Paris : Rignoux, 1857), 57.
36 “Le traitement de la fièvre puerpérale”, Depaul, 426, Cruveilhier, 548.
37 *Ibid.*, Dubois, 684–6, Danyau, 878–9.
38 *Ibid.*, Danyau, 570, Dubois, 683.
39 *Ibid.*, Dubois, 688, cf. Danyau, 572–3.
40 *Ibid.*, Danyau, 571.
41 *Ibid.*, Depaul, 836.
42 *Ibid.*, Velpeau, 749, Depaul, 836.
43 *Ibid.*, Guérard, 933.

11

Epidemiology in Transition: Tobacco and Lung Cancer in the 1950s

MARK PARASCANDOLA

Many believe that only trained investigators can plan and conduct controlled experiments whereas the man on the street can record and interpret observations of naturally occurring events.

H. Dorn

By the 1950s, epidemiologic methods and thinking had expanded beyond the mere study of epidemics to human experiments testing preventive interventions, case-control observations in hospital patients, and the long-term study of large, generally healthy cohorts. Yet there existed no single, shared vision of where epidemiology was headed. There was disagreement about who could practise epidemiology and whether the field was a proper discipline or simply an aggregation of methods.[1] The study of cancer posed unique methodological challenges, and some observers urged development of new rules of inference. Biostatisticians, clinicians, pathologists, and public health officers were conducting case-control studies of varying quality. Additionally, biostatistics made remarkable contributions to epidemiology during this period, but there were conflicting views about the role of statistics in aetiologic research. And, perhaps most important, epidemiologists were unsure about how to balance their dual roles as scientists and as protectors of public health.

The debate over tobacco and lung cancer provided a crucial test for the discipline of epidemiology. The conflict has been characterized as one between epidemiologists and laboratory scientists, where a general discomfort with statistical concepts prompted a demand for elucidation of mechanisms of causation.[2] But while scepticism about statistics was certainly influential,[3] it is far from the whole story. In reality, epidemiologists and biostatisticians themselves, whom one might have expected to have had a more favourable view of the mounting epidemiological evidence, remained divided on the issue throughout much of the 1950s. Some prominent epidemiologists and biostatisticians mounted carefully reasoned arguments that countered the case against cigarettes. Because epidemiology was going through radical changes, there existed no explicit, shared standards for evaluating evidence. Leading biostatisticians and epidemiologists acted as reformers, endeavouring to raise awareness within the medical community about standards of study design and proper interpretation of evidence. And while these reformers agreed on many key points (such as unbiased selection of cases and controls), their differences were crucial for the debate over smoking and lung cancer.

Revisiting this debate sheds light on this difficult transition that still troubles epidemiology.[4] Previous historical accounts have described the progress of research on smoking and lung cancer as well as some of the sceptical responses, but none has given sufficient attention to the historical context.[5] The (U.S.) National Cancer Institute (NCI) was building programs in epidemiology and biostatistics, and NCI researchers such as Jerome Cornfield, Harold Dorn, and Alexander Gilliam were prominent participants in the debate over smoking and lung cancer. The participation of NCI epidemiologists and biostatisticians in this debate illuminates many of the conflicts within these disciplines.

The debate over smoking and lung cancer in the 1950s occurred around four major key methodological issues. After outlining the roots of epidemiologic research at NCI, this essay explores these four aspects of the debate. First, some researchers disagreed on whether there really was an epidemic of lung cancer and what kind of evidence would be required to demonstrate that fact. Second, some prominent epidemiologists voiced concerns about the limitations of the case-control method and its potential for bias. Third, a cohort of senior biostatisticians challenged the large cohort studies conducted in the United States and the United Kingdom because they lacked the essential ingredient of a true experiment – randomization. Finally, researchers differed on how to synthesize and draw inferences from a complex and diverse body of evidence. In the end, a pragmatic approach won out, as the U.S. surgeon general's committee adopted a series of criteria for making causal inferences based largely on data from non-randomized studies.

EARLY CANCER EPIDEMIOLOGY AT THE NCI

By the mid-1930s, on the eve of the creation of the National Cancer Institute (NCI), the American public was widely aware of claims about increasing cancer death rates. Statisticians in the insurance industry, such as Frederick Hoffman at Prudential Insurance Company, had amassed statistical data documenting the growing incidence of cancer since 1900, and voluntary organizations such as the American Society for the Control of Cancer, founded in 1913, had been using these figures to bring public attention to the cancer menace.[6] In the late 1930s, NCI began publishing cancer mortality statistics for the period 1900–35 based on U.S. census data.[7] Yet there was also substantial scepticism within the medical community about whether the seemingly increasing number of cancer deaths was real or simply a statistical artifact. For example, it was possible that doctors had missed many cancers earlier but were now diagnosing them better; perhaps more cancer deaths were reported simply because people were living longer and were more likely to escape infectious diseases. Additionally, there was no adequate information on U.S. patterns of cancer incidence, and members of the medical community had little understanding of appropriate epidemiologic methods for gathering and interpreting such data. By the late 1940s, these problems became a central concern of an emerging group of epidemiologists and biostatisticians at NCI.

Harold Dorn, born in 1906 on a farm in New York state, earned his PhD in sociology from the University of Wisconsin in 1933. He spent a post-doctoral year as a Social Science Research Council Fellow at University College, London, where he attended lectures by statistical luminaries R.A. Fisher and Egon Pearson. When he returned to the United States in 1934 the Roosevelt administration was recruiting social scientists in large numbers. Dorn first took a job as a statistician with the Federal Relief Administration and in 1936 moved to the U.S. Public Health Service (PHS).[8] He designed and oversaw the (first) 10 City Cancer Morbidity survey, which interviewed hospitals and physicians in 10 major cities about living patients diagnosed with cancer.[9]

It is clear that Dorn early thought of health statistics not simply as "unique historical facts" or descriptive data, but as a basis for drawing generalizations and inferences that would guide policy choices in public health. He worried about factors in data quality and selection that could bias statistical inferences.[10] For his PhD dissertation, he had studied the effects of reporting mortality statistics by place of death rather than by place of residence – a practice that skewed urban-versus-rural death rates because seriously ill rural residents tended to die in large, city hospitals.[11] In discussing the rationale for the 10 city survey, Dorn and his co-authors explained that only "careful epidemiological investigation of cancer in representative population groups" could answer certain questions: "Does climate affect the occurrence of cancer? Is cancer more common among Negroes than among white persons? Which groups are attacked most frequently? Do persons living in the open country have more or less cancer than persons living in cities?"[12]

The NCI began to expand its field studies and biostatistics activities after the Second World War and in 1948 hired Alexander Gilliam to head its new Epidemiology Section.[13] Gilliam, born in 1904, received a medical degree in 1931 from the University of Virginia and a doctorate in public health in 1934 at Johns Hopkins School of Hygiene and Public Health, where he studied under epidemiologist Wade Hampton Frost. He joined the PHS's Commissioned Corps as an assistant surgeon and served at various locations, including the Division of Infectious Diseases at the National Institutes of Health (NIH), in Bethesda, Maryland. During the war, he worked in North Africa, China, Burma, and India as a member of the United States Typhus Commission.[14] When he arrived at NCI in 1948, he hoped to apply his experience with infectious diseases to cancer. His early project report forms, prepared with colleague Benno K. Milmore, describe ongoing research in epidemiologic methods that aimed at "[a]daptation and modification of standard epidemiological methods already of demonstrated usefulness in communicable diseases research, and extension and application of these methods to cancer study."[15] Though little remembered, Gilliam was a visible figure and served as president of the American Epidemiological Society in 1957 and chair of the Epidemiology Section of the American Public Health Association in 1952–3.[16]

In his early work at NCI, Gilliam, like Dorn, focused on reforming practices of estimating and reporting rates of cancer incidence. He made efforts to measure incidence in various racial groups and devoted substantial effort to pointing out the shortcomings of estimates appearing in the medical literature. For example, he responded to a report on rates of secondary metastases in breast cancer patients. The rates that the researchers calculated were invalid, he argued, estimated from a series of women who voluntarily sought follow-up care; those who had metastases would, it seemed, be more likely to return to the doctor because of symptoms.[17] Similarly, he claimed that statistics on leukemia and lymphoma reported for various groups and labelled as "incidence" were often based solely on the number of patients who voluntarily showed up at a particular hospital or clinic.[18]

IS THERE AN EPIDEMIC?

While Dorn and Gilliam shared many of the same concerns about the quality of data sources and inferences about risk, they ended up on opposing sides in the debate over whether the increase in lung cancer mortality was real or a statistical artifact. By the mid-1950s, some researchers, Dorn included, called lung cancer a "pandemic".[19] But NCI epidemiologists Gilliam and Benno K. Milmore objected to this alarmist use of "a word which has generally been reserved in epidemiological literature to describe such world-wide scourges as the 1918–19 influenza pandemic or the Black Death of the Middle Ages."[20] Gilliam and Milmore insisted that the disease had probably gone undiagnosed in earlier times and that improvements in diagnosis were largely responsible for the observed increase. Such a high rate of error "would appear preposterous at first glance but when looked at more closely may not be unreasonable at all." Moreover, during the same period that saw a "frightening" increase in mortality from lung cancer, a substantial decline in mortality attributed to tuberculosis occurred. Because tuberculosis was so frequent, Gilliam estimated, even a moderate (11 per cent) error rate in diagnosis before 1914 could account for the entire increase in cancer deaths. Additionally, the introduction of antibiotics might have "permitted the survival until correct diagnosis" of patients who would formerly have died of some other respiratory disease, before the "underlying" cancer of the lung could be discovered.[21]

Gilliam's interpretation, however, faced some substantial challenges. It failed to account for the dramatic differences between sex and age groups. For example, between 1914 and 1950 the age-adjusted mortality rate for lung cancer increased 25 times for white males and only 6.5 times for white females. Gilliam's view assumed that either in 1914 or in 1950 physicians were far better at diagnosing lung cancer in one sex than in the other. Moreover, on Gilliam's hypothesis one would also have to assume a sex difference in the diagnosis of tuberculosis. In response to these objections, Gilliam admitted that some of the increase in lung cancer might be real, but he continued to insist that "the magnitude of increase is nowhere near as great as recorded mortality suggests."[22]

Gilliam and Milmore were also hopeful: "It is common practice to make dire predictions of the future position of cancer of the lung as a cause of death if present trends continue.[23] But both men emphasized that, while mortality appeared to be rising (whether the increase was real or not), the *rate* of increase was declining.[24] Thus, as at the tail end of an epidemic, the mortality rate would eventually level out and, after that point, start to decline by 1983 for men and by 1960 for women. "No matter what method of projection is employed, a peak with subsequent decline <u>must</u> follow a declining rate of increase."[25] As late as

1962 Gilliam continued to insist that the "epidemic" would level out.[26] Moreover, the rate of increase was greater for non-whites than for whites. This racial difference seemed consistent with the idea that "improvements in medical practice and death certification in recent years have undoubtedly accelerated more rapidly among these races than among the white," presumably because those standards were much lower to begin with.

Dorn acknowledged that "the period of most rapid rise in the death rate has been passed",[27] but he was convinced that the increase was real and important. He cited the sex and age differentials, which posed problems for Gilliam, as "[m]y reasons for believing that the major part of the increase of mortality ... cannot be accounted for by improved methods of diagnosis."[28] Additionally, he believed that only a much higher 1914 error rate, 96 per cent, would justify Gilliam's hypothesis. "With all due credit to advances in medical knowledge during the past third of a century, this conclusion hardly seems warranted."[29]

Gilliam's arguments were not unusual at the time with regard to cancer. Much of the cancer epidemiology work conducted in the 1940s and into the 1950s aimed to use surveys of cancer incidence and mortality data to identify patterns by geography, race, time, and other factors. However, a number of epidemiologists worried about whether these observed patterns, particularly rising cancer rates, were real or artifactual.[30] For example, a debate about apparently rising leukemia incidence and mortality was prompting epidemiologists to puzzle over whether the rise was real or merely due to improvements in diagnosis and increased referrals to specialty clinics.[31] Gilliam had also previously argued that an apparent upward shift in age selection of polio was an artifact of changing mortality rates that differed by age.[32] The case for collection of higher-quality data on morbidity and mortality was coming from a number of statisticians in federal and state governments.[33]

Dorn became head of the new NCI Biostatistics Branch in 1948 and began bringing in statisticians who would make essential contributions to epidemiologic methods during the 1950s. The group included Jerome Cornfield, Samuel Greenhouse, William Haenszel, Nathan Mantel and Marvin Schneiderman. Most had not had any medically related training before arriving at the NCI, having studied demography, economics, mathematics, or sociology.[34] Their work was to be particularly important for the interpretation of case-control studies, starting with Jerome Cornfield's 1951 paper that introduced a method for deriving prevalence rates from such data.[35]

SELECTION AND THE CASE-CONTROL STUDY

Clinical and public-health researchers had used case-control methods sporadically since the 1920s for aetiologic research on cancer.[36] However, early applications of the case-control method were often crude – failing, for instance, to adjust for age differences between cases and controls or attempting to calculate cancer attack rates directly from hospital case series.[37] Dorn wrote in 1955 that "by turning the pages, almost at random, of many medical journals, one can find articles in which the author comments on the difference in the average age, sex ratio, or some other characteristic of his series of cases when compared with some other published series and speculates about the reasons for this difference without taking into consideration that the simplest explanation might be that the corresponding populations from which the two series of cases were drawn had different characteristics."[38] These naïve comparative studies became a target for reformers such as Dorn and Gilliam.

In 1950, five hospital-based case-control studies of the relationship between smoking and lung cancer were published, marking the start of a boom era for case-control investigations. These researchers, some of whom had epidemiologic and statistical training, began to improve on some of the weaknesses of earlier studies by adjusting for or matching on age, using routinely collected smoking information (to protect against interviewer bias), and/or addressing possible sources of confounding.[39] For example, Doll and Hill looked for signs of information bias in their data and also considered whether differences in social class and place of residence could explain the differences in smoking habits between cases and controls. Two of the papers came from pathology laboratories.[40]

The most difficult challenge for these researchers was ensuring that they had selected their cases and controls appropriately. Some emphasized that comparisons in case-control studies should mimic, as closely as possible, the experimental ideal, where two comparison groups are similar in all respects, except for the presence or absence of the disease being studied.[41] This comparability, which randomization helped to protect, was crucial for causal inference. But Berkson had previously described how this comparison could be biased in a hospital-based case-control study when both the exposure and the disease under study independently affect the probability of hospitalization.[42] Berkson first presented his argument at a meeting of the American Statistical Association in 1938 and finally published it in 1946 in *Biometrics,* where it was unlikely to reach clinical investigators. But his challenge gained a renewed urgency in the tobacco debate.

Gilliam was particularly critical of case-control comparisons, which he warned were full of "jokers" (spurious associations) – a term that he picked up from Frost.[43] Referring to his own unpublished data, Gilliam claimed to have found associations between lung cancer and marriage, brown eyes, and prior history of cysts.[44] Gilliam lamented that the literature on chronic-disease epidemiology was filled with reports that compared the characteristics of different case series to make generalizations about risk differences. He wrote about the "constant search of the epidemiologist for significant difference in risk" and complained that "such misuse is in large part responsible for a great deal of present confusion in epidemiologic evidence."[45] He directly cited a few obscure examples. For instance, he challenged a South African researcher who concluded that Bantu gold-mine labourers had a far higher incidence of liver cancer than a white population because 90.5 per cent of cancers in autopsied Bantu patients at a local hospital were liver cancer. Hospital autopsy series provided large numbers of subjects and allowed for more accurate diagnosis, but relative frequencies derived from them were akin to "clinical impression rather than constituting established fact." At worst, and especially in a "medically backward group," such comparisons "may lead to considerable distortion of fact."[46] Gilliam's earlier work on experimental field tests of a polio vaccine, which relied on volunteers, had made him acutely aware of selection effects.[47]

Moreover, researchers who used Cornfield's procedure for estimating relative risk on the basis of case-control studies required the further assumption that the cases and controls were representative of the populations from which they supposedly came. Gilliam, for one, believed that the requirement that samples be representative of the population from which they derived had "never yet been met in *any* case history study of cancer."[48] Despite these concerns, Gilliam collaborated with two NCI biostatisticians, Jerome Cornfield and Doris Sadowsky, on a case-control study of smoking using records collected for an earlier NCI study set up to test a variety of cancer aetiology hypotheses. They admitted that their cases and controls, like those in other studies, could not represent all cases and non-cases. But the consistency, they argued, between a number of well-conducted case-control studies under different circumstances did suggest a real association. Their conclusion, however, was not inconsistent with Gilliam's claims about the rising incidence of lung cancer. They noted that cancer of the larynx was also consistently associated with smoking, but there was no epidemic of that cancer.

The answer to these problems, argued Dorn and Gilliam, was to do cohort studies in a defined population. Only prospective studies could directly measure risk and thereby provide trustworthy estimates of the magnitude of harm posed by an exposure. "There is no substitute for measuring as precisely as possible the risk of a disease among members of a defined population," Dorn insisted. He described the variation in relative risk estimates across four studies of cervical cancer and their inconsistency with incidence rates. In theory, he noted, case-control studies with representative samples should provide the same conclusions as a cohort study, but in practice "there is no way of being sure of this without a prospective study."[49] Gilliam explained that it was possible to make groups representative on known factors, such as age, race, and sex, but "[u]ntil information is accumulated about all of the important characteristics associated with the disease, however, one is unable to estimate accurately just how representative the sample is."[50] Dorn conducted a retrospective cohort study of smoking among 250,000 U.S. veterans in co-operation with the Veterans Administration, which became a crucial piece of the growing body of evidence.[51]

Other experts were more optimistic, though appropriately cautious, about preventing and detecting selection bias. Some urged use of stratified probability sampling, rather than matching.[52] They argued for testing for consistency among subgroups. For example, pathologist Robert Schrek of the Veterans Administration and his co-authors recommended that investigators should test likely confounders, or "secondary factors" (such as race and age), to see if they differed between cases and controls such that they might explain the observed association between smoking and lung cancer.[53] Colin White and John Bailar downplayed the differences between cohort and case-control studies, suggesting that selection bias could occur in both.[54] Arthur Kraus, a biostatistician in the New York State Department of Health, challenged "oversuspiciousness" of case-control studies – use of background knowledge and judgment could determine where Berkson's bias was a true threat.[55] Similarly, Morton Levin argued that consistent findings across studies and the observed dose-response relationships made selection bias unlikely.[56] Levin had led one of the lung-cancer case-control studies published in 1950; he had trained in epidemiology under Frost, like Gilliam, but he was to take a very different position in the tobacco debate.

EXPERIMENTS AND CAUSAL INFERENCE

The method of the case-control study was not the only point of contention in the 1950s. In fact, several prominent biostatisticians were also highly critical of the large cohort studies that followed. In some respects their arguments, calling for experimental studies and attention to biological hypotheses, resemble the response that we might expect from statistically naïve laboratory researchers. But in this case, involving statistical luminaries such as R.A. Fisher, we cannot chalk it up to uninformed scepticism about statistics. "Now I should be the last person to attack evidence for being merely statistical," Fisher acknowledged. The problem was not that the evidence was statistical, but that the particular statistical links shown were open to various interpretations.

Fisher has become infamous for his stance in the tobacco debate, and several hypotheses have emerged to explain his actions.[57] But independent of any underlying motivations, he did offer thoughtful arguments rooted in methodological concerns shared by other medical statisticians. Fisher suggested that a genetic trait could be a common cause, responsible for making some people both dependent on cigarettes and also more susceptible to lung cancer. The central weakness in the evidence, according to him, was the lack of a randomized experiment, which was the only way to definitively rule out the common-cause hypothesis. The focus on 'statistically significant' associations in the epidemiologic literature frustrated him in the absence of attention to aspects of experimental design.[58]

Fisher had reason for concern. The place of recently developed randomized controlled trials in medical research was still somewhat in doubt.[59] While simple procedures such as the test of statistical significance had worked their way into medical research, medical researchers had not wholeheartedly adopted Fisher's theory of statistical inference. Moreover, Fisher's system evaluated evidence from a single study only, rather than from a diverse body of evidence, and this further reinforced for him the need for a crucial experiment. Fisher was not the only person who took seriously the possibility of a common cause; some prominent epidemiologists thought the suggestion serious enough to warrant empirical study.[60]

Berkson was more explicit about the limitations of statistics –"if biologists permit statisticians to become arbiters of biologic questions, scientific disaster is inevitable." But his ultimate aim, like Fisher's, was the proper use of statistics. Berkson also deplored the simplistic application of tests for statistical significance without attention to aspects of experimental design that would tend to prove or disprove a specific causal model. Knowledge of biological mechanisms was important not as an end in itself, but because it suggested experiments. "[T]he most important consideration with respect to a theory is not whether it appears plausible, but whether it suggests experiments, and what experiments are suggested."[61] Jacob Yerushalmy, a biostatistician at Berkeley, proposed similar arguments in response to studies showing a link between maternal smoking and infant mortality. He argued that the data were equally consistent with competing interpretations – that either the smoking or the constitution of smokers could explain an association between maternal smoking and low birth weight. Non-randomized studies simply were helpless to resolve the conflict. Yerushalmy made it clear that the problem was not with the statistical form of the results. "The evidence may not be convincing, but not because it is 'only statistical,' rather because the evidence is nonstatistical in the sense that the method of study which produced the evidence violates the basic principles for valid statistical inference."[62] Statisticians also saw that selection effects, such as Berkson had described for hospital-based case-control studies, could operate in cohort studies as well, because both smoking and study participation were voluntary (and recruitment rates for unhealthy smokers might be different from those for unhealthy non-smokers).[63]

There was a tension between the earlier germ-theory model of disease causation and an emerging multi-causal model for complex chronic diseases such as cancer.[64] As many researchers acknowledged, there was not a single, specific causal agent identified yet for lung cancer. This was not an insurmountable problem from the perspective of most epidemiologists and biostatisticians. The fact that there was not a one-to-one deterministic relationship between smoking and lung cancer – that not all smokers developed lung cancer and some non-smokers did – was not at issue. In fact, these theorists explicitly defined a cause in probabilistic terms, as a factor that increases the probability of disease, rather than in terms of necessity and sufficiency.[65] However, some investigators still hesitated to consider cigarettes as a cause even in this latter sense. Gilliam, for example, urged that epidemiologists should search for "essential causes" of disease – specific chemical agents that were analogous to infectious micro-organisms. For example, he wrote, "it is now known that neither low income nor a diet of corn bread and blackstrap [molasses] had any direct role in causing pellagra, although there was a high degree of association."[66] While epidemiology had led to practical control measures for pellagra, it was the identification, in the chemical laboratory, of the specific nutrient lacking in pellagra victims' diets that marked the discovery of the cause of the disease.

An influential 1959 paper by Yerushalmy and Carroll E. Palmer, a commissioned PHS officer with expertise in biostatistics, faulted epidemiologic studies of cancer and urged that they should follow "the more rigorous methods long in use by bacteriologists." Bacteriologists had a set of rules – Koch's postulates – for drawing aetiologic conclusions about infectious agents. But for chronic diseases there were only vectors, such as cigarette smoke, that somewhere contained specific carcinogens, and statistical methods were particularly important in studying these hidden causes. Yerushalmy and Palmer, of course, saw tremendous value in statistical methods. But in this case "conventional statistical techniques cannot be utilized without modification, because the fundamental requirement of group comparability, ordinarily achieved through randomization, is not satisfied."[67]

To help rule out spurious associations, Yerushalmy urged that investigators test for the "specificity" of an association. He was not imposing a germ-theory model on cancer, accepting only specific agents as causes; instead he based his rationale in statistics. He and Herman Hilleboe, of the New York State Department of Health, argued that researchers, even before reaching the stage of causal inference, must determine whether the association observed is what it seems. They should ascertain whether "the association between two variables is in fact between the variables investigated and does not merely reflect relationships with a broader group, of which one or the other of the variables forms a part."[68] Thus, is there really an association between cigarette smoking and lung cancer, or is that link merely a byproduct of a cluster of correlations, as poverty is associated with many health outcomes? Yerushalmy and others proposed that these multiple correlations were an indication of some sort of selection bias.[69]

HIERARCHIES OF EVIDENCE AND THE STUDY GROUP

In the late 1950s, as researchers increasingly used epidemiologic studies to investigate the causes of lung cancer and other chronic diseases, they sought to find their proper role in relation to other disciplines and other methods of aetiologic research. There were, of course, different ways to design an epidemiologic study, and not all seemed equally trustworthy. For instance, epidemiologists and biostatisticians all explicitly agreed that an experiment offered the strongest evidence that any single study could offer.[70] Epidemiologists and biostatisticians put substantial effort into categorizing different epidemiologic study designs and outlining their strengths and weaknesses. Ultimately, they sought to further the use of epidemiology; by admitting that some forms of study were less than perfect, they could defend those designs that improved on the weaker ones. Thus, while biostatisticians who were sceptical of the evidence implicating cigarettes, such as Berkson, Fisher, and Yerushalmy, had emphasized the absence of a crucial experiment that would provide a true test of the constitutional hypothesis, those who defended the new epidemiologic studies took what they considered a more pragmatic approach. Additionally, opinions differed on the standard of proof required in aetiologic research because some epidemiologists emphasized vigorous method while others took a more pragmatic view of solving problems in public health.

In contrast to biostatisticians clearly committed to the former, the dissenters who strongly supported the causal link between cigarettes and lung cancer downplayed the role of experimentation. Even a randomized controlled experiment did not guarantee the validity of a causal inference, they argued, particularly when one wanted to generalize that inference outside the particular experiment. Cornfield and Hammond both explained that randomization by itself is insufficient for inference without additional judgments and assumptions on the part of the experimenter. As Hammond explained, in an experiment "[t]he cause of the effect on the dependent variable was the totality of conditions sufficient to produce it."[71] Thus the experimental intervention consisted of not only the experimental drug, for example, but the manner of its delivery. Thus drawing generalizations about the intervention's effectiveness in other situations could be risky.

These participants also maintained that the differences between study designs, while real, had been overstated.[72] Cornfield acknowledged that while experimental studies offered greater control, "[t]here are no such categories as first-class evidence and second-class evidence."[73] The difference was one of degree rather than of kind, and these researchers used the consistency between case-control and cohort findings to further this argument. There was no single, crucial experimental design that would trump all other forms of evidence. Instead, a number of participants emphasized the need to synthesize a diverse body of evidence and look at the interrelationships between findings.[74] As Lilienfeld stated, "[t]he plausibility of the causal hypothesis is assessed, not in terms of the results of one particular study or a 'crucial experiment,' but in terms of the totality of available biologic evidence."[75] These researchers therefore focused on gathering evidence that would refute the specific arguments of Berkson, Fisher, and other sceptics; these included studies of smoking patterns and lung-cancer epidemiology to evaluate potential bias.[76]

Proponents of the cigarette link proposed their own guidelines for drawing causal inferences from a body of epidemiologic evidence. They held the strength of an association to be important because a strong non-causal association required a strong confounder to explain it, and weak associations were more likely to be artifacts of selection bias. (The reasoning went, "such an obvious fact could hardly escape the attention of any conscientious investigator."[77]) In contrast, Yerushalmy had rejected strength of association as a criterion for inference because its evaluation was necessarily subjective; "there is no rational way to decide how large a difference there must be before we accept it as indicating a cause–effect relationship".[78] Additionally, some argued that the lack of specificity of smoking as a cause of lung cancer was not a source of worry, because the association between smoking and lung cancer in particular was so dramatic relative to other adverse effects.[79] Some researchers believed that biological plausibility substantially reinforced causal inferences. However, it meant not that biological mechanisms had to be completely worked out – only that findings should be consistent with current medical and biological knowledge.[80] Additionally, because of the complex nature of cancer causation and the many differences between animal models and humans, negative animal experiments were of little relevance to human cancer aetiology.[81]

Proponents also advocated what they saw as a more pragmatic approach to causal inference that differed from the rigid experimental model promoted by Fisher – one that explicitly applied a less rigorous (or, at least, not impossible) standard of proof before public health action.[82] For example, Brian MacMahon, Thomas Pugh, and Johannes Ipsen in their influential 1960 textbook urged that when experimental evidence is unavailable "complete evidence will never be at hand, and it may be imprudent to await it."[83] Researchers from the American Cancer Society, the American Heart Association, NCI, and the National Heart Institute banded together as the Study Group on Smoking and Health (the group included Cornfield, Haenszel, Hammond, Lilienfeld, and Wynder) and produced two review articles, in 1957 and 1959. These reviews summarized the evidence from epidemiological, pathological, and animal studies, explained how the evidence answered the particular concerns raised by sceptics such as Fisher and Berkson, and concluded that public health action was warranted.[84]

CONCLUSION

At least two distinct approaches to aetiologic research were in conflict in this debate, one rooted in experimental science and Fisher's theory of statistical inference and another in the more pragmatic concerns of public-health practice. So what factors determined where individuals fell in this division? Most of the epidemiologists and biostatisticians who were proponents of the smoking-and-lung-cancer hypothesis belonged to a younger generation. NCI statisticians such as Cornfield, Haenszel, and Mantel were not steeped in Fisher's experimentalism. Indeed, they arrived at NCI as mathematical statisticians without prior experience in medical or biological research, and while at NCI they aided laboratory scientists, clinical trialists, and epidemiologists alike. Thus, it is not surprising that they would give more attention to devising ways to get more use out of existing data rather than to worrying about the origins of those data. In contrast, Dorn, Gilliam, and Palmer had first-hand experience with the challenges of gathering health and mortality data, which probably made them more cognizant of the shortcomings of those data. Additionally, ideological differences probably exerted some influence as well. While Berkson and Fisher showed visible resentment towards the declarations of public-health officials, Cornfield, Haenszel, Levin, Lilienfeld, and Shimkin all spoke about the obligation of public-health officials to take precautionary actions.

That said, no simple dichotomy will account for all the nuances of this complex debate, and the similarities between these participants were as important as their differences. All the participants acted as reformers, voicing concern about improper use of epidemiologic concepts and methods in the medical literature. For example, Lilienfeld, like Gilliam and Dorn, worked to educate medical researchers about proper selection of cases and controls,[85] and Hill, like Fisher, strongly advocated randomization and criticized excessive focus on tests of statistical significance, while also defending the observational approach.[86]

The more pragmatic approach largely won out. The surgeon general's 1964 report employed a set of criteria for judging a diverse body of evidence that incorporated key elements of the earlier debate (such as the strength, specificity, and consistency of the association),[87] and Hill's subsequent list of causal criteria has become a classic.[88] Berkson and Fisher became increasingly marginalized as a consensus emerged about tobacco, and their rhetoric grew increasingly spiteful. Yet, despite this seeming victory, epidemiologists continued to re-examine similar themes (such as balancing the rigours of science with the obligations of public health) in an ever-unfolding debate about the scope and direction of the discipline. They continue to do so to this day.[89]

NOTES

1 Editorial, "What and Who Is an Epidemiologist?" *American Journal of Public Health* 32 (1942), 414–5; C.-E.A. Winslow, "What Is Epidemiology?" (editorial), *American Journal of Public Health* 38 (1948), 852–6; J.E. Gordon, "Epidemiology – Old and New," *Journal of the Michigan State Medical Society* 49 (1950), 194–9; "The Epidemiologic Method" (editorial), *New*

England Journal of Medicine 254 (1956), 1044–5; Thomas Parran, "Nationwide Need – Epidemiologists," *Journal of the American Medical Association* 163 (1957), 742–3.

2 Allan M. Brandt, "The Cigarette, Risk, and American Culture," *Daedalus* (fall 1990), 162–3; Paolo Vineis and Neal Caporaso, "Tobacco and Cancer: Epidemiology and the Laboratory," *Environmental Health Perspectives* 103 (1995), 156–60.

3 "Experimental Links between Tobacco and Lung Cancer" (editorial), *British Medical Journal* (3 May 1958), 1050–1.

4 Sander Greenland, "Re: 'Those Who Were Wrong'" (letter), *American Journal of Epidemiology* 132 (1990), 585–6; Jan P. Vandenbroucke, "Those Who Were Wrong," *American Journal of Epidemiology* 130 (1989), 3–5.

5 Colin White, "Research on Smoking and Lung Cancer: A Landmark in the History of Chronic Disease Epidemiology," *Yale Journal of Biology and Medicine* 63 (1990), 29–46; Richard Doll, "Fifty Years of Research on Tobacco," *Journal of Epidemiology and Biostatistics* 5 (2000), 321–9; J. Clemmesen, "Lung Cancer from Smoking: Delays and Attitudes, 1912–1965," *American Journal of Industrial Medicine* 23 (1993), 941–53; Ernst L. Wynder, "Tobacco as a Cause of Lung Cancer: Some Reflections," *American Journal of Epidemiology* 146 (1997), 687–94.

6 James T. Patterson, *The Dread Disease: Cancer and Modern American Culture* (Cambridge, Mass.: Harvard University Press, 1987).

7 M. Gover, *Cancer Mortality in the United States. I. Trend of Recorded Cancer Mortality in the Death Registration States of 1900, from 1900 to 1935*, Public Health Bulletin No. 248 (Washington, DC: Government Printing Office, 1939).

8 Harold L. Stewart, "The Making of a Biometrician: Harold Fred Dorn, 1906–1963," in R.J.C. Harris, ed., UICC Monograph Series, vol. 9, Ninth International Cancer Congress (Berlin: Springer-Verlag, 1967); "Obituary," *American Statistician* 17 (1963), 53.

9 Harold F. Dorn. "Illness from Cancer in the United States," *Public Health Reports* 59 (1944), 33–48, 65–77, 97–115; Joseph W. Mountin, Harold F. Dorn, and Bert R. Boone, "The Incidence of Cancer in Atlanta, Ga., and Surrounding Counties," *Public Health Reports* 54 (1939), 1255–6.

10 Harold F. Dorn and Samuel A. Stouffer, "Criteria of Differential Mortality," *Journal of the American Statistical Association* 28 (1933), 402–13; Harold F. Dorn, "The Incidence and Future Expectancy of Mental Disease," *Public Health Reports* 53 (1939), 1991–2004; Harold F. Dorn, "The Relative Amount of Ill-Health in Rural and Urban Communities," *Public Health Reports* 53 (1938), 1181–95.

11 Harold Fred Dorn, "The Effect of Allocation of Non-Resident Deaths upon Official Mortality Statistics," PhD dissertation, University of Wisconsin–Madison, 1933; Harold F. Dorn, "The Effect of Allocation of Non-

Resident Deaths upon Official Mortality Statistics," *Journal of the American Statistical Association* 27 (1932), 401–12.

12 Harold F. Dorn, "Illness from Cancer in the United States," *Public Health Reports* 59 (1944), 33–4; Mountin et al., "The Incidence of Cancer in Atlanta, Ga., and Surrounding Counties."

13 John R. Heller, "The National Cancer Institute: A Twenty-Year Retrospect," *Journal of the National Cancer Institute* 19 (1957), 147–90.

14 "Dr. Alexander Gilliam, Former NCI Scientist, Dies of Cancer Dec. 12," *NIH Record*, 15 Jan. 15, 1964; "Dr. A.G. Gilliam Dies: Expert on Epidemiology," *Evening Star*, Washington, DC, 14 Dec. 1963.

15 "Project Report Form, NCI-056," in *Analysis of Program Activities, National Institutes of Health, National Cancer Institute*, vol. 1 (Bethesda, Md: National Institutes of Health, U.S. Public Health Service, 1954).

16 Alexander Gilliam, Biographical File, Alan Mason Chesney Medical Archives, Johns Hopkins Medical Institutions, Baltimore, Md.

17 Alexander G. Gilliam, "A Note on Estimates of the Rate of Development of Metastasis in Patients with Cancer of the Breast," *Surgery, Gynecology, and Obstetrics* 94 (1952), 641–4.

18 Alexander G. Gilliam, "Age, Sex, and Race Selection at Death from Leukemia and the Lymphomas," *Blood* 8 (1952), 693–702.

19 Harold F. Dorn, "The Increase in Cancer of the Lung," *Industrial Medicine and Surgery* 23 (1954), 253–7; Johannes Clemmesen, "Bronchial Carcinoma – A Pandemic," *Danish Medical Bulletin* 1 (1954), 37–46.

20 Alexander Gilliam, "Some Aspects of the Lung Cancer Problem," *Military Medicine* 116 (1955), 163 and 166.

21 Alexander G. Gilliam, Benno K. Milmore, and J. William Lloyd, "Trends of Mortality Attributed to Carcinoma of the Lung: Possible Effects of Faulty Certification of Deaths to Other Respiratory Diseases," *Cancer* 8 (1955), 1130–6; Benno K. Milmore, "Trend of Lung-Cancer Mortality in the United States: Some Limitations of Available Statistics," *Journal of the National Cancer Institute* 16 (1955), 267–84.

22 Gilliam et al., "Trends of Mortality Attributed to Carcinoma of the Lung," 1136.

23 Gilliam et al., "Trends of Lung Cancer Mortality," 623.

24 Gilliam, "Some Aspects of the Lung Cancer Problem," 166.

25 Gilliam et al., "Trends of Lung Cancer Mortality," 628, 627.

26 Alexander G. Gilliam, "Some Considerations on the Prevention of Cancer," in *Cancer Control* (Ann Arbor: University of Michigan School of Public Health, 1962).

27 Dorn, "Morbidity and Mortality from Cancer of the Lung," 554.

28 Harold F. Dorn, "Memorandum to Harold Stewart, January 29, 1954," in folder "Dorn, H. F. 1954," box 9, Harold Leroy Stewart Papers, 1946–78,

msc 228, History of Medicine Division, National Library of Medicine, Bethesda, Md.

29 Dorn, "The Increase in Cancer of the Lung," 257.

30 Morton L. Levin, "Some Epidemiological Features of Cancer," *Cancer* (Sept. 1948), 489–97.

31 M.S. Sacks and I. Seeman, "A Statistical Study of Mortality from Leukemia," *Blood* 2 (1947), 1–14; A.G. Gilliam and W.A. Walter, "Trends of Mortality from Leukemia in the United States, 1921–55," *Public Health Reports* 73(1958), 773–84; A.G. Gilliam and B. MacMahon, "Geographic Distribution and Trends of Leukemia in the United States," *Acta Unio Intern Contra Cancrum* 16 (1960), 1623–8; J.V. Cooke, "The Occurrence of Leukemia," *Blood* 9 (1954), 340–7; B. MacMahon, "Geographic Variation in Leukemia Mortality in the United States," *Public Health Reports* 72 (1957), 39–46; M.B. Shimkin, "Hodgkin's Disease: Mortality in the United States, 1921–1951; Race, Sex, and Age Distribution; Comparison with Leukemia," *Blood* 10 (1955), 1214–27.

32 Alexander G. Gilliam, "Changes in Age Selection of Fatal Poliomyelitis," *Public Health Reports* 63 (1948), 677–84.

33 I.M. Moriyama, "Needed Improvements in Mortality Data," *Public Health Reports* 9 (1952), 851–6; H.L. Dunn, "The Survey Approach to Morbidity and Health Data," *Public Health Reports* 67 (1952), 998–1002; H.F. Dorn, "Some Problems for Research in Mortality and Morbidity," *Public Health Reports* 71 (1956), 1–5; H.F. Dorn, "A Classification System for Morbidity Concepts," *Public Health Reports* 72 (1957), 1043–8; M.L. Levin, "Cancer Reporting in New York State," *Blood* 44 (1944), 880–3.

34 J.H. Ellenberg, M.H. Gail, and N.L. Geller, "Conversations with NIH Statisticians: Interviews with the Pioneers of Biostatistics at the United States National Institutes of Health," *Statistical Science* 12 (1997), 77–81; Samuel W. Greenhouse, "Some Reflections on the Beginnings and Development of Statistics in 'Your Father's NIH,'" *Statistical Science* 12 (1997), 82–7.

35 Jerome Cornfield, "A Method of Estimating Comparative Rates from Clinical Data: Applications to Cancer of the Lung, Breast, and Cervix," *Journal of the National Cancer Institute* 11 (1951), 1269–75; "Industrial Cancer Data Collection Methods (Conference Report)," *Public Health Reports* 69 (1954), 192–3; Nathan Mantel and William Haenszel, "Statistical Aspects of the Analysis of Data from Retrospective Studies of Disease," *Journal of the National Cancer Institute* 22 (1959), 719–48.

36 Herbert L. Lombard and Carl R. Doering, "Cancer Studies in Massachusetts. 2. Habits, Characteristics, and Environment of Individuals with and without Cancer," *New England Journal of Medicine* 198 (1928), 481–7; Jane E. Lane-Claypon, *A Further Report on Cancer of the Breast, with Special Refer-*

ence to Its Associated Antecedent Conditions, Reports on Public Health and Medical Subjects No. 32 (London: Ministry of Health, 1926).

37 A.C. Broders, "Squamous-Cell Epithelioma of the Lip: A Study of 537 Cases," *Journal of the American Medical Association* 74 (1920), 656–64; E.A. Potter and M.R. Tully, "The Statistical Approach to the Cancer Problem in Massachusetts," *American Journal of Public Health* 35 (1945), 485–90.

38 Harold F. Dorn, "Some Applications of Biometry in the Collection and Evaluation of Medical Data," *Journal of Chronic Diseases* 1 (1955), 638–64.

39 Ernst L. Wynder and Evarts A. Graham, "Tobacco Smoking as a Possible Etiologic Factor in Bronchiogenic Carcinoma," *Journal of the American Medical Association* 143 (1950), 329–36; M.L. Levin, H. Goldstein, and P.R. Gerhardt, "Cancer and Tobacco Smoking: A Preliminary Report," *Journal of the American Medical Association* 143 (1950), 336–8; R. Schrek, L.A. Baker, G.P. Ballard, and S. Dolgoff, "Tobacco Smoking as an Etiologic Factor in Disease. I. Cancer," *Cancer Research* 10 (1950), 49–58; C.A. Mills and M.M. Porter, "Tobacco Smoking Habits and Cancer of the Mouth and Respiratory System," *Cancer Research* 10 (1950), 539–42; R. Doll and A.B. Hill, *British Medical Journal* (30 Sept. 1950), 740–8.

40 Schrek et al., "Tobacco Smoking as an Etiologic Factor in Disease"; Mills et al., "Tobacco Smoking Habits and Cancer of the Mouth and Respiratory System."

41 Jacob Yerushalmy and Carroll E. Palmer, "On the Methodology of Investigations of Etiologic Factors in Chronic Diseases," *Journal of Chronic Disease* 10 (1959), 33; Joseph Berkson, "Limitations of the Application of Fourfold Table Analysis to Hospital Data," *Biometrics* 2 (1946), 47–53.

42 Berkson, "Limitations of the Application of Fourfold Table Analysis to Hospital Data."

43 Kenneth F. Maxcy, "Introduction," in Maxcy, ed., *Papers of Wade Hampton Frost, MD: A Contribution to Epidemiological Method* (New York: Commonwealth Fund, 1941).

44 Alexander G. Gilliam, "Opportunities for Application of Epidemiologic Method to Study of Cancer," *American Journal of Public Health* 43 (1953), 1250.

45 Alexander G. Gilliam, "Epidemiology in Noncommunicable Disease," *Public Health Reports* 69 (1954), 908.

46 Alexander G. Gilliam, "A Note on Evidence Relating to the Incidence of Primary Liver Cancer among the Bantu," *Journal of the National Cancer Institute* 15 (1954), 196; Charles Berman, "Primary Carcinoma of the Liver in the Bantu Races of South Africa," *South African Journal of Medical Science* 5 (1940), 54–72.

47 A.G. Gilliam and R.H. Onstott, "Results of Field Studies with the Brodie Poliomyelitis Vaccine," *Public Health Reports* 51 (1936), 160–71; Alexander G. Gilliam, "Efficacy of Cox-Type Vaccine in the Prevention of Natu-

rally Acquired Louse-Borne Typhus Fever," *American Journal of Hygiene* 44 (1946), 401–10.

48 Gilliam, "Opportunities for Application of Epidemiologic Method to Study of Cancer," 1250.

49 Harold F. Dorn, "Some Problems Arising in Prospective and Retrospective Studies of the Etiology of Disease," *New England Journal of Medicine* 261 (1959), 579.

50 Gilliam, "Epidemiology in Noncommunicable Disease," 910; Gilliam and Onstott, "Results of Field Studies with the Brodie Poliomyelitis Vaccine."

51 Harold F. Dorn, "Tobacco Consumption and Mortality from Cancer and Other Diseases," *Public Health Reports* 74 (1959), 581–93.

52 Colin White, "Sampling in Medical Research," *British Medical Journal* (12 Dec. 1953), 1284–8; Abraham M. Lilienfeld, "On the Methodology of Investigations of Etiologic Factors in Chronic Diseases – Some Comments," *Journal of Chronic Disease* 10 (1959), 41–6; Colin White and John C. Bailar, "Retrospective and Prospective Methods of Studying Association in Medicine," *American Journal of Public Health* 46 (1956), 35—44.

53 Schrek et al., "Tobacco Smoking as an Etiologic Factor in Disease."

54 White and Bailar, "Retrospective and Prospective Methods of Studying Association in Medicine."

55 A.S. Kraus, "The Use of Hospital Data in Studying the Association between a Characteristic and a Disease," *Public Health Reports* 69 (1954), 1211–4.

56 Morton L. Levin, "Etiology of Lung Cancer," *New York State Journal of Medicine* (15 March 1954), 769–77.

57 Paul D. Stolley, "When Genius Errs: R.A. Fisher and the Lung Cancer Controversy," *American Journal of Epidemiology* 133 (1991), 416–33; Stephen J. Gould, "The Smoking Gun of Eugenics," *Natural History* (Dec. 1991), 8–16.

58 Sir Ronald Fisher, "Cigarettes, Cancer, and Statistics," *Centennial Review* 2 (1958), 151–66; "Alleged Dangers of Cigarette-Smoking" (letters), *British Medical Journal* 2 (6 July 1957), 43, and 2 (3 Aug. 1957), 297–8; "Lung Cancer and Cigarettes" (letter), *Nature* 182 (12 July 1958), 108.

59 Harry M. Marks, *The Progress of Experiment: Science and Therapeutic Reform in the United States, 1900–1990* (Cambridge: Cambridge University Press, 1997); J. Rosser Matthews, *Quantification and the Quest for Medical Certainty* (Princeton, NJ: Princeton University Press, 1995).

60 Abraham M. Lilienfeld, "Emotional and Other Selected Characteristics of Cigarette Smokers and Nonsmokers as Related to Epidemiological Studies of Lung Cancer and Other Diseases," *Journal of the National Cancer Institute* 22 (1959), 259–82; Clark W. Heath, "Differences Between Smokers and Nonsmokers," AMA *Archives of Internal Medicine* 101 (1958), 377–88.

61 Joseph Berkson, "Smoking and Lung Cancer: Some Observations on Two Recent Reports," *Journal of the American Statistical Association* 53 (1958), 28–38.

62 Jacob Yerushalmy, "The Relationship of Parents' Cigarette Smoking to the Outcome of Pregnancy – Implications as to the Problem of Inferring Causation from Observed Associations," *American Journal of Epidemiology* 93 (1971), 455; Jacob Yerushalmy, "Mothers' Cigarette Smoking and Survival of Infant," *American Journal of Obstetrics and Gynecology* 88 (1964), 505–18; sometimes Yerushalmy went even further and claimed that studies tended to *disprove* the direct causation hypothesis. Jacob Yerushalmy, "Cigarette Smoking and Infant Survival" (letter), *American Journal of Obstetrics and Gynecology* 91 (1965), 883–4.

63 K.A. Brownlee, "A Note on the Effects of Nonresponse on Surveys," *Journal of the American Statistical Association* 52 (1957), 29–32; Anthony Ciocco, "Statistical Considerations and Evaluations of Epidemiologic Evidence," in G. James and T. Rosenthal, eds., *Tobacco and Health* (Springfield: Charles C. Thomas, 1962); Jacob Yerushalmy, "Statistical Considerations and Evaluation of Epidemiological Evidence," in G. James and T. Rosenthal, eds., *Tobacco and Health* (Springfield: Charles C. Thomas, 1962), 208–30.

64 Alfred S. Evans, *Causation and Disease: A Chronological Journey* (New York: Plenum Medical Book Company, 1993); J.E. Gordon, "The Twentieth Century – Yesterday, Today, and Tomorrow (1920–)," in F.H. Top, ed., *The History of American Epidemiology* (St Louis: C.V. Mosby Company, 1952), 114–67.

65 E. Cuyler Hammond, "Cause and Effect," in Ernest L. Wynder, ed., *The Biologic Effects of Tobacco* (Boston: Little, Brown, and Co., 1955); Ernest L. Wynder, "An Appraisal of the Smoking–Lung Cancer Issue," *New England Journal of Medicine* 264 (1961), 1235–40; Yerushalmy and Palmer, "On the Methodology of Investigations of Etiologic Factors in Chronic Diseases," 39; R.A. Fisher, "Indeterminism and Natural Selection," *Philosophy of Science* 1 (1934), 99–117.

66 Gilliam, "Epidemiology in Noncommunicable Diseases."

67 Yerushalmy and Palmer, "On the Methodology of Investigations of Etiologic Factors in Chronic Diseases."

68 J. Yerushalmy and H.E. Hilleboe, "Fat in the Diet and Mortality from Heart Disease: A Methodologic Note," *New York State Journal of Medicine* 57 (1957), 2343–52; Yerushalmy, "Statistical Considerations and Evaluation of Epidemiological Evidence."

69 Joseph Berkson, "Smoking and Cancer of the Lung," *Proceedings of the Staff Meetings of the Mayo Clinic* 35 (1960), 369, 376.

70 Abraham M. Lilienfeld, "Epidemiologic Methods and Inferences," in H. Hilleboe and G. Larimore, eds., *Preventive Medicine: Principles of Prevention*

in the Occurrence and Progression of Disease (Philadelphia: W.B. Saunders Company, 1959), 662–82; Austin Bradford Hill, "Observation and Experiment," *New England Journal of Medicine* 248 (1953), 995–1001; Hammond, "Cause and Effect," 193; Brian MacMahon, Thomas F. Pugh, and Johannes Ipsen, *Epidemiologic Methods* (Boston: Little, Brown and Company, 1960), 15; Alexander G. Gilliam, "Opportunities for Application of Epidemiologic Method to Study of Cancer"; Study Group on Smoking and Health, "Smoking and Health," *Science* 125 (1957), 1129–33.

71 Hammond, "Cause and Effect," 190; Jerome Cornfield, "Statistical Relationships and Proof in Medicine," *American Statistician* (Dec. 1954), 20.

72 Dorn, "Some Applications of Biometry in the Collection and Evaluation of Medical Data," 655; White and Bailar, "Retrospective and Prospective Methods of Studying Association in Medicine"; M.L. Levin, A.S. Kraus, I.D. Goldberg, and P.R. Gerhardt, "Problems in the Study of Occupation and Smoking in Relation to Lung Cancer," *Cancer* 8 (1955), 932–6; Jerome Cornfield and William Haenszel, "Some Aspects of Retrospective Studies," *Journal of Chronic Diseases* 11 (1960), 529.

73 Cornfield, "Statistical Relationships and Proof in Medicine," 20.

74 Haenszel, "Epidemiological Tests of Theories on Lung Cancer Etiology," 163, 170; Cornfield, "Statistical Relationships and Proof in Medicine," 21; Cornfield and Haenszel, "Some Aspects of Retrospective Studies," 529–30; Wynder, "An Appraisal of the Smoking–Lung Cancer Issue," 1238; Morton L. Levin, "Etiology of Lung Cancer," *New York State Journal of Medicine* (15 March 1954), 769–77; Samuel J. Cutler, "A Review of the Statistical Evidence on the Association between Smoking and Lung Cancer," *Journal of the American Statistical Association* 50 (1955), 267–82.

75 Abraham M. Lilienfeld, "On the Methodology of Investigations of Etiologic Factors in Chronic Diseases – Some Comments," *Journal of Chronic Diseases* 10 (1959), 46.

76 William Haenszel and Michael B. Shimkin, "Smoking Patterns and Epidemiology of Lung Cancer on the United States: Are They Compatible?," *Journal of the National Cancer Institute* 16 (1956), 1417–41; William Haenszel, Michael B. Shimkin, and Harold P. Miller, *Tobacco Smoking Patterns in the United States*, Public Health Monograph No. 45 (Washington, DC: U.S. Department of Health, Education, and Welfare, 1956); William Haenszel, Michael B. Shimkin, and Nathan Mantel, "A Retrospective Study of Lung Cancer in Women," *Journal of the National Cancer Institute* 21 (1958), 825–42.

77 Hammond, "Cause and Effect," 184; Lilienfeld, "Epidemiologic Methods and Inferences," 109; Cornfield and Haenszel, "Some Aspects of Retrospective Studies," 530;

78 Yerushalmy, "Statistical Considerations and Evaluation of Epidemiological Evidence," 227.

79 Lilienfeld, "On the Methodology of Investigations of Etiologic Factors in Chronic Diseases – Some Comments," 43.
80 Ibid.; Wynder, "An Appraisal of the Smoking–Lung Cancer Issue," 1238.
81 Dorn, "Cancer Morbidity Surveys: A Tool for Testing Theories of Cancer Etiology," 615–6; Lilienfeld, "Epidemiologic Methods and Inferences," 111; Wynder, "An Appraisal of the Smoking–Lung Cancer Issue," 1238.
82 Hammond, "Cause and Effect"; Wynder, "An Appraisal of the Smoking–Lung Cancer Issue," *New England Journal of Medicine* 264 (1961), 1241–5; Cornfield, "Statistical Relationships and Proof in Medicine"; Abraham M. Lilienfeld, "Epidemiologic Methods and Inferences," in H. Hilleboe and G. Larimore, eds., *Preventive Medicine: Principles of Prevention in the Occurrence and Progression of Disease* (Philadelphia: W.B. Saunders, 1959); L. Breslow, L. Hoaglin, G. Rasmussen, and H.K. Abrams, "Occupations and Cigarette Smoking as Factors in Lung Cancer," *American Journal of Public Health* 44 (1954), 171–81.
83 MacMahon, Pugh, and Ipsen, *Epidemiologic Methods.*
84 Study Group on Smoking and Health, "Smoking and Health"; Jerome Cornfield, William Haenszel, E. Cuyler Hammond, Abraham M. Lilienfeld, Michael B. Shimkin, and Ernst L. Wynder, "Smoking and Lung Cancer: Recent Evidence and a Discussion of Some Questions," *Journal of the National Cancer Institute* 22 (1959), 173–203.
85 Abraham M. Lilienfeld, "Selection of Probands and Controls," *American Journal of Human Genetics* 6 (1954), 100–4.
86 Austin Bradford Hill, "The Clinical Trial," *British Medical Bulletin* 7 (1951), 279; Hill, "Observation and Experiment."
87 *Smoking and Health: Report of the Advisory Committee to the Surgeon General of the Public Health Service,* PHS Publication No. 1103 (Washington, DC: Department of Health, Education, and Welfare, 1964).
88 Austin Bradford Hill, "The Environment and Disease: Association or Causation?" *Proceedings of the Royal Society of Medicine* 58 (1965), 295–300.
89 Milton Terris, "The Scope and Methods of Epidemiology," *American Journal of Public Health* 52 (1962), 1371–6; A.M.-M. Payne, "The Scope and Methods of Epidemiology," *American Journal of Public Health* 52 (1962), 1502–4; George L. Saiger, "A Critique on the Methods and Scope of Epidemiology" (letter), *American Journal of Public Health* 53 (1963), 1696–1700.

PART FOUR

Reducing Uncertainty and the Politics of Health

12

William Farr and Quantification in Nineteenth-Century English Public Health

MICHAEL DONNELLY

> [U]nder Farr's skilful guidance ... evolved a body of epidemiological information which laid bare the amount and conditions of prevalence of epidemic diseases, which gave ignominious publicity to the areas of excessive mortality, and which made it possible to obtain accurate information as to the social, industrial and domestic circumstances associated with disease.[1]
>
> Sir Arthur Newsholme

This paper draws on the career of Dr William Farr (1807–1883) to illustrate several uses of quantification in mid-nineteenth century public health in Britain.[2] Farr served as compiler of abstracts, and later as superintendent of statistics, at the General Register Office of England and Wales, from 1839 until his retirement in 1879. From that position he and his coworkers had unprecedented opportunities to compile, diffuse, and analyse vital statistics. Many of the practices and techniques that Farr adopted left a lasting imprint on public health medicine in England and elsewhere.

A DISTINCTIVE ERA

After outlining the context of Farr's innovations, this essay looks at his early work on vital statistics, his discovery of statistical regularity, and his development of a baseline, "regular" mortality.

To explain what is distinctive about Farr's use of quantification, I begin schematically, contrasting the early and mid-nineteenth century with what followed and with what preceded it. I am dealing here with vital statistics before the diffusion of germ theory and well before bacteriology. What drove investigations in epidemiology at this time were ideas of "miasma" or other non-specific social and environmental influences on health and disease. In Chadwick's phrase, "all smell is disease." The English sanitary program, as a response to those "smells," was likewise non-specific, and the medical historian Shryock has suggested that "public health almost ceased to be a medical field – sanitary programs could be, and often were, directed by statisticians and engineers, rather than by physicians."[3]

"Statistics" had a different meaning in this period. Nowadays we think of it as a branch of mathematics, a kit of techniques for managing masses of information. A current-day practitioner would characterize statistics as concerned with the measurement of uncertainty;[4] it provides techniques for validating observations in experimental and non-experimental science. The statistician is thus an underlabourer who tries to offer guarantees for data and to clarify, or formalize, the logic of drawing causal connections between phenomena. In sum, the self-characterization of a modern statistician is *methodological.* Statistics in that sense goes back by and large only to the late-nineteenth century, to the mathematical advances of Galton, Pearson, Yule, and so on.

I focus here on a period that antedates most of what we nowadays take for granted as foundations for statistics. But then what did "statistics" mean in the early- and mid-nineteenth century? It was arguably the original empirical social science. About 1840 a statistician would have characterized the field not in methodological but in *substantive* terms. Dr William Guy, for instance, writing in 1839, described statistics simply as "the application of the numerical method to the varying conditions and social relations of mankind."[5] In early and mid-century, the etymology of the term was still very much alive: statistics was state-istics. The approach of this science involved amassing and collating facts and attempting to discern patterns among them. The tools were by and large arithmetic.

In contrast to a later era, Farr's generation belongs in a sense to the prehistory of modern mathematical statistics. By contrast with what came earlier, Farr's generation built on and greatly extended the statistical approach of the political arithmeticians of the late-seventeenth century. John Graunt's *Natural and Political Observations* (1662) analysed the London bills of mortality, making a number of ingenious inferences from the figures. He found, for instance, that the number of deaths in London (leaving apart epidemic years) tended to be fairly regular, that urban death rates exceeded rural rates, and that the ratio of male to female births was roughly 108 to 100. Graunt was using statistics as "an instrument of observation in order to bring out ... phenomena 'perceptible only to the reason.'"[6] Edmund Halley published his famous *Life Table* in 1693, based on fuller information (on births and deaths in Breslau from 1687 to 1691) than had been available to Graunt a generation earlier. These were important first steps in vital statistics and demography, but, as Cullen notes of eighteenth-century developments, "seeds were often laid down which were long in germinating and even failed for lack of nourishment so that replanting had to occur later."[7] One obstacle was the absence of reliable data for vital statistics – a problem not systematically tackled in England until the establishment of the General Register Office (GRO) after 1837.

FARR AND VITAL STATISTICS

Before taking up his post at the GRO, Farr had already distinguished himself as a leading proponent for vital statistics. In 1837 he contributed an essay on "Vital Statistics" to McCulloch's *Account of the British Empire*[8] – an essay, as Arthur Newsholme recalled, "not extravagantly described ... as 'the foundation of a new science,' the alphabet of which had been framed in the commentaries of Captain John Graunt (1620–1674)."[9] That 1837 piece contains many of the themes and concerns that Farr would develop over a long career – notably, his appreciation of life tables and their varied possible uses as tools of investigation – purposes far broader than those of contemporary actuaries.

The life table, in Farr's words, describes "the march of a generation through life."[10] The conception is straightforward: a cohort of individuals begins its walk through life together; some members (quite a few) disappear soon; others die off at later stages. The life table captures those events, based on painstaking reconstruction from mortality data. If 1,000 started together, the table shows how many would die at each succeeding year of their age.

What made Farr's use of life tables so productive was an additional assumption – that vital phenomena contained regularities and that observations of them formed series, which one could describe mathematically. If vital phenomena were law-abiding, one could seek statistical laws to describe them and demonstrate such laws by comparing an observed series with a computed one.[11]

A striking early application of these assumptions was a series of studies of epidemic disease that Farr published in the late 1830s. Applying principles similar to those underlying life tables, he constructed sickness tables of epidemics and their course. No one had done this before the 1830s. Indeed it hadn't occurred to people to think in terms of "laws" of sickness, whose existence Farr set out to demonstrate.[12] He was from the beginning of his career confident that

Table 1 Sickness table for smallpox

Day	*Sick*	*To recover*	*To die*	*Terminating*	*Recovering*	*Dying*
0						
5	10,000	6,589	3,411	317		317
10	9,683	6,589	3,094	1,370	46	1,324
15	8,313	6,543	1,770	1,185	54	1,131
20	7,128	6,489	639	578	265	313
25	6,550	6,224	326	769	639	130
30	5,781	5,585	196	976	898	78
35	4,805	4,687	118	1055	1088	47
40	3,750	3,679	71	922	894	28
45	2,828	2,785	43	694	677	17
50	2,134	2,108	26	515	513	2
55	1,619	1,595	24	390	388	2
60	1,229	1,207	22	295	293	2
65	934	914	20	225	223	2
70	709	691	18	170	168	2
75	539	523	16	129	127	2
80	410	396	14	98	96	2
85	312	300	12	75	73	2
90	237	227	10	57	55	2
95	180	172	8	44	42	2
100	136	130	6	34	32	2
105	102	98	4			

Source: William Farr, "On a Method for Determining the Danger and the Duration of Diseases at Every Period of their Progress," *British Annals of Medicine* 1 (1837), 72–9.

definite laws regulated epidemic disease – a specific case of larger regularities in vital phenomena.

In one study he constructed such a sickness table for smallpox cases, drawing records from the London Small-pox Hospital. In place of the life table's years of life, he constructed an axis for days of sickness, at five-day intervals from the fifth to the hundred-and-fifth day. The table records not only the numbers of those dying over each five-day period, but the numbers recovering and those remaining sick. For each successive five-day period during the course of the epidemic, Farr then compares the numbers dying and recovering, or, as he puts it, the chances of recovery or death at different phases of the epidemic (Table 1).

At the end of the fifth day, for instance, out of 10,000 who are sick, 6,589 will recover and 3,411 will die – a probability of recovery of 6,589/10,000 or nearly 66 to 34. At the end of the twentieth day the chances of recovery rise to 6,489/7,128, or about 9 in 10. Farr's claim is that he has discovered ("deduced") two laws at work – a law of mor-

Table 2 Deaths in epidemic (mean deaths in consecutive quarters of reporting) versus regular series

Deaths observed in the decline of the epidemic

1	2	3	4	5	6	7
4,365	4,087	3,767	3,416	2,743	2,019	1,631

Deaths in a regular series

1	2	3	4	5	6	7
4,364	4,147	3,767	3,272	2,716	2,156	1,634

Source: William Farr, Second Annual Report of the Registrar-General, 96 (Parliamentary Papers, 1840), XVII, 19.

tality in smallpox and a law of recovery. Thus he concludes that "there is a law governing the terminations of diseased action; that this law is of a peculiar nature, never before discovered in the relations of vital phenomena; and that it may be investigated, or applied so as to yield a great variety of important results, without any more than an elementary knowledge of arithmetic."[13] Moreover, his reading of the table suggested that the "law" regulating smallpox is "as precise as any of those which guide the heavenly bodies in their courses."

In related papers Farr projected the mortality and recovery curves for a variety of epidemics, of cholera as well as smallpox. He reported, for instance, the pattern of mortality in another smallpox epidemic, laying out "deaths observed in the decline of the epidemic" over time, and then constructed a parallel geometric series, demonstrating an admirable fit between the two (Table 2). As Eyler notes, "The fact that epidemics could be described by geometric series suggested the possibility of predicting their future course."[14] In 1840, when smallpox deaths again began to rise, Farr demonstrated that the rate of increase in the prior epidemic was a close predictor of the pattern in the current one (Table 3).

In each case he fit a curve to chart the epidemic's progress – a curve like a projectile's, or otherwise, a "regular curve." Alluding to Farr's results, William Guy constructed a physical analogy: "the obstacles which oppose the increase of population, act precisely in the same way as the resistance that is offered to a moving body by the medium in which it moves. The curve, too, which represents the mortality of small-pox at the several periods of its duration, is, like the curves which represent increasing and decreasing material forces, a regular one."[15] Somewhat fancifully, Guy described such curves as determined by the interaction of increasing and decreasing forces,

Table 3 Deaths by smallpox, 1839–40

	Registered	Rate of increase in prior epidemic (1837)
13 weeks Oct.–Dec. 1839	60	60
13 weeks Jan.–Apr. 1840	104	99
13 weeks Apr.–July 1840	170	163
13 weeks July–Oct. 1840	253	267

Source: William Farr, "Note on the Present Epidemic of Smallpox, and On the Necessity of Arresting its Ravages," *Lancet*, 1 (1840–41), 352.
Note: observed and calculated series describing rise of epidemic.

analogous to a projectile's momentum against the gravitational pull exerted on it.

STATISTICAL REGULARITY

The key here – a very familiar theme in this period of statistical enthusiasm – was Farr's confidence in having discovered statistical regularity in phenomena; disease, like life and death, is law-like, at least when the effects of disease are observed in the aggregate in populations. The "regular curve" is itself a satisfying result, as if it were confirmation of the lawfulness of phenomena.

Whatever one would make of such apparent regularities now, their discovery undoubtedly fuelled enthusiasm for statistics. The idea of regularity (stability in rates of phenomena) was not new; indeed eighteenth-century demographers had commented extensively on observed regularities in births, deaths, and marriages. What changed dramatically, however, were the scope and scale of regularities that statisticians looked for and expected to find. In some respects this was probably an artifact of the "avalanche of printed numbers" described by Ian Hacking.[16] The appearance of continuous annual series of data (not merely periodic enumerations) seemed to reveal more and more regularities in vital and social phenomena, more and more instances of rates of phenomena proceeding stably over time. It was like witnessing, as many observers noted, the emergence of new order from the midst of chaos.

Like others in the statistical movement, Farr was caught up in the enthusiasm. The clearest indication of his difference from the past is his new confidence or faith in regularities, as revealed in the abundant data, the avalanche of printed numbers, that Farr himself helped produce and diffuse. Despite the traditional elements in Farr's thinking, notably the commonplaces of his environmentalism,[17] the scale and scope of vital statistics opened up new possibilities.

Farr's basic tools were simple rates – rates of death, sickness, birth, marriage, fertility. The numerators in such ratios he drew from the registration data, the denominators from the census. Both sets of figures were gathered in the same geographical areas, and the sets were reasonably compatible (increasingly so after the 1841 census). Farr concerned himself self-consciously both with the numerators (finding and identifying cases) and with the denominators (populations and subpopulations). In finding cases, for instance, early in his career at the GRO he noted problems in classifying medical returns when the diagnosis of disease was so uncertain. It was important to gather more systematic details from death certificates, but that also required some consistency in the nomenclature of disease: "The advantages of a uniform statistical nomenclature, however imperfect, are so obvious, that it is surprising no attention has been paid to its enforcement in Bills of Mortality. Each disease has, in many instances, been denoted by three or four terms ... vague, inconvenient names have been employed, or complications have been recorded instead of primary diseases. The nomenclature is of as much importance in this department of inquiry as weights and measures in the physical sciences, and should be settled without delay."[18]

Farr also stressed centralized surveillance of health returns. Information returned from individual physicians in various locales might in the aggregate reveal patterns difficult for those physicians to discern in their dispersed practices. The influenza epidemic of 1847 in London provides a dramatic example. In early 1848, as the epidemic declined, Farr retraced mortality rates week by week over the last months of the previous year. Mortality rates were fairly stable through late October and into early November, which Farr took to be a baseline for mortality in that season (Table 4). In late November and into December there was a sharp increase in total deaths – "excess mortality" which was marked for deaths attributed to influenza, as well as to other respiratory ailments (bronchitis, pneumonia, and asthma).

Farr's collating of the figures led him to suspect considerable misreporting: "In some of these cases the inflammation specified was the primary disease, in others secondary, and in many it was purely influenza – mis-reported."[19] Through the course of the epidemic, death certificates attributed only 1,147 deaths to influenza. Farr's estimate was almost 3,200. In effect he was criticizing physicians rather

Table 4 Deaths, by cause, influenza epidemic, London, 1847

Week ending	*Total deaths*	*Influenza*	*Bronchitis*	*Pneumonia*	*Asthma*
30 Oct.	934	1	36	62	12
6 Nov.	1,052	2	49	68	12
13 Nov.	1,098	4	58	79	12
20 Nov.	1,086	4	61	95	12
27 Nov.	1,677	36	196	170	77
4 Dec.	2,454	198	343	306	86
11 Dec.	2,416	374	299	294	78
18 Dec.	1,946	270	234	189	52
25 Dec.	1,247	142	107	131	14
1 Jan.	1,599	127	138	148	26
Totals					
24 Oct.–27 Nov.	4,181	11	204	304	48
28 Nov.–1 Jan.	11,339	1,147	1,317	1,238	333
Average					
24 Oct.–27 Nov.	1,045	3	54	76	12
Excess					
28 Nov.–1 Jan.	5,068	1,131	1,011	782	261

total excess respiratory deaths = 3,185
total excess non-respiratory deaths = 1,883

Source: Reconstructed from *Tenth Annual Report of the Registrar-General* by Alexander Langmuir, 8, *International Journal of Epidemiology* 5 (1976), 16.

sharply: "There is a strong disposition among some English practitioners, not only to localize disease but to see nothing but a local disease."[20] What the example illustrates is a more general capability that health authorities were developing, an intelligence apparatus to survey the health of the body politic. Local physicians were the source of much of the information, but because of their acquaintance only with local conditions, they played a distinctly subsidiary role.[21]

Farr's most celebrated contributions dealt with denominators in the cases-to-population ratios, with information about populations derived principally from the census. Farr was a consultant on the 1841 and subsequent censuses, helping to, among other things, produce better data on the age structure of the population and fuller details on occupations. His favoured approach in investigating populations was to examine differential morbidity and mortality – comparing, for example, the experience of different occupational groups or of different geographical units in the country. In his 1851 report, for instance, "drawing attention to the excessive mortality among butchers, greater than in any other class except innkeepers, he asks why? is it diet? or excessive drinking? or exposure to heat and cold? or the effluvia from decaying matter? here setting out some of the lines of an exhaustive inquiry into occupational mortality."[22]

"REGULAR" MORTALITY

Farr's basic approach for studying differential mortality was to establish a baseline of "regular" mortality (eventually a standardized death rate) against which to compare higher rates. The aim was to estimate and localize excess or preventable mortality – for instance, geographical units where rates rose above regular mortality because of presumptively remediable evils. In sum, this was investigation to identify targets for preventive medicine. Farr's aim was already clear in his first contribution to the annual reports of the registrar-general (in 1839) – a letter to the registrar-general printed as an appendix. Cullen aptly calls it Farr's "manifesto":[23]

> In exhibiting the high mortality, the diseases by which it is occasioned, and the exciting causes of the disease, the abstract of the registers will prove, that while a part of the sickness is inevitable, and a part can only be expected to disappear before progressive amelioration, a considerable proportion of the sickness and deaths may be suppressed by the general adoption of hygienic measures which are in actual but partial operation. It may be affirmed without great risk of exaggeration, that it is possible to reduce the annual deaths in England and Wales by 30,000 and to increase the vigour (may I add the industry and wealth?) of the population in an equal proportion.[24]

"This is not," Cullen comments, "the voice of a man seeking answers to new questions but that of a man wishing to state accurately his theses about the nature of urban society and demonstrate them to the public by irrefutable, government-collected statistics."[25] Much of Farr's work in fact has this character of finding confirmation for beliefs stated in advance.

Geographical variations in death rates had of course long been a staple of epidemiological thinking. Farr's contemporary Thomas Edmonds had presented a striking set of findings inscribed graphically on the map of England and Wales. He drew a line from Brighton in the southeast to Liverpool in the northwest, noting that along that line clustered the highest mortality rates; conversely the lowest rates clustered in geographical areas away from the Brighton–Liverpool line.[26]

Table 5 Annual mortality in London and in the Home Counties, 1838–44

	Annual deaths at all ages to		*Annual deaths <5 years to*	
	1,000 females living	*1,000 males living*	*1,000 girls living*	*1,000 boys living*
Surrey	18	19	41	48
Sussex	18	19	42	50
Hampshire	18	20	44	52
Kent	19	21	46	57
Berkshire	20	20	46	53
London	23	27	80	93
Lewisham	16	18		

Source: William Farr, "Excessive Urban Mortality, London, 1838–44," *Tenth Annual Report of the Registrar-General* (Parliamentary Papers, 1849, XXI).

Farr brought greater complexity and detail to such analyses in dozens of tables that he compiled comparing mortality in different geographical and administrative districts. In his 1848 report, for instance, Farr compared mortality in London and in the Home Counties. The crude mortality rate in London, 27 males dying annually per 1,000 males living, considerably exceeded the 20 males on average dying annually per 1,000 in the Home Counties. The differences appeared far sharper still in child mortality, with 80 girls under 5 years old dying in London per 1,000 girls compared with an average of 44 per 1,000 in the Home Counties (Table 5). In a more detailed comparison of mortality in London and in the countrified district of Lewisham, Farr calculated the "excess of deaths by causes peculiar to London": 43 per cent of the children under 5 dying in London, and 24 percent of the adults aged 25–65, were in his terms excess deaths (see Table 6).

In a later refinement of the tools for such comparisons, Farr introduced the "healthy district" mortality rate. Over the decade 1841–50, about one-tenth of the registration districts had annual mortality rates below 17 per 1,000. Using this rate as an index of "regular" mortality in the 1850s, Farr constructed a standard against which to measure the "insalubrity" of other districts. The "healthy districts" served as a sanitary yardstick. In one of many subsequent studies, Farr tabulated deaths in 30 large towns and compared those results with estimations of the deaths that would have occurred had townspeople died at the

Table 6 Excess mortality of London, compared with Lewisham, 1849

Age	*Deaths in London*	*Deaths that would have happened if the mortality had been the same as in Lewisham*	*Excess of deaths in 7 years by causes peculiar to London*
0–5	139,612	80,632	59,980
5–25	40,830	35,706	5,124
25–62	109,145	83,447	25,698
>65	52,464	44,343	8,121
Totals	342,051	244,128	97,923

Source: William Farr, *Tenth Annual Report of the Registrar-General* (Parliamentary Papers, 1849, XXI).

same rate as residents of the healthy districts. The difference between the two columns of figures would hence represent the excess mortality of the towns (Table 7).

Farr's methods also led him on occasion into dead-ends or less-than-fruitful investigations. His studies of cholera outbreaks are an often-cited example. Farr tried persistently to discern patterns in the mortality of cholera. In studies focused on London, his most apparently successful effort connected cholera deaths with the elevation of respective districts above the level of the Thames (Table 8). Cholera deaths in fact concentrated more in low-lying areas, but the association was in some respects positively misleading.[27] Moreover it was unlikely to lead to the more detailed house-to-house neighbourhood research that John Snow undertook.

A more egregious example of the limitations of Farr's work was his effort to relate density of population with mortality. In the fifth annual report (1843), Farr tried to provide a mathematical expression of such a relationship. He ranked the metropolitan districts by population density and by female mortality rate, finding that the mortality increased proportionally to the sixth roots of the densities (Figure 1). The association revealed something, but just what? In a related commentary on population density, Farr showed good sense about how density could spread disease: "The mere aggregation of people together in close apartments generates or diffuses the zymotic [epidemic] matter. Thus, placing lying-in women in close proximity to each other, or mix them up with the patients of a general hospital and they die of puerperal fever; place many wounded men in a ward where

Table 7 Deaths in 30 large town districts, 1851–60

Ages	*Deaths*	*Deaths in healthy districts*	*Excess mortality*
All ages	711,944	384,590	327,354
0	338,990	135,470	203,520
5	31,319	19,290	12,029
10	14,240	11,020	3,220
15	43,807	37,550	6,257
25	48,625	36,150	12,475
35	50,071	30,320	19,751
45	49,638	26,680	22,958
55	49,763	27,020	22,743
65	47,445	31,510	15,935
75	30,583	22,920	7,663
85+	7,463	6,660	803

Source: William Farr, *Supplement to the Twenty-Fifth Annual Report of the Registrar-General* (Parliamentary Papers, 1865, XIII), xxvi.
Note: Full title adds: "and also the deaths that would have occurred in the 10 years if the Mortality had been at the same rate as prevailed in the 63 Healthy Districts (1849–53)."

Table 8 Mortality of cholera in England, 1848–9

Elevation of district in feet	*No. of "terrace" from bottom*	*Cholera deaths per 10,000*	*Calculated series*
<20	1	102	102/1 = 102
20–40	2	65	102/2 = 51
40–60	3	34	102/3 = 34
60–80	4	27	102/4 = 26
80–100	5	22	102/5 = 20
100–120	6	17	102/6 = 17
...			
340–360	18	7	102/18 = 6

Source: William Farr, *Report on the Mortality of Cholera in England, 1848–49* (London, 1852), lxv.
Note: Full title adds: "The elevation of the soil in London has a more constant relation with the mortality from cholera than any other known element."

cleanliness is neglected, and erysipelas, pyaemia, gangrene spring up; imprison men within narrow walls, or crowd them in rooms and typhus breaks out."[28] Similarly, "To limit the operation of zymotic diseases overcrowding in towns must be absolutely prohibited: the mere accumulation of masses of living people within narrow limits either generates or insures the diffusion of epidemic disease."[29]

Figure 1 Density, mortality, and death rates

Relation between density and mortality

d and d′ = density of population in two places

m and m′ = mortality of population in two places

$m' : m :: \sqrt[6]{d'} : \sqrt[6]{d}$

Thus, death rates

Calculated	18.90	19.16	20.87	25.92	28.08	37.70	38.74
Observed	16.75	19.16	21.88	24.90	28.08	32.49	38.62

Source: William Farr, *Fifth Annual Report of the Registrar-General* (Parliamentary Papers, 1843, XXI).

The question is how, or if, Farr's law of density and mortality could advance understanding. Farr recognized that population density was only an indirect measure. As Eyler notes, "districts with similar population densities might have atmospheres of varying degrees of purity, depending on the provisions for drainage, ventilation, and other sanitary facilities."[30] Other commentators have seen this example running up against or beyond the limits of Farr's method. Newsholme, for example, considers it an example of "the inherent weakness of the statistical method": "Conditions cannot be controlled as in a physical or chemical experiment, and the factors involved nearly always are multiple. We may draw inferences of a general character from a series of related facts of adequate magnitude, but a complex thus investigated remains a complex, and the inference drawn is subject to the possibility that one member of a complex bundle has been given undue prominence over the remaining members of the bundle."[31] Farr's methods did not equip him to tease apart such complexes in order to establish causation. The numerical method was a powerful instrument for identifying and framing problems, but much less so for solving them.

By the end of his long career Farr's approach was, not surprisingly, backward-looking. Advances in bacteriology and new statistical techniques would moreover shift the directions of epidemiology in the 1880s and later. None the less Farr left a considerable legacy – the more remarkable considering the tools ("the simplest rules of arithmetic") at his disposal. In Newsholme's considered judgement, Farr's work was "the most fruitful example extant of the application of vital statistics to social welfare."[32]

NOTES

1 "The Measurement of Progress in Public Health," *Economica* 3 (1923), 188.

2 John Eyler's *Victorian Social Medicine: The Ideas and Methods of William Farr* (Baltimore, Md.: Johns Hopkins, 1979) provides an invaluable survey and discussion of Farr's career.

3 Richard Shryock, "Quantification in Medical Science," in Harry Woolf, ed., *Quantification* (Indianapolis: Bobbs-Merrill, 1961), 97.

4 The last phrase occurs in the subtitle of Stephen Stigler's *The History of Statistics: The Measurement of Uncertainty before 1900* (Cambridge, Mass.: Harvard University Press, 1986).

5 William Guy, "On the Value of the Numerical Method as Applied to Science, but Especially to Physiology and Medicine," *Journal of the Statistical Society of London* 2 (1839), 35.

6 Shryock, "Quantification," 95.

7 M.J. Cullen, *The Statistical Movement in Early Victorian Britain: The Foundations of Empirical Research* (New York: Barnes & Noble, 1975), 8.

8 "Vital Statistics; or, the Statistics of Health, Sickness, Diseases, and Death," in J.R. McCulloch, ed., *A Statistical Account of the British Empire: Exhibiting its Extent, Physical Capacities, Population, Industry, and Civil and Religious Institutions* (London, 1837), 2, 567–601.

9 "Measurement of Progress," 188.

10 Farr, *Fifth Annual Report of the Registrar-General*, 37 (Parliamentary Papers, 1843, XXI).

11 John Eyler has suggested persuasively that Farr drew key components of his thinking from a British actuary, Thomas Edmonds. See Eyler, "The Conceptual Origins of William Farr's Epidemiology," in Abraham Lilienfeld, ed., *Times, Places, and Persons: Aspects of the History of Epidemiology* (Baltimore, Md.: Johns Hopkins, 1979), 1–21.

12 See Ian Hacking, *The Taming of Chance* (Cambridge: Cambridge University Press, 1990), 47–54.

13 "On the Law of Recovery and Dying in Small-Pox," *British Annals of Medicine* 1 (1837), 143.

14 Eyler, "Conceptual Origins," 11.

15 Guy, "On the Value of the Numerical Method," 38.

16 Hacking, *Taming of Chance*, 3.

17 Margaret Pelling agrees that "Eyler ... is undoubtedly correct in regarding Farr's belief in the regularity of diseased as of healthy functions, as one of the most fundamental of his assumptions." She none the less argues that, "Given Farr's concentration on the application of this belief to the phenomena of the rise and fall of disease in the individual, and later in the group or population, it seems likely that he owed it as much

to Hippocrates, Sydenham, and the English school of topography as to the French statisticians"; see *Cholera, Fever and English Medicine 1825–1865* (Oxford: Oxford University Press, 1978), 88. This seems to downplay unduly the specific contributions of the "numerical method" to Farr's way of thinking.

18 *Fourth Annual Report of the Registrar-General,* Appendix, 234 (Parliamentary Papers, 1842, XIX).

19 William Farr, *Vital Statistics: A Memorial Volume of Selections from the Reports and Writings of William Farr,* ed. Noel A. Humphreys (London: Offices of the Sanitary Institute, 1885), 332.

20 Ibid.

21 See Alexander Langmuir, "William Farr: Founder of Modern Concepts of Surveillance," *International Journal of Epidemiology* 5 (1976), 13–8.

22 Newsholme, "Measurement of Progress," 193.

23 Cullen, *The Statistical Movement,* 36.

24 *First Annual Report of the Registrar-General,* Appendix (P), 64–5 (Parliamentary Papers, 1839, XVI).

25 Cullen, *The Statistical Movement,* 37.

26 Edmonds, "On the Law of Mortality in Each County of England," *Lancet* 1 (1835–6), 364–71, 408–16.

27 See Eyler, *Victorian Social Medicine,* 114–22, for a detailed analysis of Farr's cholera studies.

28 *Fifth Annual Report of the Registrar-General,* 321 (Parliamentary Papers, 1843, XXI).

29 Ibid.

30 Eyler, *Victorian Social Medicine,* 133.

31 Newsholme, "Measurement of Progress," 197.

32 Ibid., 186.

13

La santé publique et ses instruments de mesure. Des barèmes évaluatifs américains aux indices numériques de la Société des Nations, 1915–1955

LION MURARD

"Plus les conditions d'existence sont misérables, plus l'emploi du savoir médical devient affaire d'organisation[1]." Émis depuis le Peking Union Medical College au milieu des années 1930 par le "bolchevik médical" de la Fondation Rockefeller, John B. Grant, confirmé par le même Grant depuis l'All-India Institute of Hygiene and Public Health de Calcutta au milieu des années 1940, le propos se recommande à l'évidence d'une approche comparative, et implicitement politique, de la médecine comme science sociale[2]. Que s'élèvent les niveaux de vie, la santé suivra, sous réserve d'une conversion des "faits" scientifiques en termes de politique et d'organisation[3]. La nouveauté de l'argument est là : non pas tant dans la primeur conférée à la gestion de la *santé* sur celle de la *maladie*[4], que dans l'intérêt porté à la constitution d'une discipline administrative qui mette au jour les liaisons enterrées entre ignorance, *malgovernance*, pauvreté et maladie, mesure les variables en jeu et les rende gouvernables. Saisie sous cet angle, l'articulation à l'instant évoquée entre science et politique n'a guère retenu la curiosité de l'historien. À bon droit requise par la "raison statistique", la confiance dans les chiffres ou la poursuite de l'objectivité dans la vie publique[5], l'attention s'est peu tournée vers cette autre face d'une "histoire concrète de l'abstraction[6]" qu'illustrent dans des registres divers les tableaux standardisés de recueil des informations cliniques d'un Pierre Louis[7], les formulaires-types d'une Florence Nightingale[8], ou encore les "topographies médicales" et autres monographies descriptives des collectivités que romança Balzac dans son *Médecin de campagne*[9]. Non pas de simples modes de présentation de savoir, mais de véritables matrices formelles qui en déterminent partiellement le contenu[10].

ÉCHANGES TRANSATLANTIQUES : L'ESSOR D'UNE SCIENCE ADMINISTRATIVE APPLIQUÉE À LA SANTÉ

Ce qui suit s'intéresse à la naissance dans l'Amérique des années 1920 d'un instrument d'administration locale, l'Appraisal Form for Community Health Work, puis à son adoption dans les années 1930 par la Société des nations, sous forme d'un recueil d'"Indices de vie, de milieu et de santé". Avec le barème américain apparaît un document chiffré voué à la mesure des performances administratives par une note objective[11]. Un mètre étalon du rendement des services sanitaires, et un surgeon du taylorisme, le nouvel outil témoigne de l'engouement de la sociologie naissante pour une matière qui, mieux que tout autre volet des politiques publiques, paraît justiciable d'une approche coût-bénéfice. Le premier président de la Fondation Rockefeller, le sociologue rural George E. Vincent, avait tranché : la santé publique "se prête d'elle-même à la mesure objective[12]". Le niveau général de l'activité sanitaire s'élèverait-il sensiblement si l'on donnait à connaître *urbi et orbi* les savoir-faire éprouvés dans des localités pilotes en ces matières? Inspiré du General Register Office britannique, ce défi fait la raison d'être du Comité de pratique administrative de l'American Public Health Association (APHA)[13]. Mise au point d'un schéma organi-sationnel standard, d'un budget type et de barèmes pour l'évaluation quantitative des services rendus : le Comité n'aura de cesse d'apprécier la valeur des services sanitaires des États et des municipalités, leur rendement, leurs lacunes, enfin les ressources budgétaires qu'il y aurait lieu de leur affecter. Aussi bien est-ce d'orgueil que brûle en 1944 le *moving spirit* de toute l'entreprise, Charles-Edward Winslow (1877–1957) : "L'administration de la santé publique est largement fondée dans ce pays sur l'œuvre accomplie par le Comité de pratique administrative que j'ai présidé quinze ans d'affilée[14]."

Entre-temps, cependant, s'amorce sous le nom d'"indices de vie et de santé" une sorte de reconfiguration transnationale des barèmes "étendant leur propos pour inclure des éléments tels que les services médicaux, le logement et l'alimentation – tous items exclus des formulaires américains[15]". Conceptualisé en 1935 et dans les années suivantes où, mise sur la touche du grand jeu diplomatique, la SDN moribonde assiste à "l'effondrement graduel de ses institutions politiques[16]", le recueil d'indices illustre à merveille la stupéfiante extension de ses activités prétendument "techniques", humanitaires, d'envergure presque universelle. Ainsi de l'audience conquise par son service de renseignements épidémiologiques : 72 % de la population de la planète couverte en 1937[17]. Rien d'étrange, dans ces conditions, que Genève fasse (pour citer l'un des concepteurs des indices en 1936) "un usage extensif de l'expérience américaine des 15 dernières années", ni que l'APHA soit à son tour "influencée par les plans que nous avons projetés[18]". Curieuse de méthodes susceptibles d'offrir une vue à vol d'oiseau des conditions locales, l'organisation internationale brûle de s'en remettre à des indices numériques pour débrouiller l'écheveau des facteurs géographiques, économiques et sociaux agissant sur la santé publique. Le directeur médical de la SDN, Ludwik Rajchman (1881–1965), s'en ouvre à l'automne 1938 : "Comme les statistiques de mortalité et de morbidité sont à cet égard notoirement insuffisantes", l'Organisation d'hygiène a engagé des études destinées à mettre au point "un système d'indices calculés de façon à donner un aperçu d'ensemble de l'état de santé d'une région, urbaine ou rurale[19]".

Ce "bilan de l'exploitation du 'capital vie et bien-être' dans une collectivité donnée[20]" était éminemment élaboré. Une sorte de "fin stéthoscope à même de nous faire entendre le battement de cœur d'une collectivité[21]", les indices se présentent comme une véritable histoire sans paroles encourageant les "comparaisons internationales, ou fréquemment même intra-nationales[22]". L'ambition de ces tableaux sans aucun texte descriptif? Saisir et représenter les facteurs influant sur les collectivités vivantes, et plus encore en mesurer la variation, le dynamisme. Au lieu des figurations chiffrées, en quelque sorte inertes, des annuaires statistiques, au lieu des notations impressionnistes, touffues, détaillées, des *surveys*, le recueil genevois prétend *construire* des grandeurs "agrégées", de véritables "indices" rendant compte de "la variation de certaines quantités et ainsi, tout au moins dans une certaine mesure, de la Vie collective, si mouvante et si difficilement saisissable, dont on peut alors entrouvrir le grand Livre[23]". Prétention quelque peu démesurée, sans doute – en tout cas frappée par l'éclipse de la mémoire historique – mais qui, planifiée et conduite comme une "entreprise commune[24]" à l'Organisation d'hygiène de la SDN et au Milbank Memorial Fund, nous intéresse, pour reprendre un mot de Winslow, comme "un idéal type de la coopération internationale[25]".

LE COMITÉ DE PRATIQUE ADMINISTRATIVE DE L'AMERICAN PUBLIC HEALTH ASSOCIATION (1920–1956)

Vivifié par l'esprit de Wall Street, l'effort tous azimuts déployé par la *progressive era* pour fixer des normes en matière d'assistance, de logement ou de conditions de travail, n'en soulignait que davantage l'incapacité des administrations urbaines à rendre ne serait-ce qu'un minimum de services. Vrai, il a quelque chose de saisissant, le portrait tracé par l'économiste Irving Fisher d'un monde à ce point souillé que "le cours de l'Ohio déroule mille miles de fièvre typhoïde, et celui de l'Hudson une *cloaca maxima* depuis Albany jusqu'à l'Océan" – une lande disgraciée où, "sur 80 000 000 de nos concitoyens, 8 000 000 périront sous peu de tuberculose", cependant qu'en Californie "la peste bubonique a si bien pris pied qu'on a requis le concours des forces armées[26]". Autoflagellation, autocompassion : il ne faut pas s'étonner du besoin nouvellement ressenti d'une "mesure quantitative des performances locales[27]", non plus que des emprunts faits aux procédures en vogue dans le commerce et l'industrie. Barbares, ces autorités locales que ne retient guère la traduction sociale de découvertes médicales majeures. Barbares, et davantage encore "inexcusablement aveugles à leur propre intérêt économique", puisque la bactériologie les dote d'un corps de connaissances si opératoire, paraît-il, que "la détermination du taux de mortalité moyen est entre leurs mains[28]".

Aussi n'était-ce qu'un cri : que ces mêmes édiles se débarrassent de tout empirisme, substituent au monde de l'à-peu-près celui de la mesure, et œuvrent pour des résultats pratiques et durables. Une sorte d'établissement commercial à vocation sociale, le gouvernement local serait "forcé d'adopter de bonnes habitudes", la première consistant à remplacer ses budgets hors d'âge, désordonnés, fourre-tout, par une comptabilité plus moderne. Le vaisseau amiral du City Manager Movement, le Bureau de la recherche municipale de New York parraine en 1908 la première exposition consacrée outre-Atlantique à la gestion des finances locales et multiplie les rapports sur la gestion des services comptables ou sur le rendement de services plus opérationnels tels les travaux publics, la police et la lutte contre les incendies. "100 % d'efficacité, 100 % d'Américanisme[29]".

L'astreinte à une obligation de résultats dans les limites d'une certaine enveloppe budgétaire – c'est ce flambeau que reprennent aux alentours de la Grande Guerre les *sanitarians* eux-mêmes par la voix de Charles V. Chapin (1856–1941), surintendant à la santé de Providence (Rhode Island) : "Il n'est probablement pas aux États-Unis un seul grand département d'hygiène municipale opérant selon des principes logiques", tranche en 1915 sa monumentale dissertation sur le sujet. "La plupart d'entre eux sont mal équilibrés. Bien des choses sont faites qui comptent peu pour la santé des administrés, et beaucoup d'autres délaissées qui sauveraient bien des existences[30]". De quoi jeter "la plus grande consternation[31]" dans les rangs d'une

American Public Health Association qui, pauvre en hommes et en moyens, désespère de devenir un point de ralliement dans sa discipline. Quelques brillants météores sur fond d'arriération profonde : c'est un tableau violemment contrasté qu'offre alors une nation partagée entre les rêves de succès dans l'arène internationale et la conscience aiguë de son provincialisme. "Aucune norme[32]", pleurnichait encore au lendemain de la Victoire le président de l'APHA – partout le caprice et la diversité.

Une machinerie sanitaire si peu assurée de ses destinées qu'on l'eût plutôt dite "le ballon de foot des politiciens[33]" – le déboire n'eût guère agité l'Amérique officielle si ne s'en était irrité un tiers acteur de longue main disposé à former les masses à l'allongement de la durée de la vie, savoir le monde de l'assurance-vie. Gaspillage, ce mot insultait à son éthique quantitative. Dès 1909, aussi bien, la Metropolitan Life Insurance Company lançait pour ses millions de modestes salariés détenteurs d'une police d'assurance une pleine brassée de services sociaux confiés à un travailleur social réputé de la Russell Sage Foundation, ancien directeur de la New York City's United Hebrew Charities, Lee K. Frankel (1867–1931)[34]. L'assistait Louis I. Dublin (1882–1969), un biostatisticien attiré par les travaux de la British Biometric School[35], qui, né en Lituanie, élevé dans cette "Babel de bruit et de saleté" qu'était le Lower East Side, avait en charge le Statistical Bureau de la Metropolitan. Assureur et assuré ne partageaient-ils pas un commun intérêt? Si l'assuré pouvait être amené à comprendre qu'en prenant soin de sa santé, "son portefeuille en bénéficierait à la longue[36]", il en retirerait un avantage direct en s'épargnant quantité de maladies, souffrances et décès prématurés, l'assureur "profitant pour sa part d'une moindre mortalité" parmi les cotisants[37]. S'ensuivraient pour la Metropolitan une croissance phénoménale de son service gratuit d'infirmières-visiteuses et l'explosion consécutive de budgets sociaux qui se chiffreraient en millions de dollars. Éminemment concernés par le statut de l'hygiène et des métiers afférents, Frankel et Dublin n'avaient du reste guère balancé à lier leur sort à celui de l'APHA, le premier mettant l'association sur ses pieds en qua-lité de trésorier : 500 membres en 1890, seulement 700 en 1912, 3 400 en 1919, quand il fut élu président; le second recommandant pour sa part le 17 mai 1920 l'installation d'un comité spécial appelé à améliorer le *modus operandi* des administrations locales en en "mesurant le rendement[38]" d'un bout à l'autre du continent.

Un surgeon du City Manager Movement, donc, le Committee on Municipal Health Department Practice installé par l'APHA le 20 septembre 1920 tirait son concept originel de la proposition phare émise par Chapin, suggérant d'exprimer l'activité des services, leurs accomplissements, "en termes de notes ou de scores numériques qu'il serait loisible de combiner en une note unique globale[39]". "Éviction de la politique de l'œuvre sanitaire", l'intitulé de l'article publié par W.S. Rankin, le premier directeur des opérations du Comité, en indique le dessein central, ordonnateur : standardisation, normalisation techniciste ne désignent, sous sa plume, autre chose qu'une prometteuse "élévation de l'activité sanitaire du plan politique au professionnel[40]". Nous le suggérions à l'instant, jamais cependant l'instauration de normes numériques n'eût été sérieusement poursuivie si la Metropolitan, aiguillonnée par sa Welfare Division, n'avait financé de ses deniers l'intégralité du budget requis. Rebaptisé "Committee on Administrative Practice" (CAP) en octobre 1925 pour correspondre à l'élargissement de son rayon d'action aux États et comtés ruraux après que le Milbank eut joint ses petites économies à celles de la Metropolitan, ce comité pionnier conjugue les talents les plus divers. À la présidence, riche de ses "dix générations de New Englanders[41]", Charles-Edward A. Winslow, professeur et président du département de santé publique de Yale, le premier hygiéniste d'envergure à saisir l'intérêt d'une "économique sanitaire[42]". Au secrétariat, Louis Dublin, travailleur social à ses heures et la cheville ouvrière de l'entreprise.

UN INDICE NUMÉRIQUE DE L'EFFICACITÉ DES SERVICES

"À quel rang se situe ma ville?" À l'unisson d'un William Farr orchestrant les rivalités de clocher entre les "districts en bonne santé" et les autres, Chapin avait annexé à son enquête-inventaire une cotation des activités majeures – statistiques vitales, laboratoire, contrôle des maladies transmissibles, etc. – sur la base d'un total de 1 000 points pour un programme idéal complet. Non content de suggérer le classement des cités selon leur mérite sanitaire, il s'aventurait à montrer comment une telle évaluation pouvait être conduite, formalisant ainsi une sorte de norme du désirable à l'aune de laquelle les localités mesureraient leur retard éventuel. C'est cet effort de discrimination entre procédures fécondes et inutiles que prolonge le CAP dans son enquête exhaustive sur l'administration sanitaire des 83 plus grandes villes des États-Unis ("le premier survol comparatif des pratiques jamais effectué dans le monde"), lequel, daté de juillet 1923 et publié sous forme de *Bulletin 136* du Public Health Service américain[43], dégage aussi les grandes lignes d'un "programme normatif standard à l'échelle d'une collectivité[44]".

Puisé aux "méthodes précises des hommes d'affaires[45]", et tout particulièrement au barème évaluatif adopté en 1916 par les compagnies d'assurance contre les incendies pour estimer les risques et établir leurs contrats en conséquence, le formulaire mis au point à compter de 1923–24 est d'abord un appareil d'enregistrement des données selon un protocole uniforme, agencé de manière à permettre au médecin-fonctionnaire d'apprécier les forces et les faiblesses des unités en mouvement sur son champ de bataille. Répandu dans la plus vive excitation en deux versions – *Appraisal Form for City Health Work* (1925, révisé en 1926, 1929, 1934) et *Appraisal Form for Rural Health Work* (1927, amendé en 1932) – puis refondu à l'été 1938 dans une version unique sous l'intitulé *Appraisal Form for Local Health Work*, le barème ne prétend pas mesurer l'état de santé collectif, mais "les résultats immédiatement atteints" tels que la pertinence des statistiques obtenues et analysées, le nombre de vaccinations réalisées, de nourrissons surveillés, ou de malformations découvertes et corrigées parmi les écoliers. "Se découvre en un coup d'œil le statut dévolu par une ville à la protection de sa santé[46] (*tableau 1*)".

Soit la salubrité en général, section valant 80 points sur les 1 000 possibles. Robert-Henri Hazemann (1897–1976), un fellow de la Fondation Rockefeller formé à la Johns Hopkins aux biostatistiques, la décrit en ces termes :

Le premier article concerne l'inspection sanitaire. La note 10 est accordée pour 3 000 visites annuelles pour 100 000 habitants. Le deuxième article se rapporte à l'eau, avec 35 points au maximum, dont 30 si l'eau est conforme aux normes de laboratoire établies à Washington. Les piscines ont droit à 5 points au maximum dont 1 si la douche et le lavage au savon sont appliqués à tous les baigneurs avant l'entrée dans la piscine. L'éducation de la collectivité en matière d'assainissement donne droit à 5 points, dont 2 si l'on distribue annuellement plus de 150 brochures de propagande pour 100 000 habitants, 1 point si les auditoires aux conférences spéciales groupent au moins 3‰ de la population, et 2 points si les journaux publient au moins deux articles par an[47].

S'agit-il, dans un tout autre domaine, des visites faites à domicile par des infirmières scolaires? "La norme est de 400 visites par an pour 1 000 enfants des écoles élémentaires. 400 visites valent 10 points; 200 visites ne valent que 4 points; pour moins de 100 visites, la note est 0[48]." L'ivresse du détail (*tableau 2*) …

En possession d'un pareil instrument, le planificateur local paraît armé pour rationaliser ses services (songeons que dans les années 1930, le commissaire à la Santé de New York est à la tête de plus de 2 500 employés), et plus encore pour résister victorieusement aux compressions de crédits faites à l'aveugle. Délicieuse, l'affaire de ce maire qui, “apprenant que sa cité occupait un rang médiocre en fait de prévention contre la diphtérie et qu’il en irait tout différemment pour peu qu’on alloue 175 dollars à l’achat de toxine antitoxine, dégagea immédiatement la somme nécessaire sur des fonds spéciaux[49]”. Avec le barème apparaissent un instrument de travail, une grammaire de l’intérêt général et, indissolublement, un outil de combat. Car la valeur numérique collectivement accordée à telle ou telle activité en marque la plus ou moins grande urgence. Et dans le mouvement même qui lui fait “tenir tête à la démagogie”, le fonctionnaire sanitaire s’affirme comme autorité souveraine. Père du premier centre de santé en France et bientôt chef du cabinet technique du ministre de la Santé du Front populaire, Robert-Henri Hazemann le voit bien, lui qui, soulignant en 1936 combien le formulaire américain “standardise” les réponses, en dégage toute l’efficace : il “permet aux hygiénistes de s’y retrouver”, “oriente les hommes politiques” et invite “l’opinion publique à s’établir sur des bases techniques[50]”. C’est dire qu’il sert la volonté de puissance d’un corps professionnel et, dans l’exacte mesure où il y parvient, concourt à l’utilité publique ...

LA VALEUR ÉCONOMIQUE DE LA VIE HUMAINE

Appliqué au suivi des activités majeures (éducation sanitaire, tuberculose, cancer, protection maternelle et infantile, etc.)[51], l’*Appraisal Form* classe les localités selon leur “capacité à acheter de la sécurité sanitaire[52]”. Judicieusement investi, un modeste dollar *per capita* permettrait au calcul de Dublin de “ne courir aucun risque[53]”, d’aucuns moins placides portant à deux dollars par tête la somme nécessaire à l’exécution d’un programme adéquat[54]. Peu importe au demeurant, tant la conquête de l’opinion dans un âge où la santé paraît monnayable passe avant toute chose par la promesse de dividendes. Dividendes positifs : existence prolongée, confort de vie; négatifs : maladies et morts évitées – avantages assez tangibles en tout cas pour soutenir l’engouement de la presse à l’endroit de statistiques qui, savamment distillées, constituent autant de *news* sujettes à cimenter la confiance placée dans l’expertise locale[55]. Le conseiller de l’homme de la rue, comme l’assure dès 1925 l’épidémiologiste britannique Wade H. Frost (1880–1938, alors professeur invité à la Johns Hopkins), le médecin de la santé publique ne se distingue guère d’un conseiller fiscal auquel la collectivité confie la gestion de certaines obligations publiques et autres bons du Trésor : à charge pour lui de les placer en sorte qu’ils rapportent “les profits les plus élevés en fait de santé”. Son capital provenant entièrement du public, il se fera un point d’honneur d’indiquer ses raisons pour opérer tel ou tel placement et de donner quelque estimation chiffrée des bénéfices attendus. Il ne saurait pas davantage se fâcher si ce même public souhaite disposer de temps à autre d'un compte-rendu l'informant des profits effectivement tirés[56].

"Business" et bienfaisance mêlés, la santé publique s'avère "l'objet d'un calcul[57]". L'exact pendant de ces services collectifs que sont le pavage des rues, la construction des routes et l'entretien de sapeurs-pompiers, elle rapporte au demeurant infiniment plus qu'elle ne coûte. Remis en honneur par W.S. Rankin en Caroline du Nord (1920–1924), ce pont aux ânes de la pensée actuarielle manque de force probante. Un excellent placement, n'en plaident pas moins Louis Dublin et Alfred Lotka dans *The Money Value of a Man* (1930), "l'hygiène paie" et "quoiqu'il soit impossible de chiffrer en dollars et en cents les profits tirés de l'argent investi, il ne fait aucun doute que le bénéfice soit considérable[58]". En charge de l'évaluation des démonstrations de méthode que mène le Milbank dans diverses localités de l'État de New York pour reproduire sur une plus vaste échelle la célèbre démonstration antituberculeuse de Framingham, dans le Massachussets, Winslow n'a pas de ces précautions de langage. Confiant dans la table Dublin-Lotka de transcription des taux de mortalité en termes monétaires, il se mêle de chiffrer les économies réalisées en 1931 à Syracuse, dans l'État de New York, sur la diarrhée infantile (126 nourrissons sauvés à 7 000 dollars, soit 90 0000 dollars), les mala-dies transmissibles aiguës (70 existences à 10 000 dollars, 700 000) ou la tuberculose (1 574 000 dollars) (*tableau 3*)[59]. Conversion des activités en dollars et des dollars en services rendus : on touche à cette sorte de perfection dans l'utilitarisme qu'évoquait Dickens dans ses *Temps difficiles.*

LES CONCOURS INTER-VILLES DE PRÉSERVATION DE LA SANTÉ

N'approchons-nous pas d'un moment où les compagnies d'assurance sur la vie, sur les accidents ou la maladie, useront de la technique du barème pour "distinguer dans leurs primes entre les cités pourvues de services efficients *[business-like]* et celles mal équipées[60]?", s'interroge le CAP dans l'édition de 1929 de son *Appraisal Form.* Prophétie réalisée, puisque le Comité entre alors dans sa seconde phase, celle des concours inter-villes. Cette année-là en effet, l'aile marchante de l'APHA couronne dix années de recherches opiniâtres par l'inauguration, de concert avec la Chambre de commerce des États-Unis, du premier *Health Conservation Contest*, futur *National Health Honor Roll.* Forte du soutien financier d'un groupe de compagnies d'assurance-vie (Prudential, Equitable et Metropolitan), la Chambre de commerce s'appuie sur le CAP pour lancer à l'échelle nationale "une compétition inter-villes de préservation de la santé sur le modèle de ces concours de prévention des incendies qui se sont révélés si utiles par le passé". Événement mémorable, comme s'empresse de l'écrire Winslow dès l'automne 1928 au directeur du Milbank, John Kingsbury (1876–1956), en ce qu'il offre "une occasion unique pour stimuler l'activité sanitaire à travers l'ensemble du pays et traduire l'expérience des démonstrations du Milbank en termes de pratique générale[61]".

Le creuset dans lequel les médecins-hygiénistes avaient mis en commun leurs trésors d'expérience, le CAP se présente volontiers comme "une agence de diffusion pour les démonstrations du Milbank", la rampe de lancement d'une entreprise dont la visée "n'était pas d'aider le comté de Cattaraugus, non plus que Syracuse ou Bellevue-Yorkville, mais de s'en servir comme d'autant de leviers du changement de la pratique sanitaire aux Etats-Unis[62]". C'est dire les perspectives ouvertes par ces championnats annuels. Les *Appraisal Forms* qui avaient migré vers le monde des œuvres (Fiche d'évaluation du rendement des œuvres sociales, 1924[63]) essaiment vers le monde des affaires, le directeur médical de l'American Telephone and Telegraph Company soumettant par exemple un "barème évaluatif d'un service de médecine du travail" à l'APHA (1932), et de là à l'American Management Association (1933)[64]. Preuve que le temps était enfin venu d'en appeler à ces méthodes pour majorer le rendement de la machinerie sanitaire tout entière. Ce à quoi s'emploierait une Chambre de commerce à laquelle Dublin ne cesse de susurrer qu'"un bon dossier sanitaire est, pour une ville, un atout économique de premier ordre[65]". Orgueil civique et intérêt commercial piqués au vif, 108 cités participent ainsi au premier *contest* en 1929, 171 en 1931 et 97 en 1934. La compétition élevée à la hauteur d'un sport national grâce à des financements de la Metropolitan et d'autres, s'étend cette même année 1934 aux comtés ruraux grâce à un concours additionnel de la Fondation W.K. Kellogg.

Tout ceci se reflète dans la croissance prodigieuse du budget du CAP : un demi million de dollars drainés en 1935, un million en 1956, à la dissolution du Comité. "Ce qui avait commencé comme une aventure étriquée en 1920, financée par la seule Metropolitan Company, se métamorphosa en une large opération grosse d'effets inespérés sur la santé publique[66]."

EXPERTISE TRANSNATIONALE ET ACTION SANITAIRE LOCALE

Au fondement d'un "système international d'indices de santé", la crise de 1929 met cruellement en lumière le caractère non comparable de l'information courante sur l'incidence relative du chômage ou des privations sur la santé des populations. Incomplétude et inexactitude des données. "Nous sommes fort éloignés de statistiques démographiques internationales," s'était déjà attristé Edgar Sydenstricker (1881–1936), le premier statisticien du Public Health Service américain (USPHS), après qu'il se fut fait détacher en 1923 à la Société des nations naissante pour en organiser sous le parrainage de la Fondation Rockefeller le service des renseignements épidémiologiques et des statistiques sanitaires[67].

C'est cette demande d'un langage commun qui prend résolument corps à l'orée des années 1930, lorsque s'accuse à Genève le divorce entre des statistiques officielles qui, pays après pays, "révèlent un état de santé meilleur que jamais", et le sentiment largement répandu que "la crise devait avoir des effets délétères[68]". "Ce qu'il faudrait, s'inquiète à l'automne 1932 la Section d'hygiène par la voix de l'Américain Frank Boudreau, c'est un outil statistique qui plonge au cœur du mystère", un étalon composite capable d'être d'un vrai secours pour les administrations nationales menacées par le couperet des restrictions budgétaires, en ce qu'il "soulignerait autoritairement la folie de coupes sombres dans les services au moment même où leur action s'avère indispensable[69]".

Ainsi conduite à envisager un système complet d'appréciation des conditions sanitaires, la Section d'hygiène met ses pas dans ceux d'Edwin Chadwick, de Lemuel Shattuck, et plus encore dans ceux de John S. Billings, ce médecin militaire dont le minutieux formulaire pour un *survey* des États-Unis (1875) comportait 500 à 600 questions, du climat ou de la densité démogaphique aux déchets en passant par les amenées d'eau potable et l'évacuation des eaux usées[70]. Environ 500 indices de santé, de milieu et d'action médico-sociale : tel est précisément le chiffre auquel s'arrête en décembre 1936 le *Bulletin* de l'Organisation d'hygiène de la Société des nations dans sa première publication sur le sujet, instantanément reprise en janvier 1937 dans le *Milbank Quarterly* avec une préface de Winslow[71]. Dû à Ludwik Rajchman[72], directeur médical de la SDN, le pluriel indique assez qu'il ne s'agit point là d'un de ces indicateurs synthétiques comme se plaît parfois à en imaginer le démographe (tel Hersch rapportant en 1920 l'inégalité devant la mort à un "indice d'aisance[73]") ou le statisticien (tel Roesle préconisant en 1933 le calcul d'un "indice de santé" pour les chômeurs et leurs familles[74]). Indices, et non indice, l'esprit serait plutôt celui des *Indices numériques de la civilisation et du progrès* d'Alfredo Niceforo[75], transposés de la saisie d'une civilisation dans l'espace et le temps à la caractérisation numérique d'un certain "capital vie et bien-être", ainsi que des facteurs susceptibles de l'influencer : conditions naturelles, économiques et sociales, d'une part, rendement des services sanitaires, de l'autre, en interaction[76].

Quelque instructive que fût la traduction monétaire que donne de ses patients efforts le fonctionnaire d'hygiène, le critère ultime du succès, comme le signifiait dès 1926 Edgar Sydenstricker à l'intention du Milbank Memorial Fund, ne saurait reposer que sur "un critère et un seul, et c'est la santé des populations" : non pas la somme de travail abattue, tant d'enfants pesés et repesés, tant de visites d'infirmières-visiteuses, mais, consignés sous forme d'indices numériques, "les changements ou contrastes enregistrés dans l'état de santé lui-même[77]". Une pierre dans le jardin du CAP ...

LE SUIVI DE L'ÉVOLUTION VIVANTE D'UNE COMMUNAUTÉ DONNÉE

Printemps 1935, donc, dans ce (rare) moment propice que découpe le New Deal dans les sombres années 1930, Ludwik Rajchman forme le dessein d'un étalon transnational et, "désireux d'accroître la contribution de l'Amérique[78]" aux activités dites "techniques" de la SDN, consulte sur le sujet Isidore Falk (1899–1984), chercheur associé au Milbank[79]. Un choix mûrement pesé : statisticien sanitaire mué en économiste de la santé, hier l'élève de Louis Dublin et "le protégé de Winslow[80]" au sein du Comité sur les coûts des soins médicaux, puis le bras droit de Sydenstricker à la direction scientifique du Milbank, Falk par ces temps de *rush* sur Washington vient d'être appelé en compagnie du même Sydenstricker au Comité sur la sécurité économique (29 juin 1934) pour y plancher sur le Social Security Act (14 août 1935), dont la préparation l'amène en Europe courant mai pour s'y familiariser avec les institutions sanitaires et celles d'assurance-maladie. Prié à cette occasion par Rajchman de se concentrer sur les indices, ce progressiste attentif aux dimensions socio-économiques de la santé peaufine au gré de ses déplacements en Écosse et en Angleterre, à Copenhague, Stockholm, Vienne, Prague, Bratislava, Bruxelles et Nancy, deux memoranda préliminaires. Des discussions qui s'ensuivent, et en accord avec le directeur médical de la SDN, sort un arrangement "purement dicté", paraît-il, "par un désir de comparabilité avec l'*Appraisal Form* américain[81]" : 3 grands thèmes (vitalité et santé, conditions sanitaires, pratiques administratives) et 44 sous-thèmes groupant 500 indices qui se peuvent tour à tour condenser en une liste *détaillée* (pour de brèves enquêtes périodiques intensives), une liste *abrégée* pour l'examen de routine (incluant environ 100 indices), voire une *courte* liste de 60 indices (suffisante, paraît-il, pour offrir "une vue d'avion de la situation dans son tout")[82]. Sont alors envisagés comme terrains possibles d'expérience le Danemark ou la Suède, certaines régions françaises, l'Angleterre ou l'Écosse. Cela sous la caution de Sydenstricker[83] (*tableau 4*) ...

Du barème aux indices, cependant, la traversée de l'Atlantique se solde par une double inflexion. Dans la visée, tout d'abord. Bien près de céder à ce péché mignon de l'Amérique qu'est "l'excès de standardisation[84]" (la présentation de l'*Appraisal Form* aux *sanitarians* britanniques ne suscite d'ailleurs pas grand écho[85]), le calibrage des pratiques se borne aux tâches administratives : 30 infirmières-visiteuses pour une ville de 100 000 habitants, 8 visites pour chaque nouveau cas de coqueluche, etc. "Inversement, les indices sont destinés à couvrir tout objet en relation signifiante, ou présumée telle, avec la santé[86]." Mutation d'importance : non plus "anatomie des services[87]", mais mise en forme structurale d'un état de santé, l'accent se déplace pour intégrer la critique des données, et plus encore la notion toute nouvelle de "diagnostic synthétique" des situations. *Critique* des données, au sens où les indices ne marquent aucune considération particulière pour le taux de mortalité devenu "un index statistique extrêmement raffiné aux dépens de sa valeur comme outil d'aide à la décision[88]". *Diagnostic,* ou bilan, que l'observation régulière des mœurs, des coutumes et de l'état économique de la collectivité considérée permet d'éprouver et de réviser au besoin[89]. Prend corps, en somme, et c'est la seconde inflexion d'importance, une approche "problème-solution[90]" sujette à encourager les autorités locales à penser en termes de "choses à faire", *hic et nunc,* plutôt que d'un agenda standard[91].

CONJONCTURE

Et comment ne pas songer au glissement parallèle qui s'opère au même moment, du baromètre au modèle, dans cette discipline économique naissante qu'est la conjoncture? Le début du siècle avait vu naître aux États-Unis plusieurs organismes-conseils tels la Babsonian Statistical Organisation, ou le Brookmire Economic Service, qui, désireux de disposer d'une sorte de baromètre des affaires, s'efforçaient par tâtonnements de combiner des données chiffrées en un indice tendanciel de la marche générale des faits économiques. Strictement empirique, cette prévision à court terme essaimait à l'Université Harvard où prit corps en 1917 le premier observatoire conjoncturiste voué à la construction d'un baromètre à partir de séries statistiques. Appliquée avec plus de souplesse à Berlin par l'Institut für Konjunkturforschung d'Ernst Wagemann à compter de 1925[92], la méthode, toutefois, essuya des échecs de plus en plus cinglants : les prévisions de Harvard sans cesse démenties, son baromètre bloqué au beau fixe à la veille de la catastrophe de 1929, les instituts de conjoncture à peine nés changèrent leur nom en celui d'instituts de recherche économique (Moscou 1930, Berlin 1938) et s'essayèrent à la construction de modèles appliqués à l'interprétation causale. Médecine ou mécanique, non plus météorologie[93].

C'est ce principe peu à peu abandonné d'une détermination automatique du tonus économique au moyen d'un instrument préfabriqué, qui, nous l'avons vu, s'était transporté dans le domaine de l'administration sanitaire. Au croisement de la guerre des nombres et de la bataille de l'opinion, le barème apprécie les écarts observés à partir d'un niveau de performance considéré comme normal. L'exemple vient de plus loin : du General Register Office britannique quantifiant, pour ainsi dire, la négligence des principales cités du royaume à partir des données de l'état civil, et donnant à l'exercice une tournure politique en priant les Victoriens de consulter chaque semaine à leur petit déjeuner "le baromètre de la santé nationale comparée[94]". Assurée de son caractère scientifique pour peu qu'elle procède à la façon de l'astronomie, la santé publique, à en croire William Farr, dicterait ses lois au politique à qui elle servirait de "thermomètre" socio-biologique, ou "biomètre[95]". Une métaphore que filera à son tour l'American Child Health Association, soulignant à l'intention du fonctionnaire d'hygiène la similarité du barème avec "le spectromètre du physicien et de l'astronome[96]".

Baromètre, thermomètre, spectromètre, ce jeu de renvois à la médecine, à la physique ou à l'astronomie est évidemment révélateur d'une certaine fragilité de la démarche – "un exemple unique d'autoévaluation d'un service public[97]", comme le dit joliment Winslow, mais peu fait sans doute (à raison de son caractère autogéré) pour se prêter à ce débordement du local au fédéral ("un plan d'envergure nationale") que brûlent d'engager les New Dealers. Par l'entremise du CAP, claironne le même Winslow en 1935, un groupe de professionnels de la chose publique s'est déterminé à mettre en commun ses connaissances pour élever aussi haut que possible les niveaux de scientificité : "Partis d'un méli-mélo d'entreprises toutes locales et accidentelles, ils ont haussé la pratique administrative à la hauteur d'un programme national concerté[98]." Peut-être. Mais le ton est autrement féroce chez Sydenstricker qui insinue début 1936, en sa double qualité de patron de l'USPHS Office of Statistical Investigations et de directeur scientifique du Milbank, que les standards véhiculés par le Comité n'ont pas toujours été "correctement calibrés", ni même "continûment testés quant à leur efficacité réelle". Pire, "la liste des procédures en usage pourrait être reconsidérée dans son intégralité à la lumière d'un scepticisme de bon aloi[99]." Éclatants, daube également son plus proche collaborateur, Falk, les défauts d'un schéma préconstruit auquel "certains (de nombreux?) médecins-fonctionnaires ajustent leurs façons de faire en sorte d'accroître au maximum leurs notes pour le minimum d'efforts et de frais[100]". L'insatisfaction n'épargne pas le CAP lui-même où J.W. Mountin (1891–1952), directeur en herbe de l'USPHS Office of Studies of Public Methods (1931), regrettait dès 1929 que le formulaire "ne jette la moindre lueur ni sur les besoins financiers ni sur ceux en personnel", faute de quoi l'on ne pouvait établir "si la médiocrité de tel ou tel score était due à la mauvaise organisation des services ou à l'avarice de la communauté considérée[101]". Jusqu'au Commonwealth Fund qui trouvera les barèmes "moins pertinents comme un tableau d'affichage des résultats [*scoreboard*] que comme un guide pour l'analyse du travail accompli sur l'année[102]". Car enfin, les preuves sont là, que rendra publiques le *National Survey* conduit en 1935–36 auprès de 2,5 millions de personnes[103] : "Le peuple américain n'est pas en aussi bonne santé qu'il serait en droit de l'être" – d'où il appert que "la politique consistant à se reposer sur les municipalités et les États du soin de la santé publique a ignominieusement échoué[104]".

Jamais une nation n'avait paru si avertie des questions de santé, et cependant le cinquième à peine de sa population rurale jouissait d'une prévention digne de ce nom. "C'est avec la plus mauvaise grâce, tempête Sydenstricker, qu'on s'extorque les plus maigres crédits" – un fiasco qui ne pouvait manquer de rejaillir sur le CAP, créateur et gardien des barèmes. Stouman et Falk n'ont pas de mots assez cruels à son encontre : déplorant que le but principal des *Appraisal Forms* ait été de "susciter une émulation mutuelle dans des domaines déjà choisis comme prometteurs de résultats", les concepteurs des indices se recommandent plutôt de Billings soulignant dès 1875 "l'influence qu'exercent sur la santé publique l'urbanisme, l'habitation et le surpeuplement, tous facteurs qui dans son propre pays ne sont guère encore considérés comme des faits d'intérêt public", pour conclure sarcastiquement : "Il ne semble pas qu'on puisse voir là [dans l'œuvre du CAP] une continuation directe de l'idée originale du Dr Billings", savoir la collecte de "renseignements sur lesquels on pouvait fonder des plans plutôt qu'organiser des concours[105]".

NEW HAVEN

Foin des notes et des normes idéales! Le recueil d'indices "diffère considérablement des formulaires américains[106]" en ce qu'il ne vise pas tant à apprécier l'activité des départements de santé publique qu'à évaluer l'état de santé d'une communauté donnée – l'ironie voulant que la première étude expérimentale suggérée par Rajchman à l'automne 1935 en guise de "préalable pour que le recueil soit soumis aux 'sanitarians' européens[107]" eût pour cadre une ville américaine de taille moyenne, la petite patrie de Winslow et sa terre d'élection pour ses expériences communautaires en tout genre : New Haven[108]. C'est à ce dernier qu'est adressé Knud Stouman (1889–?), le statisticien défrayé par le Milbank pour mener l'enquête-inventaire : "Vous travaillerez de manière plus productive avec le professeur Winslow à New Haven qu'avec le staff du CAP[109]", lui suggère Falk, un conseil pour le moins révélateur de certaines tensions...

De nationalité danoise, l'intéressé n'avait pu cacher son "immense joie" à être rappelé aux États-Unis après 17 ans et demi d'absence : "Probablement le dernier membre du corps expéditionnaire américain à retourner en Amérique[110]", Stouman, qui possédait une certaine expérience des services statistiques danois et britanniques, avait été employé par la Prudential Insurance Company sur les tables de mortalité. Engagé volontaire, et devenu l'assistant de Louis Dublin au sein de la Croix-Rouge américaine en Italie, il reste à Rome jusqu'à son recrutement par la Ligue des Sociétés de la Croix-Rouge comme directeur du département des statistiques sanitaires, titre qu'il conserve après son transfert à la SDN, sur recommandation de Winslow, le 1er septembre 1921. De ce transfert, soit dit en passant, résulte un certain retard dans la révision décennale des nomenclatures nosologiques que lui avait confiée Jacques Bertillon, malade, cette même année 1921[111]. À parcourir sa conférence donnée à la Yale Medical School le 17 janvier 1936, on se demande du reste s'il ne se serait pas satisfait d'une simple nomenclature d'indices de santé, d'un catalogue sans valeur explicative calqué sur la classification par Bertillon des causes de décès[112] – hérésie aux yeux d'un Falk qui conçoit la statistique comme la science d'un ordre à *faire,* et prétend construire à partir des données chiffrées des *grandeurs agrégées*[113] : "Le Dr Stouman semble oublier que ces indices n'ont pas été conçus en fonction de l'information accessible, immédiatement disponible[114]." Qu'importe au demeurant, puisque le brusque décès de Sydenstricker en mars 1936, à la veille de la conférence annuelle de la Milbank sur "La Mesure en santé publique", clôture inopinément la partie américaine de l'aventure.

DE L'HYGIÈNE À LA VIE COLLECTIVE

Héritage de la crise économique, Paul Weindling le souligne à bon droit, les indices relèvent d'un courant de pensée "holistique" en matière de soins[115]. Ventres creux et greniers pleins, la Conférence européenne sur l'hygiène rurale de juin 1931 donne ainsi à connaître, pour citer Andrija Stampar, que "la santé marche de pair avec la diffusion de l'enseignement, de l'agriculture, des sciences vétérinaires et de l'économie domestique[116]." Monde meilleur ou Ordre nouveau nazi : le contexte est ici déterminant, d'une montée des tensions internationales. Mark Mazower l'a montré, les "États-providence fascistes" auront enseigné aux démocrates qu'il ne suffisait point, pour s'assurer la loyauté des peuples, de leur octroyer des libertés individuelles[117]. Vouée à "une égalisation des classes devant la santé[118]", la médecine sociale participe dans cet esprit d'une thérapeutique des crises, ou "médecine préventive des guerres[119]".

LE MARIAGE DE L'AGRICULTURE ET DE L'HYGIÈNE

Alimentation, santé et revenu soudés en un bloc, les années 1935 et suivantes n'auraient de cesse de placer le niveau d'existence à la base de tout progrès réel de la santé. Emblématique est à cet égard le rapport de l'Organisation d'hygiène signé en juin 1935 par E. Burnet et W.R. Aykroyd sur "l'alimentation et l'hygiène publique", qui, tenant une meilleure diète pour "un facteur de croissance et de productivité", n'assigne plus tant aux gouvernements le soin de prévenir des maladies évitables par une alimentation minimum que de susciter la santé par une alimentation optimum. Les vitamines politisées, pour ainsi dire, l'"hygiène défensive" le cédait à une "hygiène créatrice de santé[120]" – en l'espèce, à une politique de l'alimentation bénéfique aux millions de consommateurs mal nourris comme à ces millions de producteurs appauvris qui croulent sous leurs excédents prétendus. En phase avec les réflexions d'un Frank L. McDougall, futur directeur de la FAO qui, "guidé et inspiré par John Boyd Orr[121]", plaide lui aussi pour "une association délibérée des questions agricoles et sanitaires[122]", le document Aykroyd-Burnet prend résolument le contre-pied de la seule proposition concrète avancée par la Conférence mondiale économique et monétaire de 1932 – restreindre la production, créer la rareté et attendre la montée des prix – pour affirmer que "la crise économique qui a été longtemps considérée comme une crise de surproduction doit être considérée plutôt comme une crise de sous-consommation[123]".

Répandus en ce printemps 1935 où Rajchman charge Falk des indices, des concepts de cette sorte arrachaient au laboratoire la nouvelle science de la nutrition pour la porter sur la place publique. Enseignement populaire ménager, budgets-nourriture calculés en calories-francs, cantines scolaires, coopératives, il ne serait bientôt bruit dans les couloirs de Genève que d'aliments riches en vitamines, de pouvoir d'achat et de relance de la consommation. Coup sur coup, sur proposition du premier délégué de l'Australie, Stanley M. Bruce (inspiré par son conseiller économique, F.L. McDougall), l'Assemblée générale invite la Société des nations en septembre 1935 à "marier la santé publique et l'agriculture[124]" et, derechef, en septembre 1937, oriente son activité vers "le relèvement des niveaux de vie, spécialement dans les populations paysannes de l'Europe orientale[125]". Conjurer par la prospérité le spectre de la guerre approchante? Voilà qui précipite la mue de la SDN en une ligue économique, une agence de planification globale apte à rapprocher le fermier incapable de vendre ses produits de la ménagère incapable de les acheter ...

Qu'advenait-il des "indices de vie, de milieu et de santé", dans cette sphère de la haute politique? Retour d'URSS où, fait exceptionnel, s'était réuni du 22 au 28 juin 1936 sous la présidence du danois Thorvald Madsen le Bureau du Comité d'hygiène[126], Rajchman se félicite de l'intérêt considérable qu'éveillent les indices aux États-Unis, à Stockholm et à Copenhague, pour ajouter en référence à l'étude conduite à New Haven : "Winslow et moi ne doutons guère qu'une enquête similaire pourrait être utilement menée dans quelques quartiers urbains et suburbains soigneusement choisis de Moscou et de Leningrad[127]." Espoirs déçus, non pas tant pour cause de (re)glaciation stalinienne que pour la primeur dorénavant donnée par Rajchman et consorts au "relèvement général économique et social des régions rurales[128]". "Rajchman et consorts" est du reste trop peu dire, l'Assemblée générale pénétrée des vertus d'une "médecine keynésienne" pour adoucir les dissensions internationales n'ayant de cesse d'encenser l'œuvre de l'Organisation d'hygiène comme la base même de l'ensemble des travaux poursuivis par la SDN. Rejointes par l'Espagne et les Pays-Bas, treize délégations d'Amérique latine demandent ainsi cette même année 1936 la convocation d'une conférence des pays d'Amérique sur l'hygiène rurale, cependant que s'initie aux diverses expériences indiennes ou chinoises de reconstruction rurale la Commission préparatoire à la Conférence intergouvernementale des pays d'Orient qui se réunira sur le même sujet à Bandoeng du 3 au 13 août 1937.

Prescience inquiète du criant échec de la *Zwischeneuropa* à se consolider d'elle-même, vision moralement absolue d'une paysannerie intelligente et prospère comme "l'assise d'une démocratie durable[129]" : c'est cet "esprit de Genève" dernière manière qu'exprime à sa façon Jacques Parisot (1882–1967), titulaire de la chaire de médecine sociale à Nancy, appelant depuis Moscou, toujours en juin 1936, à "pénétrer dans l'intimité" de la vie paysanne, "améliorer le sort des habitants des campagnes", "lutter contre leur exode, préparer le retour à la terre[130]". Rien de vertigineux, comme l'ordre du jour de la Conférence européenne sur la *vie* rurale (et non, comme en 1931, sur l'*hygiène* rurale) dont le Bureau lors de cette même session moscovite décide la tenue.

I. Ambiance rurale : culture paysanne, art paysan et folklore, crédit agricole, réforme agraire, mouvement coopératif, repeuplement des campagnes, aménagement rural, planification communautaire, transports, électrification, administration locale.
II. Alimentation et production des denrées alimentaires.
III. La maison rurale et ses dépendances.
IV. L'éducation du paysan : éducation générale, ménagère, technique, hygiénique.
V. Le paysan au travail : nouvelles méthodes d'agriculture, industries rurales.
VI. Le paysan au repos : organisation des loisirs, éducation physique, bibliothèque, TSF, cinéma.
VII. Politique médico-sociale : protection maternelle et infantile, contrôle des naissances, crèches et jardins d'enfants en milieu rural, paludisme, alcoolisme, personnel sanitaire, sage-femmes, *feldscher* ...

C'est au succès de cette conférence qui, la situation internationale l'eût-elle permise, se serait tenue en juillet 1939, qu'étaient invités à concourir les indices[131].

LA "MISSION AUTRICHIENNE" DE LA SDN

A.J.P. Taylor l'a montré, la mission suprême des Habsbourg avait été de veiller à ce que le cœur de l'Europe ne fût ni russe ni allemand[132]. À leur manière, les indices participent précisément d'une tentative désespérée pour ranimer au tout dernier instant ces États agricoles de l'Est européen que la crise attirait dans le champ magnétique des fascismes. La page américaine tournée à l'automne 1936, c'est en Hongrie que les indices revivent début 1937 grâce au concours financier du Milbank après que Bela Johan (1889–1983), sous-secrétaire d'État à l'Intérieur et ancien directeur de l'Institut d'hygiène de Budapest, se fut avoué désireux "d'exprimer sous forme concise l'état de santé d'un district rural, et d'y mesurer ultérieurement le fruit de nos efforts[133]". De longue date préoccupé par "le coût d'un service d'hygiène rurale par tête d'habitant[134]", celui que la Fondation Rockefeller tient pour le meilleur administrateur sanitaire européen s'ouvre alors à la Section d'hygiène de son désir de donner aux indices une application concrète, de préférence en terrain rural. Propos relayé au Comité d'hygiène où Parisot, porté le 1er novembre 1937 à la présidence en remplacement de Madsen, demande que l'on donne suite aux récentes suggestions de Stanley Bruce en faveur de méthodes simples d'évaluation des progrès de la santé publique – et donc que l'on mette sans plus tarder sur le métier la question des indices qui, confiée aux directeurs des écoles et instituts d'hygiène européens réunis ce même mois à Genève, prendrait une couleur austro-hongroise prononcée[135].

Rien d'évocateur, justement, comme la liste des nations disposées en novembre 1937 à une application expérimentale des indices : Belgique, France, Pays-Bas, qu'appuie le bloc des États successeurs : Hongrie, Pologne, Roumanie, Tchécoslovaquie, Yougoslavie, et même Turquie[136]. Absence des États-Unis, le Surgeon General Hugh S. Cumming se retirant de la course après s'être dit intéressé[137]. Splendide isolement de l'Angleterre où Major Greenwood se montre fort sceptique[138], paraît-il, et William Jameson plus réservé encore à l'endroit d'une question qui, selon lui, ne relève pas de l'École d'hygiène de Londres mais du ministère de la Santé[139]. Mêmes réserves de la part du Danemark, de la Suède et de la Lettonie, qui comptaient pourtant parmi les 12 nations (sur 28 participantes) disposées à préparer pour la Conférence une monographie sur l'état de santé de leurs populations rurales. À l'Europe agricole, en somme, le soin des indices : les francophones, à peu de choses près, et la défunte "internationale verte" à l'Est.

"Winslow aime le rapport hongrois", avait fait savoir Falk à Stouman; "preuve est faite que le système des indices se prête de lui-même à la technique des enquêtes rurales[140]." On ne s'étonne pas si cette même réunion de novembre 1937 à Genève, où pour la première fois officie sous la présidence du belge René Sand une sous-commission des indices (R.-H. Hazemann assurant le secrétariat), envisage d'en poursuivre l'étude "sous l'angle de l'hygiène rurale" en complétant les questions par des notions de géographie humaine, d'économie rurale, de travail social, d'urbanisme et de sanitation[141]. En dépit de l'opposition de Stouman ("Le formulaire de Nancy est un aide-mémoire pour des *surveys* et ne saurait être tenu pour un système d'indices[142]"), sont ainsi intégrés au recueil certains points du formulaire d'enquête utilisé en Lorraine dans le cadre du diplôme d'hygiène : maison paysanne, éclairage, ventilation, fumiers, mouches, moustiques et rongeurs, hygiène alimentaire, contrôle des légumes verts, maladies communes à l'homme et aux animaux, heures de travail, organisation des loisirs, surveillance et contrôle du sport, population militaire et de passage, divorces, etc.[143]. Une sorte de retour à l'esprit des topographies médicales[144], mais sans aucun texte narratif : "objectives, parce que numériques[145]." Et de fait, Bruxelles mis à part, où Stouman conduit à l'été 1937 un ultime *survey*[146], l'étude expérimentale des indices fuirait la grande ville.

"L'OBSERVATION *IN SITU* DU MODE DE VIE DES PAYSANS[147]"

Car enfin, comment perdre de vue les affinités électives, en un temps où plus de la moitié de l'Europe est rurale, qui "tirent" la médecine sociologique vers la "géographie de plein vent[148]"? Vers l'enquête de terrain, l'excursion, le voyage à la Montesquieu… tous apprentissages "aussi indispensables au futur fonctionnaire sanitaire que l'observation clinique pour le futur médecin[149]". Mœurs, coutumes, état économique de la collectivité placée sous sa sauvegarde, l'hygiéniste doit les connaître à fond : témoins les inventaires sanitaires dressés à l'aube des années 1930 dans plusieurs communes rurales de Seine-et-Marne par cet ancien *fellow* de la Rockefeller, concepteur en banlieue parisienne d'"indices de pauvreté" puis expert à la Section d'hygiène de Genève, qu'est Hazemann. Plus d'une cinquantaine de tableaux chiffrés, depuis la "Quantité de viande consommée par semaine et par personne" à la "Distance des puits aux cabinets insalubres", en passant par l'"État juridique de la propriété" ou l'"Aération nocturne" de la maison rurale[150]. Comme quoi, médecin-sociologue ou médecin-géographe, c'est tout un. On citerait aussi bien les *health surveys* inlassablement menés aux États-Unis, plus de 4 000 dans la seule entre-deux-guerres, les campagnes monographiques effectuées en Roumanie par la jeunesse étudiante dans le cadre de la loi sur le Service social, ainsi que celles conduites en Europe centrale sous l'impulsion de ces écoles d'hygiène parrainées par la Rockefeller qu'un John B. Grant en provenance de Pékin disait beaucoup plus faibles en épidémiologie que leurs homologues américaines, mais "beaucoup plus fortes en administration sanitaire[151]". Ou encore, nous en avons dit un mot, les monographies qualitatives faisant parfois près de 600 pages qu'exige Parisot de ses étudiants de l'Institut régional d'hygiène de Nancy, sur la vie et la santé dans telle ou telle cité lorraine au cours de mille ans d'histoire, ou sur l'économie agricole, eau, lait, purin, et autres instantanés de la vie paysanne[152].

Se réunissent-ils à Genève pour préciser le cadre spatial dans lequel appliquer les indices, les directeurs des écoles et instituts d'hygiène européens n'hésitent pas une seconde : ce sera "la région naturelle", concept-clé de l'école géographique française. Région naturelle, ce choix a valeur de critique indirecte de la *Wehrgeopolitik* allemande. Cette dernière, on le sait, ne pense que frontières, en parle comme autant d'isobares ethnopolitiques, et calcule de part et d'autre des quotients de pression démographique au kilomètre carré. La géomédecine, pour sa part – terme forgé en 1931 – se plaît à considérer le monde slave entre Baltique et Mer noire comme une entité épidémiologique distincte[153]. Racialisation de la santé publique, à laquelle l'effort de formalisation des phénomènes médico-sociaux mené depuis Genève nous paraît opposer une sorte de contre-modèle. Songeons seulement à ces courbes que dresse en 1939 Gustavo Pittaluga, l'ancien président de la Conférence européenne d'hygiène rurale de 1931 : courbes dites d'"isohygie", vouées à l'expression cartographique des conditions et surtout des possibilités de vie hygiénique des populations de la planète[154]. Climat, densité, us et coutumes locales dans l'alimentation, l'habitation, autrement dit "genres de vie" : on ne voit guère là de ces "indices de biologie sociale" que déploie l'école sociologique roumaine[155], par exemple.

Curieux, tout de même, ce profil épistémologique qui, dans ses tensions entre arithmétique politique et topographie descriptive, n'est pas sans rejoindre celui de la statistique soviétique, elle aussi tiraillée entre les monographies de budgets paysans et les enquêtes dynamiques agricoles conduites dans des "aires types[156]". Le nombre ou le lieu? Les indices s'interdisent de choisir. Résumé graphique de la vie d'une communauté, inventaire de ses forces et faiblesses, ils ne sont que "l'expression numérique des enquêtes monographiques[157]" et conservent à ce titre de nettes attaches empiriques : Maximilien Sorre, le seul élève de Vidal de la Blache à s'être intéressé aux rubriques de Stouman et Falk, y reconnaît d'ailleurs "les principales têtes de chapitre de toute étude de géographie rurale[158]". "Un guide pratique d'administration sanitaire rurale et générale", comme les nomme Hazemann, ils n'en épousent pas moins cette forme axiomatique qui les assimile à des protocoles d'interprétation, ou de prévision, conduisant au choix de mesures "présumées effectives[159]". Problématique de la décision, et de la décision conjecturale. Leur originalité est là, dans cet appel à l'aléatoire, au probable. Leurs concepteurs, Falk et Stouman, le soulignent au demeurant d'emblée, les indices n'ont de valeur qu'opérationnelle, expérimentale, ce sont des variables stratégiques sur lesquelles fonder des plans[160]. Aussi bien l'instrument de connaissance ne prend-il tout son sens que comme instrument d'administration, tout l'art, ici, étant de parachever la compréhension synthétique des us et coutumes d'une collectivité donnée par la formulation d'un programme logique d'action – et par exemple, d'un de ces plans régionaux à forte composante médico-sociale dont le plus célèbre, alors, est celui que développe à l'échelle de sept États américains la Tennessee Valley Authority sous l'autorité de son directeur de la santé publique, E. L. Bishop[161]. Comme si, mariée à l'agriculture, la médecine sociale s'inscrivait naturellement dans une politique d'aménagement du territoire…

UN IDÉAL TYPE DE COOPÉRATION INTERNATIONALE...

Avisant Rajchman des révisions en cours du barème rural de l'APHA, qui s'apprête à "incorporer une courte liste d'indices de santé", Falk en décembre 1937 laisse libre cours à son enthousiasme : "Ainsi avons-nous bouclé le cercle. Le concept des indices s'est à l'origine développé par adaptation de la technique du barème. À présent, la technique des indices fait retour vers les barèmes pour les modifier à son tour[162]." Circularité des influences, débouchant sur une sorte de greffe méthodologique? On le croirait assez à parcourir les éloges prodigués à quelque temps de là par W.F. Walker, président de l'Appraisal Form Committee, à la liste d'indices incluse en 1938 dans le nouveau formulaire : une liste choisie, paraît-il, pour de "brefs résumés, tout préparés [*readily made*], des conditions et besoins sanitaires[163]". Ou la curieuse brochure de l'APHA intitulée *Health Practice Indices* comparant en 71 diagrammes pour l'année 1944, par exemple, 243 services locaux aux États-Unis et au Canada : "Ces données analysées sur la base d'une distribution des activités par moitié et par quart du tableau [le coût par tête d'habitant, notamment] sont d'une grande utilité au fonctionnaire local pour dresser son propre programme[164]." Et cependant, ledit Walker, en sa qualité de directeur de la division des études sanitaires du Commonwealth Fund, se refuse à financer plus avant ce qui n'est encore qu'un "outil expérimental pour des relevés et comparaisons périodiques[165]". Comme quoi, Sydenstricker disparu, les illusions fondaient comme neige au soleil : "Le CAP n'a pas une haute opinion des indices[166]", avait constaté Boudreau dès son accession à la direction du Milbank, en cela précédé par Falk en personne consolant ce "pauvre Stouman" : "Rien à espérer du côté du CAP[167]."

... OU DE MÉSENTENTE CORDIALE?

Ce fossé grandissant, comment l'expliquer? Certes pas par la tonalité agraire des travaux genevois. Plus déterminés que jamais à "déclencher, appuyer et accélérer" le relèvement des campagnes, et d'ailleurs aiguillonnés en ce sens par les ministres, experts (parmi lesquels F.L. McDougall) et autres dirigeants des partis paysans qui siègent à la Commission préparatoire à la Conférence sur la vie rurale, les directeurs des écoles et instituts d'hygiène européens procèdent au printemps 1938 sous la houlette de Parisot à une "refonte des indices pour l'usage rural", refonte d'où sort une "liste minima" accompagnée de notices explicatives par Hazemann[168]. Le geste témoigne d'une certaine indépendance d'esprit face aux *sanitarians* américains plutôt occupés à mettre la dernière touche à la "fusion des barèmes urbain et rural[169]". Mais enfin, ces légères divergences techniques n'affectent pas l'opinion dominante de part et d'autre de l'Atlantique, comme quoi, "d'évidence, le problème rural demeure le grand problème non résolu de la santé publique[170]". Preuve en est la présence du secrétaire exécutif de l'APHA (et ancien commissaire à la Santé de Cattaraugus County, NY), Reginald M. Atwater, à la tête de la Commission spéciale des indices sanitaires assemblée mi-octobre 1938 sur les bords du Léman, quelques jours à peine après Munich…

La discorde ne porte pas davantage sur la visée assignée aux indices d'une "réorganisation de l'administration des régions rurales non seulement du point de vue médical, mais général[171]". L'étude des services, de leur ratio de performance au regard de la performance standard, avait fait la raison d'être du CAP. Ce qui, dans l'essai d'application mené à New Haven, pique un instant sa curiosité, tient précisément dans la promesse ébauchée d'un protocole d'enquête "utilisable en tout point du pays[172]". On conçoit par là le regain d'intérêt provoqué outre-Atlantique par les développements hongrois du printemps 1938, lorsque, convaincu que la méthode de "reporting" des 160 centres de santé du pays était inadéquate, le directeur de l'Institut d'hygiène de Budapest dresse une liste de 48 indices choisis pour uniformiser les rapports mensuels des principaux médecins de la santé publique : empruntant à la liste des 68 indices dressée par Stouman dans le district de Mezökövesd (*tableau* 5), J. Tomcsik leur adresse ainsi en mars sa liste abrégée pour qu'ils établissent sur cette base homogène leur rapport annuel de 1937, d'où pourrait être extrait un rapport national[173]. Octobre 1938 sur ces entrefaites verra la Commission Atwater établir non plus seulement une série d'indices révisés convenant aux régions rurales, mais bien le "Schéma d'un rapport type sur l'état de santé des populations et ses facteurs[174]" intégrant dans ses divers chapitres des indices numériques choisis.

Avancée significative. Conçu comme "un moyen de stimuler l'hygiéniste sur des questions aussi importantes que les mouvements démographiques, la mortalité infantile ou les cas de fièvre typhoïde[175]", ledit *Schéma* n'eût guère été, à l'américaine, que l'instrument d'une norme technique. Mais, d'un outil appelé à nous donner "d'une extrémité de l'Europe à l'autre" une "vue panoramique de la vie journalière des travailleurs de la terre[176]", on est en droit d'attendre davantage. D'abord, qu'il encourage les "comparaisons expéditives"[177] dans l'espace entre différentes localités et dans le temps pour la même localité. Ensuite, qu'il dégage différents types d'organisation sanitaire idéale eu égard à l'environnement géographique, climatique, culturel, et même politique. Enfin, qu'il concourt à cette "standardisation automatique des pratiques[178]" qu'échoue à assurer à grande échelle la simple démonstration de méthode. Avancée, au sens où l'essai d'axiomatisation ne se satisfait plus ici de refléter les meilleures pratiques – Folk High Schools danoises, dopolavoro italien, coopératives yougoslaves et autres "agents sanitaires de village" chinois – mais s'interroge sur leur reproductibilité.

Que penser à cet égard du souverain mépris manifesté par le directeur de l'Institut de Varsovie au terme d'un délicat essai d'application des indices dans le district de Plock, 135 000 habitants ("New Haven ne peut servir d'exemple ou de référence pour notre pays[179]"), sinon qu'il conforte cette assertion d'Arthur Newsholme, qui fut comme une révélation pour un John B. Grant en Chine, selon laquelle on ne saurait planifier quoi que ce soit en santé communautaire sans songer en premier lieu à la viabilité économique du programme? Étude des prix de revient des services d'hygiène, de leur coût par tête d'habitant[180]... Aussi bien Belà Johan n'a-t-il de cesse de comparer les indices calibrés par Stouman en 1937 dans son *survey* du district de Mezokövesd aux données recueillies dans le même district par la Fondation Rockefeller en 1927, pour en tirer la leçon que la mortalité d'un coin du monde primitif et misé-rable peut être réduite d'un tiers sur une décennie pour le prix de 10 cents par tête par année. Sa conclusion – "il en coûte environ 12,20 dollars pour sauver une vie à Mezokövesd[181]" – s'inscrit à l'évidence dans le cadre de la toute récente Conférence de Bandoeng sur l'hygiène rurale (3–17 août 1937), qui avait appelé à persuader les opi-nions que les fonds consacrés à la santé constituent "un placement sage et profitable des deniers publics[182]".

Encore n'est-ce pas assez dire, tant l'adoption des pratiques les meilleures paraît liée à celle d'une "conscience locale technique[183]". La Fondation Rockefeller dans le New South américain, Andrija Stampar en Croatie, le Mouvement d'éducation des masses à Ting-Hsien et ailleurs ... Elles sont sans âge ni frontières bien définies, les ruses de Sioux déployées par un Johan dans la grande plaine hongroise pour encourager les mères à fréquenter les consultations. La plus classique : se procurer 40 wagons de sucre, denrée coûteuse, et faire savoir que les enfants présentés à la visite en recevraient deux livres par mois[184]. Ou, dans un autre registre, distribuer des semences de légumes dans l'espoir que les paysans s'efforceront de "modifier leur régime alimentaire[185]". Ses services, pour le coup, ne laissent pas d'être "particulièrement désireux de disposer d'indices capables de prouver et de mesurer l'utilité de leur travail[186]"...

MÉDECINE SOCIALE, SOCIALISÉE, SOCIALISTE

Cet étalon composite, justement, on se tromperait à en cantonner l'usage à l'Europe du cheval de trait : Hongrie, Pologne, Finlande, Cluj et Jassy pour la Roumanie; ou même à celle du cheval-vapeur : Belgique, puis France où Hazemann présente le 26 mai 1939 au Conseil supérieur de la statistique une liste de 80 indices numériques sur laquelle se caleraient les rapports annuels des inspecteurs départementaux d'hygiène[187]... Car la démarche est tricontinentale. Le directeur médical de la SDN le confirme à l'été 1938, alors que s'éloigne la Conférence de Bandoeng et que se profile celle de Mexico : le moment est venu de finaliser un rapport-type sur l'état de santé des populations, qui ne se placerait plus seulement au point de vue des campagnes européennes mais de "tous les pays ayant atteint un certain degré de civilisation sanitaire[188]". Quelque hésitation que puisse manifester le Bureau international du travail devant l'ampleur de la tâche, fait ainsi connaître Rajchman, il revient à l'Organisation d'hygiène, "aujourd'hui, d'orienter la vie rurale en Europe, mais aussi hier en Asie, demain en Amérique[189]". Vers le Schéma plus haut évoqué, "Schéma d'un rapport-type sur l'état de santé d'une collectivité, et sur les facteurs qui l'influencent[190]", convergent pour lors dix ans d'enquêtes d'allure encyclopédique sur les méthodes à suivre pour "déterminer l'état alimentaire d'une population[191]", "dégager les données fondamentales du logement sain et à bon marché", mesurer et améliorer "les niveaux d'existence[192]". Ajoutée aux études Stouman-Falk "qu'il ne s'agit pas de reprendre[193]", leur synthèse, début 1939, fera du Schéma un document "encore trop compliqué – mais un fruit déjà bien mûr[194]".

Un fruit très nettement tropical, surtout, à en croire les ultimes essais d'application conduits en ordre dispersé à Ceylan[195], en Inde après 1944 sous l'impulsion de Henry Sigerist[196], plus tard en Malaisie, à Singapour, à Panama et dans la zone du Canal sous celle d'Isidore Falk[197]. Tentatives sans lendemain mais suffisamment attentives aux correspondances cachées entre pauvreté, maladie et sous-administration, pour constituer une étape majeure sur la route du rapport Bhore (1944), du Manitoba Health Plan (1945), et par-dessus tout de la mémorable conférence organisée par l'OMS et l'UNICEF à Alma-Ata en septembre 1978. Quelque maladroits qu'ils paraissent, en effet, les indices adaptés en 1938 aux régions tropicales[198] ne laissent pas d'anticiper cette conception quelque peu touche-à-tout de la réhabilitation rurale qui trouverait son banc d'essai le plus solide non pas dans le Sud-Est européen, ni en Amérique latine, mais dans les campagnes déshéritées d'Extrême-Orient. Un système intégré qui s'enracine dans le village...

À cet endroit se creuse le fossé transatlantique. L'ossature d'un plan national de santé, au jugement d'un Sigerist en Inde, à la veille de l'indépendance? "L'électrification des campagnes[199]." On citerait aussi bien Stampar instruisant les étudiants en médecine de Harvard de l'utilité de "tarir les revendications sociales[200]" par la réforme agraire, condition *sine qua non* d'une coopération populaire à l'œuvre de santé. La médecine sociale n'est autre chose que ce mélange illicite entre des séries prétendument allergiques l'une à l'autre. Une interconnexion généralisée, que s'emploie précisément à formaliser le recueil d'indices. Voyez seulement l'insistance de Winslow lors de leur première application à New Haven pour "qu'on étoffe la section relative aux déterminants sociaux de la santé, alimentation et logement tout spécialement, [et qu'on cherche] des indices propres à exprimer le niveau culturel d'une population[201]". Ou l'attention portée par Rajchman à la qualité de la fonction publique, question dont il a pu mesurer l'extrême importance lors de ses fréquents séjours en Chine, au point de requérir l'envoi sur place d'un expert versé dans les arcanes de l'administration britannique, et d'un autre au fait du système municipal allemand[202].

Cette route sans cesse foisonnante de nouveaux chemins, justement, les États-Unis ne seraient plus disposés à l'emprunter. Entre la mesure des performances administratives et celle de la Vie collective, la différence n'est pas mince, en effet. Le "livre de raison[203]" de l'administrateur local, l'aune à laquelle il mesure l'urgence de ses tâches, l'*American Form* n'apprécie que les forces et faiblesses du département sanitaire. Genève, pour sa part, rêve d'outils par lesquels une société pourrait présumer, prévoir et assumer ses besoins, au lieu d'en être réduite à les enregistrer. Éducation, agriculture, art vétérinaire et économie domestique puissamment appariés, elle sent le soufre, cette mise en relations globalisée que ne se cachent pas de poursuivre des "indices directs et objectifs de la santé proprement dite, c'est-à-dire de l'état de bien-être[204]". Médecine sociale, socialisée, socialiste, la frontière ne laisse pas d'être des plus ténues, parfois[205].

Au vrai, cette mise en oubli des indices paraît générale. "Pas de problème plus essentiel pour l'administrateur de la santé publique que celui qui consiste à mesurer le niveau de santé de la collectivité dont il est chargé[206]", rappelle en 1955 un groupe d'étude réuni par l'OMS sur la mesure des niveaux de santé. Le propos, toutefois, n'amorce pas un nouveau cycle de réflexions, il le ferme. Développés en ordre dispersé par les divers comités d'experts de l'OMS sur la planification ou les statistiques sanitaires, par les Nations unies, la Banque mondiale et l'OCDE, multipliés comme champignons dans une littérature aussi pointue qu'aride[207], les indicateurs épidémiologiques, d'état de santé ou de niveaux de vie, manifestent à raison de leur disparité même une sorte de désenchantement grandissant à l'égard d'un système intégré dont la quête semble à jamais différée. Parmi les indices disponibles, concédait du reste l'OMS elle-même dans les années 1970, lesquels "sont tous des mesures de la maladie", "aucun ne peut être considéré comme une mesure de la santé" collective[208]. On ne saurait plus cavalièrement tourner la page ouverte à l'orée des années 1920 par le meilleur épidémiologiste américain, Sydenstricker, que consumait le désir de livrer dans ses célèbres statistiques de morbidité compilées à Hagerstown (Maryland) "un aperçu de ce que le *sanitarian* a toujours souhaité voir – une peinture de la situation sanitaire dans son tout, croquée dans la bonne perspective et sous ses vraies couleurs[209]". Elle ne retient plus guère l'attention, cette "rationalisation par le bas" des politiques publiques qu'avait parue amorcer "le bilan de l'actif et du passif du 'capital-vie' d'une collectivité donnée[210]".

Tableau 1. Le Barème évaluatif de l'activité sanitaire locale

Sections	*Formulaire urbain (1926)*	*Formulaire urbain (1929)*	*Formulaire rural (1932)*	*Formulaire urbain (1934)*	*Formulaire local (1938)*
Démographie	60	50	50	60	40
Laboratoire	70	60		45	
Éducation populaire	20	40			
Contrôle des maladies contagieuses aiguës	175	160	170	155	160
Maladies vénériennes	50	50	55	65	90
Tuberculose	100	90	100	90	90
Cancer		20			
Cardio-vasculaires		20			
Hygiène maternelle		80	90	90	90
Hygiène infantile		80	90	90	
	200				170
Hygiène préscolaire		80	90	90	
Hygiène scolaire	150	120	140	110	140
Salubrité générale	80	80	90	80	90
Lait et alimentation	75	70	75	75	80
Inspection sanitaire	20				
Programme équilibré			50	50	50
Total	1 000	1 000	1 000	1 000	1 000

Sources : C.-E.A. Winslow, "The Appraisal of Administrative Health Practice", *Journal of the Royal Sanitary Institute,* 47 (1926), 2, 142 ; "Anon., L'Appréciation des services d'hygiène au moyen de *l'Appraisal Form,* APHA, 1929", *Bulletin mensuel de l'Office international d'hygiène publique,* 23 (1931), 6, 1114 ; R.-H. Hazemann, "Application de la méthode des indices en vue de l'établissement, de l'exécution et du financement des programmes sanitaires", *Bulletin de la Statistique générale de la France,* 28 (1939), 4, 675.

N.B. "Il est à remarquer que les coefficients de l'*Appraisal Form* se rapportent à l'importance de chaque service, et non à l'importance de son objet. Ainsi, la surveillance de l'eau potable étant facile dans la plupart des villes, ce service cote un faible chiffre, bien que l'importance de l'eau potable soit de premier ordre." Anon., "L'Appréciation des services d'hygiène au moyen de *l'Appraisal Form,* APHA, 1929", *Bulletin mensuel de l'Office international d'hygiène publique,* 23 (1931), 6, 1116.

Tableau 2. Le Barème évaluatif : Contrôle de la tuberculose (total maximum 100 points)

Item	*Standard*	*Valeur*
Signalement (10 points)	2 nouveaux cas (toutes formes) signalés l'an passé pour 1 décès	10
Service des infirmières-visiteuses (25)	Nombre de visites : 5 000 pour 100 décès enregistrés l'an passé	20
	Suivi des cures post-sanatoriales : 20 % du total des visites à domicile	5
Consultations aux dispensaires (25)	Nombre de consultations : 3 000 pour 100 décès	15
	Ratio de 3 visites par malade inscrit	10
Hospitalisation (25)	25 000 journées pour 100 décès	15
	25 % de cas à leur début	10
Classes de plein air, preventoria et colonies de vacances (15)	10 enfants pour 1 000 scolarisés (dans le public et le privé)	15

Source : C.-E.A. Winslow, "The Appraisal of Administrative Health Practice", *Journal of the Royal Sanitary Institute,* 47 (1926), 2, 145-46.

Tableau 3. Accomplissements du programme de Syracuse, New York
Existences sauvées par la chute du taux de la tuberculose, bénéfices économiques afférents

Tranche d'âge	*Existences sauvées*	*Valeur estimée des gains futurs (en $)*	*Bénéfices (en $)*
Moins de 5 ans	9	10 000	90 000
5-14	8	14 000	112 000
15-19	3	20 000	60 000
20-44	46	20 000	920 000
45 et plus	49	8 000	392 000
Total	115		1 574 000

Source : C.-E.A. Winslow, *A City Set on a Hill. The Significance of the Health Demonstration at Syracuse, New York,* New York, Doubleday, Doran & Cy 1934, 357.

Tableau 4 Le Recueil des indices de santé en résumé (3 sections, 44 sous-sections)

A. Indices de vitalité et de santé
I. Population
II. Natalité
III. Mortinatalité, mortalité maternelle et infantile
IV. Mortalité générale et causes de décès
V. Morbidité
VI. Invalidité
VII. Aliénation et maladies mentales
VIII. Alcoolisme et toxicomanies
IX. Accidents
X. Suicides et Homicides
XI. Examens médicaux

B. Indices de milieu
I. Climat
II. Topographie et densité de la population
III. Distribution socio-professionnelle de la population
IV. Répartition de la richesse
V. Niveau culturel
VI. Naissances illégitimes et prostitution
VII. Habitation
VIII. Alimentation
IX. Consommation des boissons alcooliques, etc.

C. Indices se rapportant à l'activité administrative
I. Dépenses générales au titre des maladies et de la santé publique
II. Personnel sanitaire
III. Statistiques démographiques
IV. Services de laboratoire
V. Maladies contagieuses aiguës
VI. Maladies vénériennes
VII. Tuberculose
VIII. Autres maladies
IX. Infirmières-visiteuses
X. Hygiène maternelle
XI. Hygiène infantile et préscolaire
XII. Hygiène scolaire
XIII. Education physique
XIV. Assainissement général
XV. Inspection des denrées alimentaires et alimentation
XVI. Habitation
XVII. Hygiène industrielle
XVIII. Enseignement de l'hygiène
XIX. Soins aux aliénés et faibles d'esprit
XX. Hôpitaux
XXI. Assurance-maladie
XXII. Assistance médicale gratuite
XXIII. Soins aux invalides
XXIV. Protection des vieillards

Source : K. Stouman et I.S. Falk, "An International System of Health Indices", *AJPH*, 27 (1937), 4, 365.

Tableau 5. Hongrie, liste réduite des indices de santé après enquête sur place (20 indices de milieu, sur un total général de 68 indices de santé)

Indices se rapportant au milieu	
1. Température (1928–1936)	
Moyenne mensuelle maximum	22,6 °C.
Moyenne mensuelle minimum	–2,1 °C.
2. Hauteur annuelle des pluies (1901–1930)	52 cm
3. Densité de la population (1936) par km²	94,5
4. Pourcentage de la population habitant le chef-lieu (1936)	29,8
5. Pourcentage de la population habitant hors des villages (1930)	4,5
6. Pourcentage des habitants vivant de l'agriculture (1930)	81,3
7. Pourcentage des habitants se livrant au commerce (1930)	2,2
8. Pourcentage de la population agricole appartenant à la catégorie des petits paysans (1930)	28
9. Pourcentage de la population agricole appartenant à la catégorie des ouvriers agricoles non propriétaires (1930)	46,4
10. Proportion de la population agricole effectuant un travail saisonnier hors du district (1936)	37,3
11. Pourcentage des cultivateurs possédant moins de 5,6 hectares de terre	78,8
12. Proportion de la terre appartenant aux grands propriétaires (1930)	50%
13. Nombre de téléphones par 1 000 habitants	2,7
14. Nombre d'automobiles par 1 000 habitants	0,4
15. Pourcentage d'analphabétisme à l'âge de 6 ans et au-dessus (1930)	11,9
16. Fréquentation de l'école primaire (1936)	93%
17. Probabilité pour une femme célibaraire de 15 à 44 ans d'avoir un enfant, divisée par la probabilité pour une femme mariée de la même catégorie d'âge d'avoir un enfant (1936)	0,14
18. Pourcentage des maisons construites en brique de terre crue (1930)	66,6
19. Pourcentage des maisons contruites dans le rocher (1936)	5,4
20. Nombre d'habitants par maison ordinaire de paysan (pièce principale, une cuisine et une resserre) (1936)	5

Source : K. Stouman, "Les Indices de santé, essai d'application dans un district rural de Hongrie, Mezökövesd", *Bulletin trimestriel de l'Organisation d'hygiène de la SDN*, 6 (1937), 880–81.

NOTES

1 J.B. Grant, "Principles for Medicine and Public Health in the China Experiment", [1934], C. Seipp (dir.), *Selected Papers of Dr John B. Grant* (Baltimore : Johns Hopkins, 1963), 8.

2 E. Fee et T.M. Brown (dir.), *Making Medical History: The Life and Times of Henry E. Sigerist* (Baltimore : Johns Hopkins, 1997); D. Porter (dir.), *Social Medicine and Medical Sociology in the Twentieth Century* (Amsterdam : Rodopi, 1997); et du même auteur, *Health, Civilization and the State* (London & New York : Routledge, 1999); J. Eyler, *Sir Arthur Newsholme and State Medicine, 1885–1935* (Cambridge : Cambridge UP, 1997).

3 V. Berridge, "Science and Policy: The Case of Postwar British Smoking Policy," dans S. Lock, L. Reynolds et E.M. Tansey (dir.), *Ashes to Ashes: The History of Smoking and Health* (Amsterdam : Rodopi, 1998), 143.

4 J.B. Grant, *The Health of India* ("Oxford Pamphlet on Indian Affairs", 12, Bombay : Oxford U.P., 1943), 5.

5 T. Porter, *Trust in Numbers: The Pursuit of Objectivity in Science and Public Life* (Princeton : Princeton U.P., 1995); A. Desrosières, *La Politique des grands nombres : Histoire de la raison statistique* (Paris : Découverte, 1993).

6 J.-C. Perrot, *Une histoire intellectuelle de l'économie politique, XVIIe-XVIIIe siècle* (Paris : EHESS, 1992), 19.

7 J. Piquemal, "Succès et décadence de la méthode numérique en France à l'époque de Pierre-Charles-Alexandre Louis", dans *Essais et leçons d'histoire de la médecine et de la biologie* (Paris : PUF, 1993), 69–92.

8 E. Magnello, "The Introduction of Mathematical Statistics into Medical Research: The Roles of Karl Pearson, Major Greenwood and Austin Bradford Hill", dans E. Magnello et A. Hardy (dir.), *The Road to Medical Statistics* (Amsterdam : Rodopi, 2002), 99.

9 M. Bulmer, "The Decline of the Social Survey Movement and the Rise of American Empirical Sociology", dans M. Bulmer, K. Bales et K.K. Sklar, *The Social Survey in Perspective, 1880–1940* (Cambridge : Cambridge U.P., 1991), 303.

10 J. Goody, *The Domestication of the Savage Mind* (Cambridge : Cambridge U.P., 1977).

11 C.-E.A. Winslow, "Fifteen Years of the Committee on Administrative Practice, II : The Evolution of the Program", *American Journal of Public Health* (ci-après *AJPH*), 25 (1935), 12, 1305.

12 G.E. Vincent, cité dans Lewis Hackett, *History of the International Health Division,* manuscrit, Rockefeller Archive Center [ci-après RAC], 3, 908, 5, 28.

13 H.F. Vaughan, "Local Health Services in the United States: The Story of the CAP," *AJPH,* 62 (1972), 1, 95–111.

14 Cité par A.J. Viseltear, "C.-E.A. Winslow and the Later Years of Public

Health at Yale, 1940–1945", *The Yale Journal of Biology and Medicine*, 60 (1987), 460.

15 I.S. Falk à L. Rajchman, 26 février 1936, League of Nations Archives (ci-après LNA), 8A/20615/20615, R 6121.

16 F.P. Walters, *A History of the League of Nations* (London, New York, Toronto : Oxford U.P., 1952), II, 749–50.

17 P. Weindling, "Social Medicine at the League of Nations Health Organisation and the International Labour Office Compared", dans P. Weindling (dir.), *International Health Organisations and Movements, 1918–1939* (Cambridge, New York : Cambridge U.P., 1995), 141.

18 Falk à Rajchman, 26 février 1936, LNA, 8A/20615/20615, R 6121.

19 Rajchman à R. Sand, 25 octobre 1938, LNA, 8A/34605/8855, R 6106.

20 R.-H. Hazemann, Méthodes facilitant la planification de la politique médico-sociale dans les collectivités, *Vie Urbaine*, 51 (1939), 180.

21 K. Stouman, "Lecture Given at the Yale Medical School, January 17, 1936", adressée à I.S. Falk, 24 janvier 1936, Yale University Library, Manuscript Collections, Falk Papers, Series I, General Correspondence, Box 25, f. 522.

22 K. Stouman et I.S. Falk, "An International System of Health Indices: A Preliminary Report", *AJPH*, 27 (1937), 364.

23 R.-H. Hazemann, "Le Recueil d'indices sanitaires, instrument d'administration", *Annales d'Hygiène Publique, Industrielle et Sociale*, 18 (1940), 3, 90.

24 Stouman et Falk, "International System", 363.

25 C.-E.A. Winslow, "The International Appraisal of Local Health Programs", *Milbank Memorial Fund Quarterly*, 15 (1937), 1, 5.

26 Cité par G. Rosen, "The Committee of One Hundred on National Health and the Campaign for a National Health Department, 1906–1912", *AJPH*, 62 (1972), 2, 261–2.

27 C.-E.A. Winslow, "Administrative Practice", *American Public Health Association Year Book, 1930–1931*, Suppl. de l'*AJPH*, 21 (1931), 63.

28 H. Biggs, "The Administrative Control of Tuberculosis", *The Medical News*, 84, 8 (20 février 1904), 345; et "Preventive Medicine: Its Achievements, Scopes, and Possibilities", *Medical Record*, 65, 2 (11 juin 1904), 955.

29 M.J. Schiesl, *The Politics of Efficiency: Municipal Administration and Reform in America, 1880–1920* (Berkeley, Los Angeles : UCLA, 1977), 125; et S. Haber, *Efficiency and Uplift: Scientific Management in the Progressive Era, 1890–1920* (Chicago : University of Chicago Press, 1964), 51, 61–2.

30 C.V. Chapin, *A Report on State Public Health Work Based on a Survey of State Boards of Health* [1915], cité par Vaughan, "Local Health Services", 96.

31 W.G. Smillie, *Public Health Administration in the United States* (New York : Macmillan, 1949 [1935]), 420.

32 L.K. Frankel, "The Future of the American Public Health Association", *AJPH*, 9 (1919), 2, 89.

33 *Ibid.*, 90.
34 D.T. Rogers, *Atlantic Crossings: Social Politics in a Progressive Age* (Cambridge, Mass., et Londres : Belknap, Harvard U.P., 1998), 248, 262–4.
35 L.I. Dublin, "The Statistician and Institutional Policy", *AJPH*, 54 (1964), 5, 876.
36 Frankel, "Insurance Companies and Public Health Activities", *AJPH*, 4 (1914), 1, 5.
37 L.I. Dublin, *After Eighty Years: The Impact of Life Insurance on the Public Health* (Gainesville : University of Florida Press, 1966), 38.
38 L.I. Dublin, *A Family of Thirty Million: The Story of the Metropolitan Life Insurance Company* (New York : Metropolitan, 1943), 439.
39 "From Health Honor Roll to National Reporting Area", éditorial non signé (Winslow, éditeur), *AJPH*, 34 (1944), 1099.
40 W.S. Rankin, "Elimination of Politics from Public Health Work", *The Journal of the American Medical Association* (ci-après *JAMA*), 83, 17 (25 octobre 1924), 1287, 1285.
41 Winslow, "Poverty and Disease" [1948], cité par R.M. Atwater, "C.-E.A. Winslow: An Appreciation of a Great Statesman", *AJPH*, 47 (1957), 1070.
42 Selon son étudiant I.S. Falk, dans L.E. Weeks (dir.), *I.S. Falk in First Person: An Oral History* (Chicago : American Hospital Association, 1983), 12.
43 Winslow, "Administrative Practice", 63.
44 Winslow, "Fifteen Years", 1308.
45 "Moyens employés aux États-Unis pour apprécier numériquement les services d'hygiène publique", *Revue internationale des sciences administratives* (Bruxelles), 4 (1931), 625.
46 G.T. Palmer, P.S. Platt et W. F. Walker, "Eighty-Six Cities Studied by Objective Standards", *AJPH*, 15 (1925), 391.
47 R.-H. Hazemann, "Application de la méthode des indices en vue de l'établissement, de l'exécution et du financement des programmes sanitaires", *Bulletin de la statistique générale de la France*, 28 (1939), 675–6.
48 "L'Appréciation des services d'hygiène au moyen de l'Appraisal Form, APHA, 1929", *Bulletin mensuel de l'Office international d'hygiène publique*, 23 (1931), 1115.
49 Palmer, Platt et Walker, "Eighty Cities", 392.
50 R.-H. Hazemann, "Du planisme au civisme par la technique", *Le Mouvement sanitaire*, 1 (1936), 15.
51 "Work of Committee on Administrative Practice", *AJPH*, 19 (1929), 378.
52 J.A. Ferrell, "Economics of Public Health", *JAMA*, 89, 2 (9 juillet 1927), 77.
53 L.I. Dublin, "Public Health Service – A Sound Investment", *AJPH*, 21 (1931), 487.

54 C.-E.A. Winslow, "Current Tendencies in American Public Health", *Journal of the Royal Sanitary Institute* (Londres), 53 (1932), 75.
55 G.H. Van Buren, "Does the Press Want Health Statistics?", *AJPH*, 24 (1934), 329.
56 W.H. Frost, "Rendering Account in Public Health", *AJPH*, 15 (1925), 394.
57 G. Canguilhem, *La Santé, concept vulgaire et question philosophique* (Toulouse : Sables, 1990), 24.
58 L.I. Dublin et A.J. Lotka, *The Money Value of a Man* (New York : Ronald Press, 1930), 131, 135. Sur les essais de W.S. Rankin en Caroline du Nord, J. Farley, *To Cast Out Disease: A History of the International Health Division of the Rockefeller Foundation, 1913–1951* (Oxford, New York: Oxford U.P., 2004), 36–37.
59 C.-E.A. Winslow, *A City Set on a Hill: The Significance of the Health Demonstration at Syracuse,* New York (New York : Doubleday, Doran & Cy., 1934), 356–8.
60 Committee on Administrative Practice, *Appraisal Form for City Health Work* (New York : APHA, 1929), 3.
61 Winslow à J. Kingsbury, 24 octobre 1928, Yale University Library, Manuscript Collections, C.-E.A. Winslow Papers, Group 749, Series 111, Box 81, f. 1283.
62 Winslow à Kingsbury, 30 novembre 1928, *ibid.*
63 I.S. Falk et K. Stouman, "Indices de santé : Leurs rapports avec le milieu et l'action sanitaire", *Bulletin trimestriel de l'Organisation d'ygiène de la Société des Nations* (ci-après *BOH*), 5 (1936), 1003.
64 L.D. Bristol, "An Appraisal Form for Industrial Health Service", *AJPH*, 22 (1932), 1263 et suiv.
65 Dublin, "Public Health Service", 489.
66 Dublin, *Eighty Years*, 55–6.
67 E. Sydenstricker, "The Outlook for International Vital Statistics", *AJPH*, 14 (1924), 832.
68 F.G. Boudreau à G.K. Strode, 21 octobre 1932, LNA, 8A/39674/39674, R 5936.
69 Boudreau à H.S. Cumming, 28 octobre 1932, *ibid.*
70 G. Rosen, "John Shaw Billings and the Plan for a Sanitary Survey of the United States", *AJPH*, 66 (1976), 494.
71 Stouman et Falk, "Indices", *BOH*, 5 (1936), 990–1089.
72 *Ibid.*, 994 ; de même Hazemann, "Application", 684 : "C'est au Dr L. Rajchman … que l'on doit l'idée d'une telle méthode."
73 L. Hersch, *L'Inégalité devant la mort d'après les statistiques de la Ville de Paris : Effets de la situation sociale sur la mortalité* [1920], cité par A. Fagot-Largeault, *Les causes de la mort : Histoire naturelle et facteurs de risque* (Paris : Vrin, 1989), 154.

74 Selon une “Note du Directeur médical”, 24 octobre 1933, LNA, CH 1124.

75 Précédés de *La Misura della Vita* (1919), les *Indices numériques* (1921) d'A. Niceforo ont attiré l'attention de P. Lazarsfeld, “Notes on the History of Quantification in Sociology: Trends, Sources and Problems”, *Isis*, 52 (1961), 277 et suiv.

76 R.-H. Hazemann, “Commentaires concernant les indices sanitaires des districts ruraux”, Genève, 5 mai 1938, LNA, CH 1331.

77 E. Sydenstricker, “The Measurement of Results of Public Health Work”, [1926], dans R.V. Kasius (dir.), *The Challenge of Facts: Selected Public Health Papers of Edgar Sydenstricker* (New York : Prodist, 1974), 42.

78 Boudreau évoquant Rajchman dans une lettre à Winslow, 22 février 1929, Winslow Papers, Box 79, f. 1226.

79 L.E. Weeks (dir.), *I.S. Falk in the First Person*; M.I. Roemer, “I.S. Falk, the Committee on the Costs of Medical Care, and the Drive for National Health Insurance”, *AJPH*, 75 (1985), 841–8; et, sur sa “démonisation” pendant le maccarthysme, A. Derickson, “The House of Falk: The Paranoid Style in American Health Politics”, *AJPH*, 87 (1997), 1836–43.

80 J.-F. Jekel, “Health Departments in the U.S. 1920–1988: Statements of Mission with Special Reference to the Role of C.-E. A. Winslow”, *The Yale Journal of Biology and Medicine*, 64 (1991), 468.

81 Stouman à Rajchman, “Preliminary Memorandum on the Establishment of Sanitary Indices” [dactyl., 7 f.], 19 septembre 1935, LNA, 8A/20615/20614, R 6121.

82 K. Stouman et I.S. Falk, “An International System of Health Indices”, *AJPH*, 27 (1937), 364.

83 Falk à Sydenstricker, 2 octobre 1935, Falk Papers, 25, 521.

84 Winslow, “Administrative Practice”, 66.

85 C.-E.A. Winslow, The Appraisal of Administrative Health Practice, *Journal of the Royal Sanitary Institute*, 47 (1926), 133–51.

86 Stouman et Falk, International System, *AJPH*, 27 (1937), 368.

87 *Ibid.*, 364.

88 Falk, “Preliminary Memorandum on ‘Sanitary Indices’” [dactyl., 62 f.], 7 août 1935, LNA, 8A/10407/403, R 6033.

89 R.-H. Hazemann et R.M. Taylor, “Les Inventaires sanitaires”, *Revue d'hygiène*, 45 (1933), 82. Également Hazemann, “Inventaires et Bilans sanitaires”, *Revue d'hygiène et de médecine sociales* (Nancy), 18 (1939), 79–87.

90 Winslow, “Health Honor Roll”, 1102.

91 Stouman et Falk, “International System”, 369.

92 J.A. Tooze, *Statistics and the German State, 1900–1945: The Making of Modern Economic Knowledge* (Cambridge : Cambridge U.P., 2001).

93 G.-G. Granger, *Méthodologie économique* (Paris : PUF, 1956), 337–53.

94 H.W. Acland [1872], cité par J. M. Eyler, “Mortality Statistics and Victorian Health Policy: Program and Criticism”, *Bulletin of the History of Medicine*, 50 (1976), 343.

95 W. Farr, cité par K.H. Metz, "Social Thought and Social Statistics in the Early Nineteenth Century: The Case of Sanitary Statistics in England", *International Review of Social History*, 29 (1984), 267.
96 Palmer, Platt et Walker, "Eighty-Six Cities", *AJPH*, 15 (1925), 390.
97 Winslow, "Health Honor", 1100.
98 Winslow, "Fifteen Years", 1315.
99 Sydenstricker, "Economy in Public Health", dans Kasius, *Challenge of Facts*, 88–9.
100 Falk, "Preliminary Memorandum", 1935, LNA, , R 6033.
101 J.W. Mountin, "Measurements of Efficiency and Adequacy of Rural Health Service" [1929], *Selected Papers of Joseph W. Mountin* (J.W. Mountin Memorial Committee, 1956), 299.
102 "Report of the General Director [Barry C. Smith] to the Directors of the Commonwealth Fund presented at the April 8, 1943 meeting of the Commonwealth Fund's Board of Directors", RAC, CF Series 18.1, f. 105, 3546.
103 N. Krieger et E. Fee, "Measuring Social Inequalities in Health in the United States: A Historical Review, 1900–1950", *International Journal of Health Services*, 26 (1996), 407.
104 E. Sydenstricker, "Health in the New Deal", *The Annals of the American Academy of Political and Social Science*, 176 (novembre 1934), 131, 135.
105 Stouman et Falk, "Indices", 1003–4, 998.
106 *Ibid.*, 1001.
107 Falk à Sydenstricker, 5 décembre 1935, Falk Papers, 25, 521.
108 C.-E.A. Winslow, *Health Survey of New Haven* (New Haven, Conn. : Quinnipiack Press, 1928).
109 Falk à Stouman, 31 octobre 1935, Falk Papers, 25, 521.
110 Stouman à Falk, 2 novembre 1935, *ibid.*
111 Sur K. Stouman, T.D. Tuttle, "Theory vs. Practice in Vital Statistics", *AJPH*, 8(1918), 153; Dublin, *Eighty Years*, 72; A. Fagot-Largeault, "Histoire des classifications en santé", dans G. Pavillon (dir.), *Enjeux des classifications internationales en santé* (Paris : INSERM, 1998), 47.
112 Stouman, "Lecture", 1936, Falk Papers, 25, 522; une tentation récurrente, Martin Kacprzak, directeur de l'Institut d'hygiène de Varsovie, suggérant au cours d'une réunion de la sous-commission sur les indices de santé, Genève, 26 novembre 1937, de dégager "une nomenclature de véritables indices de santé, comme le Dr Bertillon l'avait réalisé pour les causes de décès", LNA, CH 1297.
113 D'une formule de G.-G. Granger, *La Science et les sciences* (Paris : PUF, 1995), 94.
114 Falk à Sydenstricker, 18 octobre 1935, Falk Papers, 25, 521.
115 P. Weindling, "From Moral Exhortation to the New Public Health, 1918–45", in E. Rodriguez-Ocana (dir.), *The Politics of the Healthy Life:*

An International Perspective (Sheffield : European Association for the History of Medicine and Health Publication, 2002), 124.

116 A. Stampar, "On the Eve of an Anniversary: International Work on the Promotion of Health", dans M.D. Grmek (dir.), *Serving the Cause of Public Health: Selected Papers of Andrija Stampar* (Zagreb : University of Zagreb, 1966), 232.

117 M. Mazower, *Dark Continent: Europe's Twentieth Cen*tury (Londres : Penguin, 1998), 79.

118 E. Burnet, "Vue d'ensemble sur la tuberculose, maladie sociale", *Revue d'hygiène*, 55 (1933), 586.

119 R. Aron, "Des comparaisons historiques", É*tudes politiques* (Paris : Gallimard, 1972), 427.

120 E. Burnet et W. Aykroyd, "L'Alimentation et l'hygiène publique", *BOH*, 5 (1935), 332.

121 W. Aykroyd, "International Health – A Retrospective Memoir", *Perspectives in Biology and Medecine*, 11 (1967), 279; on comparera le *Food, Health and Income* de J.B. Orr (1936), et le *Food and Welfare* de F.L. McDougall (1938).

122 F.L. McDougall, "The Agricultural and the Health Problems", 1934, Archives de la FAO (Rome), RG 3.1., Series D1, 4.

123 E. Burnet devant le Comité d'hygiène, PV. 22e session, Genève, 7–14 octobre 1935 [ronéo], Archives J. Parisot (ci-après AJP), Vandœuvre-les-Nancy.

124 S.M. Bruce, 11 septembre 1935, Société des nations, *Journal officiel*, Supplément 138, Actes de la seizième session ordinaire, 53.

125 J. Avenol, Note du 19 janvier 1938, LNA, 8A/31762/8855, R 6103.

126 W. Bronner (URSS), M. Kapcrzak (Pologne), N.M.J. Jitta (Pays-Bas), M.T. Morgan (Royaume-Uni), J. Parisot (France) et G. Pittaluga (Espagne) ; A. Stampar, de passage à Moscou après trois longs séjours en Chine, représentait pour sa part, en compagnie de Rajchman, la Section d'hygiène.

127 Rajchman à Falk, 2 octobre 1936, Falk Papers, 25, 421.

128 J. Parisot, "Procès-verbal de la Session du Bureau du Comité d'Hygiène, tenue à Moscou du 22 au 28 juin 1936", dactyl. [34 f.], LNA, CH/Bureau/IV/Procès-verbal, 3.

129 C.E. Rosenberg, "Science, Technology and Economic Growth: The Case of the Agricultural Experiment Station Scientist, 1875–1914", dans *No Other Gods: On Science and American Social Thought* (Baltimore : Johns Hopkins Press, 1978 [1976]), 155–6.

130 "L'Œuvre poursuivie et à poursuivre dans le domaine de l'hygiène rurale par l'Organisation d'Hygiène de la Société des Nations", Rapport présenté par le Pr J. Parisot au Bureau du Comité d'hygiène lors de la session tenue à Moscou en juin 1936, LNA, CH 1218, 14–5.

131 "Note du Pr Parisot et du Directeur médical au sujet des études ultérieures sur l'hygiène rurale, Cinquième réunion du Bureau d'hygiène, Paris, 29 octobre 1936", Genève, 8 octobre 1936, LNA, CH/Bureau/6.
132 A.J.P. Taylor, *The Habsburg Monarchy 1809–1918* (Londres : Penguin, 1990 [1948]), 74.
133 B. Johan à Boudreau, désormais directeur du Milbank, 3 février 1937, LNA, 8A/20615/20615, R 6121.
134 Johan, Commission pour l'étude des Centres de santé ruraux, PV dactyl., Genève, 28–29–30 avril 1931, LNA, R 5927.
135 J. Parisot, PV révisés de la 26e session du Comité d'hygiène, Genève, 1er–5 novembre 1937 [ronéo], AJP.
136 "Rapport sur la Réunion des Directeurs d'Instituts et Ecoles d'Hygiène tenue à Genève du 22 au 27 novembre 1937," *BOH*, 7 (1938), 184.
137 Intéressé, dit-il, car les tentatives d'établissement d'indices aux États-Unis n'ont donné que des "résultats médiocres", PV de la 25e session du Comité d'hygiène, Genève, 26 avril–1er mai 1937 [ronéo], AJP, 8.
138 Selon Morgan, 25e session du Comité d'hygiène, *ibid.*, 10.
139 W. Jameson à A. Stampar, 9 octobre 1937, LNA, 8A/25954/587, R 6048.
140 Falk à Stouman, 14 septembre 1937, Falk Papers, 25, 523.
141 Biraud et Hazemann, "Les Recueils d'indices de santé" [dactyl., 5 f.], 17 novembre 1937, AJP.
142 Stouman à Gautier, 2 mars 1938, LNA, 8A/20615/20615, R 6121; même lettre à Hazemann, 3 mars 1938.
143 Rapport sur la réunion des directeurs, 22–27 novembre 1937, *BOH*, 7(1938), 185.
144 "Aperçu général sur la politique médico-sociale à la campagne" [M. Kapcrzak, R. Sand], *BOH*, 7 (1938), 983. Sur les liens entre méthode statistique et néo-hippocratisme, J.A. Mendelsohn, "From Eradication to Equilibrium: How Epidemics Became Complex after World War I," in C. Lawrence et G. Weisz, eds., *Greater Than the Parts: Holism in Biomedicine, 1920–1950* (Oxford, New York: Oxford University Press, 1998), 303.
145 "Les Indices sanitaires. Leur place dans les rapports sur la santé publique" [Y. Biraud], *BOH*, 8 (1939), 63.
146 K. Stouman, "Indices de santé établis au cours d'une étude expérimentale de la ville de Bruxelles", *BOH*, 7 (1938), 127–77.
147 "Premier voyage d'études du Dr R.-H. Hazemann [Danemark, Suède, Lettonie, Meurthe-et-Moselle] concernant la politique médico-sociale dans les campagnes", juin 1938 [dactyl.], LNA, 8A/34168/8855, R 6104.
148 L. Febvre, cité dans G. Baudelle, M.-V. Ozouf-Marignier et M.-C. Robic, *Géographes en pratiques (1870–1945) : Le terrain le livre, la Cité* (Rennes : Presses universitaires de Rennes, 2001), 18.
149 Hazemann, "Application", 668.

150 Hazemann et Taylor, "Inventaires", 82.
151 Oral History Research Office, Columbia University, *The Reminiscences of Doctor John B. Grant*, 1961 (Glen Rock, N.J. : Microfilm, 1976), 522.
152 À titre d'exemple : L. Amidieu du Clos, *L'Amélioration des conditions sanitaires et sociales de la vie rurale : L'effort réalisé en Meurthe-et-Moselle* (1935, 368 p.); J. Bichat, *La Vie et la santé dans une cité lorraine à travers les siècles : Lunéville, 1034–1936* (1936, 608 p.).
153 P. Weindling, *Epidemics and Genocide in Eastern Europe, 1890–1945* (Oxford & New York: Oxford U.P., 2000).
154 G. Pittaluga, "Sur l'établissement des services de santé rurale dans certains pays d'Amérique et en général dans les pays à faible densité de population", *Revue d'hygiène*, 61 (1939), 198–207 sur les isohygies.
155 D. Gusti, *La Monographie et l'action monographique en Roumanie* (Paris : Domat-Montchrestien, 1937), 52.
156 A. Blum et M. Mespoulet, *L'Anarchie bureaucratique : Statistique et pouvoir sous Staline* (Paris : Découverte, 2003), 316–8.
157 "Note sur les travaux relatifs aux indices de santé" [Y. Biraud], 2 juillet 1938, LNA, 8A/20615/20615, R 6121.
158 M. Sorre, *Les Fondements de la géographie humaine*, I, *Les Fondements biologiques* (Paris : 1947), 379–80.
159 Hazemann, Méthodes, *Vie urbaine*, 50 (1939), 70.
160 Stouman et Falk, Indices, 1003–4.
161 E.L. Bishop, "The TVA's New Deal in Health", *AJPH*, 24 (1934), 1023–7, et "The Health Programme of the Tennessee Valley Authority", *Canadian Public Health Journal*, 27 (1936), 1–5.
162 Falk à Rajchman, 17 décembre 1937, LNA, 8A/20615/20615, R 6121.
163 F.J. Walker, "The New Appraisal Form for Local Health Work", *AJPH*, 29 (1939), 500.
164 Smillie, *Public Health Administration*, 420–1.
165 Stouman à Falk, 30 décembre 1938, Falk Papers, 25, 523.
166 Boudreau à Winslow, 3 mars 1937, Winslow Papers, 80, 1230.
167 Falk à Stouman, 9 février 1937, Falk Papers, 25, 523.
168 "Indices sanitaires. Commentaires concernant les indices sanitaires des districts ruraux" [R.-H. Hazemann], 5 mai 1938, LNA, CH 1331.
169 R.M. Atwater à Hazemann, 13 avril 1938, LNA, 8A/20615/20615, R 6121.
170 Winslow à G. Vincent, 6 juin 1918, Winslow Papers, 97, 1691.
171 B. Borcic, Consultation sur la politique médico-sociale à la campagne, 10–14 octobre 1938, PV provisoires [dactyl.], LNA, R 6104.
172 Falk à Rajchman, 26 février 1936, Falk Papers, 25, 421, également dans LNA, R 6121.
173 J. Tomcsik à Hazemann, 14 février 1938, LNA, R 6100, 8A/29930/8855. Et B. Johan, 28e session du Comité d'hygiène, Genève, 30 juin-2 juillet 1938, PV révisés, p. 42, où il ajoute que le rapport Stouman a été traduit et, "le 1er juin [1938], tous les fonction-

naires d'hygiène publique et médecins de communes en avaient le texte entre les mains. En outre, un grand nombre d'exemplaires seront distribués aux membres du Parlement."

174 En annexe à "Les Indices sanitaires. Leur place dans les rapports sur la santé publique" [Y. Biraud], *BOH*, 8 (1939), 64 et suiv.

175 M. Kacprzak, Sub-Committee of Experts on Rural Hygiene, Genève, 25–27 avril 1938, Summary of Proceedings, 8A/3176/8855, R 6103.

176 "Conférence européenne sur la vie rurale. Rapport de la Commission préparatoire sur les travaux de sa première session, 4–7 avril 1938", LNA, C161.M.101.

177 Hazemann, "Recueil", 88.

178 Winslow, "International Appraisal", 5.

179 Kacprzak à Rajchman, 2 avril 1938, LNA, 8A/20615/20615, R 6121; et "Indices de santé. Essai d'application sur le territoire de Plock", 25 avril 1938, CH 1325.

180 Hazemann, "Les Tendances récentes de la politique médico-sociale en Europe" [septembre 1938], *BOH*, 8 (1939), 759.

181 Johan, *Rural Health Work in Hungary* (Budapest : State Hygienic Institute of Hungary, nº 9, 1939), 225–6.

182 Première Commission de la Conférence intergouvernementale des pays d'Orient sur l'hygiène rurale, Bandoeng (Java), 3–17 août 1937, LNA, A.19.1937.III, 1311.

183 *Reminiscences of Doctor John B. Grant*, 86.

184 Johan, Consultation sur la politique médico-sociale à la campagne, Genève, 10–14 octobre 1938, LNA, CH 1374, R 6104.

185 Johan, 30e session du Comité d'hygiène, Genève, 4–6 mai 1939, Procès-verbaux, AJP.

186 Stouman à Rajchman, 1er juillet 1937, LNA, 8A/20615/20615, R 6121.

187 Hazemann, "Application", 688.

188 L. Rajchman, Comité d'hygiène, 28e session, Genève, 30 juin-2 juillet 1938, PV révisés, 40–41, AJP.

189 *Ibid.*

190 "Schéma d'un Rapport-type", 31 octobre 1938, LNA, CH 1382, avec au crayon dans sa version dactylographiée : "Note by Dr Biraud, June 10, 1938", R 6104.

191 "Aide-mémoire à l'intention des membres de la Commission préparatoire, Commission préparatoire de la Conférence européenne sur la Vie rurale, juillet 1939", Genève, 28 mars 1938, CH 1321, LNA, R 6103.

192 "Enquête préliminaire sur les mesures d'ordre national et international visant à relever le niveau d'existence. Memorandum préparé par M.N.F. Hall", Genève, 13 juin 1938, LNA, A.18.1938.II.B.

193 Rajchman, Comité d'hygiène, 28e session, Genève, 30 juin-2 juillet 1938, PV, 40–41, AJP.

194 Kacprzak à Biraud, 11 février 1939, LNA, 8A/34592/8855, R 6104.

195 S.F. Chellapal et W.P. Jacoks, *A Guide to Health Unit Procedure in Ceylon* (Colombo : Imprimerie administrative, 1937).

196 W.L. Halverston, "A Twenty-Five Year Review of the Work of the Committee on Administrative Practice," *AJPH*, 35 (1945), 1256.

197 I.S. Falk, *Health in Panama, a Survey and a Program* (1957); et *Survey of Health Services and Facilities in the Canal Zone* (1958); M.I. Roemer, "I. S. Falk," 841–8.

198 "Adaptation of the Forms of Health Indices to Tropical Areas : Note by Dr Y. Biraud, June 10, 1938", LNA, CH 1387.

199 H. Sigerist, "Report on India" [1944], in Roemer (dir.), *Henry E. Sigerist on the Sociology of Medicine* (New York : M.D. Publications, 1960), 292.

200 A. Stampar, "Observations of a Rural Health Worker", *The New England Journal of Medicine*, 218 (1938), 994.

201 Stouman à Rajchman, 6 décembre 1935, LNA, 8A/20615/20615, R 6121.

202 Note de L. Rajchman au Secrétaire général et à J. Avenol, 5 décembre, 1932, Paris, Archives du ministère des Affaires étrangères, Papiers Avenol, vol. 25, Coopération avec la Chine.

203 Hazemann, "Le Recueil d'indices", *Annales d'Hygiène*, 18 (1940), 94.

204 "Note sur les travaux relatifs aux indices sanitaires", Genève, 15 juin 1938, LNA, CH 1346.

205 L. Murard et P. Zylberman, "French Social Medicine on the International Public Health Map in the 1930s", dans Rodriguez-Ocana, *Healthy Life*, 197–218.

206 "La Mesure des niveaux de santé. Rapport d'un groupe d'étude" [1955], OMS, Série de Rapports techniques n° 137, Genève, 1957, 6.

207 *International Journal of Health Indicators, Social Indicators Research, Journal of Public Health Management and Practice, International Journal of Technology Assessment in Health Care, Journal of Evidence Based Policy and Management*, etc.

208 "Statistical Indicators for the Planning and Evaluation of Public Health Programs", Fourteenth Report of the WHO Expert Committee on Health Statistics, OMS, Série de Rapports techniques n° 472, Genève, 1971, 18.

209 Cité par Krieger et Fee, "Measuring", 397–8.

210 Hazemann, "Living Standards and Health" [dactyl., 14 p.], WHO, Study Group on the Measurement of Levels of Health, Genève, 24–28 octobre 1955, WHO/PHA/Lev. Hlth/13.

14

Statistical Theory Was Not the Reason That Randomization Was Used in the British Medical Research Council's Clinical Trial of Streptomycin for Pulmonary Tuberculosis

IAIN CHALMERS

"RANDOMIZATION WAS INTRODUCED
TO CONTROL SELECTION BIASES,
NOT FOR ANY ESOTERIC STATISTICAL REASON."[1]

An understanding of the history of controlled trials is of importance today because their history is still evolving. Although it is possible to identify treatments with dramatic effects – good and bad – without carefully controlled studies, inferences about more typical treatment effects are usually insecure unless based on studies with concurrent comparison groups, assembled in ways that reduce the likelihood that biases or the play of chance will mislead people.

The principal defining characteristics of controlled clinical trials today are the measures taken to reduce biases and the play of chance. Although several historians have been interested in "the taming of chance" – Ian Hacking's apt expression[2] – very few have focused on "beating biases."[3] Recent exceptions include Kaptchuk's history of the evolution of measures to reduce observer biases in clinical trials[4] and Harry Marks's commentary on some aspects of control of biases in clinical trials after 1950.[5]

The apparent lack of interest in bias by historians of clinical trials is particularly surprising, given the importance that they ascribe to the 1948 report of Britain's Medical Research Council (MRC) of a randomized clinical trial of streptomycin in pulmonary tuberculosis.[6] The report is notable for its exceptionally clear description of measures taken to control bias, and it rapidly became a historical landmark. At the annual meeting of the American Association of the History of Medicine in 1954, Donald Mainland, after describing the many problems that faced him as a medical statistician, declared: "all has not been darkness ... In the clinical field there appeared in 1948 a beacon or lighthouse beam – the report of the British Medical Research Council's co-operative trial of streptomycin in pulmonary tuberculosis."[7]

The report noted that allocation of patients to the comparison groups had been accomplished by reference to "a statistical series based on random sampling numbers drawn up for each sex at each centre by Professor Bradford Hill."[8] These words reflect the statistical language developed by theorists such as Karl Pearson and Ronald Fisher during the previous half-century. Against a background of interest in the history of probability and inferential statistics, some historians believe that the evolution of statistical theory played a key role in the evolution of the randomized clinical trial. Rosser Matthews,[9] for example, suggests: "The professional emergence of statistics as a codified body of knowledge and the concomitant rise of individuals trained in its methods provided the necessary conditions for the Laplacian vision of the probabilistically based clinical trial to come into being." Harry Marks[10] judges the randomized clinical trial to have been "an extension of the statistician R.A. Fisher's ideas about experimental design" and that "the statisticians' randomized controlled trial came to represent the symbol and substance of the statistical method in medicine."[11] Jean-Paul Gaudillière[12] observes: "The history of randomized clinical trials may be traced back to the biometricians' work and it seems to be a good example of 'applied statistics'. On the one hand there was a direct lineage from Pearson to Bradford Hill via Fisher and Major Greenwood ... On the other hand, it is not too difficult to argue for conceptual legacy, since the basic concepts grounding the choice of randomisation can be traced back to R.A. Fisher's work." Most recently, Eileen Magnello has stated that Karl Pearson's 1904 proposal for a clinical trial using alternation to generate the comparison groups constituted a "seminal statistical idea."[13]

I have been unable to find any evidence to support these interpretations of the origins of the MRC's randomized trial of streptomycin, and I propose an alternative history. This has little to do with statistical theory and much more to do with the more fundamental and less technical concept of a fair – that is, unbiased – test, which is a separate concern in the history of ideas about study design.

To defend this proposition, I begin by describing the two separate steps needed to achieve unbiased allocation to treatment groups in clinical trials – generating unbiased allocation schedules intended to ensure that like will be compared with like; and preventing foreknowledge of allocations among those involved in recruiting patients to clinical trials. I show that formal random allocation coexisted with alternate allocation in medicine throughout most of the twentieth century; that the word 'random' has often been used loosely, without any necessary link to the significance of random allocation in statistical theory; and that random allocation was adopted for the MRC trial of streptomycin for pulmonary tuberculosis to prevent foreknowledge of allocations among those involved in recruiting patients. I draw extensively on the writings, official and unofficial, attributed and unattributed, of the main protagonist, Austin Bradford Hill, and compare the relevant passages in successive editions of his textbook. I end by noting that the 'clinical' and 'statistical' reasons for random allocation came together only during the second half of the twentieth century.

UNBIASED ALLOCATION TO COMPARISON GROUPS: TWO SEPARATE STEPS, BOTH ESSENTIAL

Assembling comparison groups in clinical trials such that any differences in measured *and unmeasured* variables of prognostic importance are due solely to chance involves two quite separate steps, both of which are essential to ensure comparison of like with like.[14]

Generating Allocation Schedules

The first of the two steps involves using an unbiased method to decide which of the comparison groups each patient will join. One may generate allocation schedules using alternation or rotation, by tossing coins or drawing lots, or by reference to tables of random sampling numbers (the method used in the 1948 streptomycin trial) or to computer-generated lists of (pseudo-)random numbers.

Contrary to widespread belief, allocating by strict alternation does not control bias less effectively than use of random numbers.[15] Clearly, if some factor of possible prognostic importance confounds alternation, it will not control (allocation) bias. For example, if factors other than chance had influenced the day of the week on which Semmelweis's maternity hospital in Vienna admitted women, or the days on which Fibiger's hospital in Copenhagen admitted patients with diphtheria, then their use of "day of hospital admission" to construct comparison groups might have been biased.[16]

If alternation is not so correlated with potential confounders, formal random assignment (based on coin tosses, for example) controls bias no better than strict alternation in a consecutive series of people. This shared feature of the two approaches surfaces in the frequent use of the word "random" with reference to alternate allocation to comparison groups. For example, in his *Principles of Medical Statistics*, Bradford Hill noted that alternation results in "a random division of the patients among the comparison groups in a trial," as long as "no departure from this rule is allowed."[17] Indeed, strict alternation actually generates comparison groups that are more alike than groups formed using simple randomization.[18]

In the decades before and after the MRC streptomycin trial, Hill was one of many writers[19] to use "random" in a sense that is less specific than the concept proposed by statistical theorists, although Fisher and other theoretical statisticians (for example, 'Student') debated the relative merits of alternation and randomization.[20]

Preventing Foreknowledge of Allocations

Whether one uses alternation, randomization, or some other unbiased method to generate an unbiased allocation schedule, strict observance of the allocations generated is crucial. For this reason, it is essential to prevent foreknowledge of the allocations among clinicians, patients, and others involved in recruiting participants to trials and so prevent subversion of the allocation schedule (cheating!). As empirical research has amply demonstrated,[21] failure to conceal allocation schedules and adherence to them will introduce bias.[22]

Generating allocation schedules based on random numbers cannot – simply through the mystique of randomization – guarantee the avoidance of bias in assembling comparison groups in clinical trials. Quite apart from the "open invitation" to introduce bias that would result from pinning a random-allocation schedule on a noticeboard in a clinic where patients were being assessed for possible eligibility,[23] some "concealed" random allocations can be guessed, especially if organized within small blocks of unvarying size. Bradford Hill recognized this problem and drew attention to it in his discussion of a paper by Peter Armitage in 1959.[24] Of the two essential components of unbiased allocation – genesis of an unbiased sequence, and unbiased implementation of the sequence – the former remains trivially easy, while the latter will continue to pose challenges.

In the streptomycin trial "the details of the (allocation) series were unknown to any of the investigators or to the coordinator and were contained in a set of sealed envelopes, each bearing on the outside only the name of the hospital and a number."[25] The MRC streptomycin trial deserves its place in the history of clinical trials because of this and other exceptionally clear statements about precautions to minimize allocation bias.

THE EVOLUTION OF ALLOCATION SCHEDULES IN CLINICAL TRIALS

"Comparing like with like" in therapeutic experiments receives insufficient appreciation even today; but for at least two centuries some people have recognised its importance. In James Lind's 1753 account of his clinical trial of treatments for scurvy, for example, he notes that, apart from the treatments, the 12 patients whom he studied were otherwise similar: "They all in general had putrid gums, the spots and lassitude, with weakness of their knees. They lay together in one place, being a proper apartment for the sick in the fore-hold; and had one diet common to all."[26] Lind does not tell us how he allocated his twelve patients to each of the six treatments that he compared, but had he cast lots or used alternation or rotation it would not have been inconsistent with the use of these devices to make fair decisions in other contexts.[27] Other controlled comparisons reported in the eighteenth century involved giving different treatments to the same patient for alternating periods. Thus Caleb Parry reported on a series of patients, to each of whom he had given either imported Turkish rhubarb or native rhubarbs, one after the other, to assess their relative merits as aperients.[28]

In 1816, Alexander Hamilton reported having used alternation to generate parallel comparison groups in a clinical trial of bloodletting in 366 soldiers during the Peninsular War.[29] Hamilton described how sick soldiers had been "admitted, alternately" under the care of surgeons who either used or withheld venesection, but whose patients were otherwise "attended as nearly as possible with the same care and accommodated with the same comforts"[30]. His report leaves several uncertainties,[31] but it seems reasonable to speculate that he described the use of alternation to show that he had tried to generate comparable treatment groups.

By the mid-nineteenth century, the rationale for alternation was sometimes explicit. In 1854, Thomas Graham Balfour described his assessment of whether belladonna could prevent scarlet fever. He divided 151 boys into two comparison groups, "taking them alternately from the list, *to avoid the imputation of selection*" (emphasis added).[32] Balfour clearly used alternation to control bias. Although he was a distinguished statistician as well as a doctor, however, he was not a theoretical statistician in the 'Pearsonian/Fisherian' sense.[33]

There are further isolated examples of alternation up to the mid-1920s,[34] in addition to Pearson's unfulfilled proposal for an alternate allocation trial.[35] From the late 1920s on, however, there were more and more reports of alternation in clinical trials, with well over 30 published by 1948.[36] Among these, at least four took place under the aegis of the MRC's Therapeutic Trials Committee.[37] The first multi-centre, placebo-controlled trial under the MRC's aegis was organized by its Patulin Clinical Trials Committee in 1944.[38] The committee was chaired by Harold Himsworth (later head of the MRC) and included three fellows of the Royal Society, among them the medical statistician Major Greenwood. A system of "strict rotation" allocated volunteers suffering from the common cold to comparison groups. Committee Secretary Philip D'Arcy Hart observed that the method ensured "an effectively random allocation of the subjects to patulin and placebo."[39] Despite the reported use of random sampling numbers in the MRC's streptomycin trial, alternation continued, even in MRC trials,[40] and remains in use today.[41]

As already noted above, the term "random" has been and continues to be used quite loosely, without any necessary conceptual reference to its technical meaning in statistical theory. It seems improbable in the extreme, for example, that the seventeenth-century Flemish physician Van Helmont had statistical theory in mind when he proposed casting lots to decide which patients should be treated by orthodox medical practitioners, using bloodletting and purging, and which patients he should treat without these unpleasant interventions.[42] Van Helmont's proposal to cast lots to decide who would have which patients almost certainly reflected his belief that this was a way of ensuring a fair therapeutic contest, in the same way that lots had been cast over centuries to make other fair decisions.[43]

Investigators have reported drawing lots to generate comparison groups in clinical research since at least August 1927. In that month, recruitment began in an MRC-controlled trial of the effects of ultraviolet radiation on the health and development of children. The youngsters in each of seven classes were divided into three groups by "drawing lots (*method not specified*) ... so that the three large groups should be composed of children of the same ages whose school life was influenced by similar conditions."[44] Two years later, James Doull and his colleagues studied the effects of ultraviolet radiation on the health of staff members and students at Johns Hopkins.[45] Professor Lowell Reed, a mathematician colleague of the American medical statistician Raymond Pearl, allocated volunteers to the comparison groups using different-coloured dice. These were "thoroughly mixed in a sampling machine known to be practically free from systematic error. They were then withdrawn from the machine one at a time."[46] The same year, Amberson and his colleagues reported having tossed a coin to decide which of two matched groups of patients would receive gold treatment for tuberculosis.[47]

A few years later, Theobald, a British obstetrician, invited pregnant women to assign themselves at random to a vitamin-supplementation or control group: "An equal number of blue and white beads were placed in a box. Each woman accepted for the experiment was asked to draw a bead from the box. Those who drew blue beads were placed in Group A while those who drew white beads were placed in Group B. The beads drawn out were placed in a separate container."[48] Theobald acknowledged help from Egon Pearson (Karl's son, and also a statistician) in analysing the results of his study.

Despite these and other examples of random allocation in clinical trials during the 1930s, alternation remained the principal method used to achieve prospective control of biases until well after the end of the Second World War, even in studies by investigators such as Richard Doll, who were very familiar with Fisher's writings.[49]

THE ORIGINS OF FORMAL RANDOMIZATION AND THE PERSISTENCE OF ALTERNATION IN CLINICAL TRIALS

As already noted, some historians believe that the evolution of statistical theory during the first half of the twentieth century helped inspire the randomized clinical trials designed by Austin Bradford Hill and his colleagues in the 1940s. Descriptions of formal randomization in research go back at least a hundred years, however.

Some of the instances noted by others[50] did not generate comparison groups to evaluate the effects of interventions. In an experiment to assess the ability to distinguish small differences in weights,[51] Pierce and Jastrow wanted to avoid "psychological guessing of what changes the operator (experimenter) was likely to suggest." Initially, they began and ended the series of weights with the heaviest, but then they decided to begin on alternate days with the heaviest and the lightest and used a shuffled deck of cards to decide the order in which to present the different weights to the observers. A few years later, Thorndike and Woodworth[52] wanted to assess the effects of guessing and correcting estimates of the areas of pieces of paper of varying shapes, so they shuffled these so that observers "could judge their area only from their intrinsic qualities." Neither of these studies applied random allocation to generate comparison groups with a view to making causal inferences about the effects of interventions, but only to keep the assessors unaware. The same applies to the use of playing cards in all but one of the experiments to investigate telepathy reviewed by Ian Hacking;[53] in the one exception, John Edgar Coover used dice to decide whether or not a telepathic "agent" should look at a randomly selected playing card before inviting a "reagent" to guess its identity, thus providing the basis for assessing the effects of the intervention of "looking at the card."[54]

Early-twentieth-century texts sometimes mentioned the possibility of random allocation in experiments in spheres more comparable to medicine, but there is little evidence that it was adopted in practice. In 1923, William McCall, discussing the design of experiments in education, noted that "equivalence may be secured by chance, provided the number of subjects to be used is sufficiently numerous."[55] However, neither in an earlier report co-authored by him,[56] nor in any other report of an experiment in education in the early twentieth century, have I identified an unambiguous description of random allocation (or alternation, for that matter). Most of the studies to which other writers have referred appear to use matching in attempts to control bias – for example, Winch's 1908 study to assess the effects of interventions to improve memory in schoolchildren.[57]

Even among statisticians, many of whom, like Fisher, designed agricultural experiments, the origin of randomization remains far from clear. Donald Rubin[58] has noted: "Despite the early use of physical randomization by Pierce and Jastrow, the allusions to random assignments by 'Student'[59] (1923) and the mathematical results using the urn-model formulation in Neyman,[60] all writers since 1925, including Neyman, seem to agree that the first explicit recommendation to make physical randomization an integral part of experimentation was in Fisher in 1925 and in 1926.[61] This situation, with its juxtaposition of implicit suggestions and explicit contrary attribution from the same author, emphasizes to me the dangers of over interpreting, with ebullient and embellished hindsight, early writings of great men."[62]

What is not in any doubt is that Fisher's 1926 paper – "The Arrangement of Field Experiments" – and his 1935 book – *The Design of Experiments* – affected the design of experiments in agriculture and influenced (and continues to influence) the thinking of theoretical and applied statisticians far beyond that subject.[63] I have been unable to find any evidence, however, that Fisher's writings and conceptualization of the theoretical importance of randomization directly influenced the adoption of randomization in the clinical trials leading up to the MRC streptomycin trial.

Yet despite Fisher's theoretical considerations, people still used the word "random" to describe alternate allocation to comparison groups in reports of clinical trials during the 1930s and 1940s and in texts on study design, including Bradford Hill's articles and his *Principles of Medical Statistics.*[64] If Bradford Hill did not distinguish strict alternation from formal random allocation, this was not because he was statistically naïve.[65] His mentors had been Pearson, Yule and, Greenwood, and he used series of random numbers published by members of Karl Pearson's school (who had produced them principally for selecting representative samples from populations).[66]

Although Bradford Hill did not regard himself as a mathematical statistician and had little interest in statistical theory,[67] he was certainly aware of Fisher's views on the theoretical justification for random allocation. He had known Fisher personally since the 1920s (Fisher had invited him to join the staff at Rothampsted in 1929), and both men held offices in the Royal Statistical Society in the 1930s and 1940s.[68] Bradford Hill simply did not accord randomization the special status that Fisher and other statistical theorists did. His main interest was in the practical steps required in running clinical experiments, and he adopted randomisation to improve these.

Bradford Hill recognized that the circumstances of experiments in therapeutics were different in important respects from those in agriculture. Thus, in the introductory section of his book, he states: "Elaborate experiments can be planned in which a number of factors can be taken into account statistically at the same time (R.A. Fisher, *The Design of Experiments*, 2nd Edition, 1937, Oliver and Boyd, Edinburgh). It is not my intention to discuss these more difficult methods of planning and analysis; attention is confined to the type of simple experimental arrangement with which medical workers are familiar. Limitation of the discussion to that type must not be taken to mean that it is the best form of experiment in a particular case."[69] The complex (and statistically efficient) factorial experiments that Fisher had promoted in agriculture were not so readily applicable in clinical research. In agriculture, it is often possible to use already formed study samples – fields, or flocks of sheep, for example. In clinical trials it is usually necessary to assemble study samples over time – for example, patients with pneumonia admitted to hospital over a period of years. The circumstances of clinical medicine are different not only from those in agriculture, but also from those in some other spheres, such as education, where study populations such as school classes exist in their entirety at the beginning of experiments, rather than requiring assembly over time.

An even more important difference between Fisher's and Hill's experiments relates to the essential need for researchers to collaborate with autonomous professionals in clinical research. Hill was aware of the substantial challenge that this presented. Reflecting on it more than half a century later, he wrote: "In (my) articles, I had set out the need for controlled experiments in clinical medicine with groups chosen at random. At the outset, I think I pleaded that trials should be made using alternate cases. I suspect that if (and it is a very large IF) that were done *strictly*, they would be random. I deliberately left out the words 'randomisation' and 'random sampling numbers' at that time, because I was trying to persuade the doctors to come into controlled trials in the very simplest form and I might have scared them off. I think the concepts of 'randomisation' and 'random sampling numbers' are slightly odd to the layman, or, for that matter, to the lay doctor, when it comes to statistics. I thought it would be better to get doctors to walk first, before I tried to get them to run."[70]

Some commentators have called this retrospective rationalization, but it fits with the testimonies of those who came under Bradford Hill's influence as a teacher. Both Scadding[71] and Doll,[72] for example, have stated that they used alternation rather than randomization in the studies that they designed during that era probably because of Bradford Hill's exceptionally clear teaching in the 1930s. Bradford Hill believed that medicine could be improved by statistics, and so his starting point was medicine and the medical profession, rather than statistics and theoretical statisticians.[73]

Bradford Hill's achievement in reaching out to the medical profession was nicely encapsulated in a conversation that he had with John Crofton, who had just presented him for an honorary doctorate in medicine at the University of Edinburgh. Unsurprisingly, Crofton had a good deal to say about Bradford Hill's role in the evolution of controlled trials. A passage in Bradford Hill's unpublished memoir is revealing: "'John', I said, 'you know I did not invent the controlled trial. It goes back at least to Lind who tried lime juice in scurvy compared with the usual nauseating mixtures of the day'. 'I know that', Crofton replied, 'but you persuaded an extremely conservative profession which regarded change with suspicion, to accept and use them'. That was, and is, I think a fair judgement," concluded Bradford Hill.[74]

WHY RANDOMIZATION IN THE MRC'S TRIAL OF STREPTOMYCIN?

I concur with Alan Yoshioka's judgment that Bradford Hill's justifications for randomization did not have "much connection with randomisation as discussed in the statistical theory of R.A. Fisher."[75] So if Bradford Hill's use of "a statistical series based on random sampling numbers" to allocate patients in the streptomycin trial had nothing to do with statistical theory, why was randomization used?

In 1933 Bradford Hill, at the request of the MRC Therapeutic Trials Committee (which had no statistician member), prepared an internal review of an MRC trial of serum treatment for lobar pneumonia.[76] This had taken place in four centres and employed a variety of methods, including alternation, to generate control groups.[77]

Bradford Hill's report has disappeared, but Ben Toth[78] has reconstructed his views of the study from an account that Bradford Hill gave to Stephen Lock[79] and from Joan Austoker, who read the original report at MRC headquarters in the 1980s.[80] According to Lock, Bradford Hill criticized the method of allocation in the lobar pneumonia study as insufficiently robust. "He showed, for example, that in the pneumonia trials there were two groups of patients, one of people aged between 20 and 39, and the other aged 40 to 60. Roughly 35 percent of the controls were aged 40 to 60 as opposed to 24 percent of the (serum) patients."[81] Austoker and Bryder reported that Bradford Hill provided detailed criticism of the provision of controls for the trial and recommended greater effort to see "that the division of cases really did ensure a random selection."[82] Judging by the vast majority of the 51 clinical trials funded under the aegis of the Therapeutic Trials Committee (1931–39), it ignored his advice, and he had little chance of influencing its thinking as he joined it only a year before its demise.[83]

A report of the serum study appeared a few months after Bradford Hill had submitted his critique of it.[84] In 1987, Jan Vandenbroucke observed that the published document contains "a beautiful discussion of selection and comparability of treatment groups".[85] The passage to which he was referring reads as follows:

The good results of insulin on patients with diabetes or of liver treatment in pernicious anaemia are so constant that the trial of these remedies in a very few cases was enough to establish their value. With the antiserum treatment of lobar pneumonia the conditions are very different. The action of the serum is only that of a partial factor for good, and its influence may be overwhelmed by an infection that has been allowed several days to establish its dominance in the patient, or by other complicating factors that weaken the patient's resistance. In order to measure precisely what this partial benefit may be it would be necessary to take two groups of cases of identical severity and initial history and compare the sickness and the fatality in each, the one being treated with serum and the other serving as a control. But this is impracticable, for very few cases, even of "Type 1" lobar pneumonia, are quite alike, and a sufficient number of similar cases could never be got together under one observer and under similar conditions. Some American workers have sought to avoid this difficulty by using a special system of ratings for the various harmful features of the disease, thus expressing each patient's numerical value in reference to a common standard. Such differentiation seemed too intricate, and perhaps too much a matter of personal judgement, for the present inquiry. If a straightforward comparison of treated cases with controls, under the average conditions whereby patients succeed one another in the wards of a hospital, could not reveal any advantage for those treated by serum, then common sense would conclude that the use of this remedy should be disregarded in the routine of practical medicine. The method consequently agreed upon for London, Edinburgh and Aberdeen was that alternate cases of lobar pneumonia, taken simply in the order of their admission to hospital, should be used respectively for serum treatment and controls. So far as possible both were treated in the same wards and under the care of the same physicians. In the independent inquiry at Glasgow, however, the "serum" cases were treated in the Royal Infirmary, and a series of patients of the same social stratum, admitted during the same period to the Belvedere Isolation Hospital under the care of one physician, served as the control group. It is clear that there may be serious fallacies in any system which contrasts a group of serum-treated patients with a control group drawn from a different stratum of the population, or with a control group in a previous year, when the severity of the prevailing pneumonia might have been different.

Who wrote that paragraph? In 1988, I sent Jan Vandenbroucke's published comment to Bradford Hill, who replied: "I feel certain that I wrote that para and I had learned from Pearson & Greenwood & Yule (vide the references No 21 & 22)... I had applied that teaching to the M.R.C's trial of a vaccine against whooping cough and was itching to apply it in the clinical field. Streptomycin provided the opportunity."[86] Bradford Hill's reference to "that teaching" must presumably refer to alternation, which Pearson had suggested in 1904. Neither alternation nor randomization receives mention in Greenwood and Yule's 1915 article,[87] nor indeed in the first ten editions of Yule's *Introduction to the Theory of Statistics.* The eleventh edition, co-authored with Kendall and published in the same year as the first edition of Bradford Hill's *Principles of Medical Statistics,* contains sections on "random sampling," but there is no mention of random allocation to comparison groups in intervention studies. However, a section entitled "human bias" opens by declaring: "Experience has, in fact, shown that the human being is an extremely poor instrument for the conduct of a random selection. Wherever there is scope for personal choice or judgement on the part of the observer, bias is almost certain to creep in. Nor is this a quality that can be removed by conscious effort or training. Nearly every human being has, as part of his psychological makeup, a tendency away from true randomness in his choices."[88]

Bradford Hill conceded in his letter to me, "Of course later I may have been influenced by Fisher but not very much – in fact in his famous 'tea and milk' experiment I think he was wrong."[89] Bradford Hill's statistician son David Hill has explained that his father's objection "was not to Fisher's analysis of the experiment, but that he thought it would have been a better experiment if the subject had not been told that the 8 cups were to be 4 of each sort." [90] This comment is consistent with a concern to prevent foreknowledge of allocations among human participants in experiments.

The report of the whooping-cough vaccine trial, which began recruiting a few months before the streptomycin trial, states that the allocation letters A, B, C, and D were "drawn up in random order."[91] Even though the trial was not reported until three years after the streptomycin trial, however, there is no mention of "a statistical series based on random sampling numbers," which might have encouraged the view that considerations of statistical theory lay behind the reference to random allocation. Indeed, Alan Yoshioka[92] has noted that the word "random" and its derivatives appear nowhere in the MRC files relating either to the whooping-cough trial or to the streptomycin trial! The only explicit reference to Bradford Hill's scheme in the streptomycin trial is a letter referring to "a statistical process of selection," sent by Marc Daniels, the trial's clinical coordinator, to the chair of the steering committee.[93]

The lack of reference to randomization in the papers relating to the MRC's randomized trial of streptomycin contrasts with proposals for a U.S. randomized trial of streptomycin.[94] Carroll Palmer, a former member of the Biostatistics Department at Johns Hopkins, was in charge of Public Health Service field studies on tuberculosis and sought controlled studies. Palmer's proposals stated: "The cases chosen by the panel shall, by proper random device, to avoid all possibility of bias, be divided by the Central Unit into cases for treatment and cases for control."[95]

Strict observance of an allocation schedule based on alternation was substantially more probable in a placebo-controlled vaccine trial than in an open trial involving clinical judgments about use of a promising new drug for an often-lethal disease. Thus the *British Medical Journal* (BMJ) noted in its leading article that accompanied the streptomycin report that the panel set up by the trial's steering committee to assess patients' eligibility "conceivably might have been influenced in selecting or rejecting a patient if it had known beforehand whether the patient was to be allocated to the streptomycin or to the controlled group – e.g., if alternate patients had been taken. It was relieved of any such worries by an ingenious system of sealed envelopes. Once a patient had been accepted an appropriate numbered envelope was opened, and not till then was the patient's group revealed. The allocation to "S" or "C" in this form had been made at random by the statistician ... The random allocation has not only removed personal responsibility from the clinician and possible bias in his process of choosing patients, but has on the whole effectively equated the groups."[96]

Bradford Hill probably wrote the BMJ editorial. There is no relevant documentation, but Stephen Lock, a previous editor of the BMJ who knew Bradford Hill well,[97] thinks that Bradford Hill told him this. He notes in addition that it is unlikely that the BMJ's pool of editorialists had anybody else who could – or, more cogently, would – have done it, given the quarrelsome temperament of the then editor (who travelled on the same commuter train from home to London as Bradford Hill).[98]

Bradford Hill did not attend the initial meetings of the streptomycin trial's steering committee, but other members had used alternation in clinical trials.[99] Furthermore, recent testimony from two members of the group – Philip D'Arcy Hart and Guy Scadding – indicates that it adopted the randomization scheme proposed by Bradford Hill not because of statistical considerations, but, as in the patulin trial,[100] because it would help to conceal allocations until after eligible patients had irrevocably entered the study.[101] D'Arcy Hart, secretary to the committees overseeing the MRC trials of both patulin and streptomycin, asked in 1996: "Why has [the patulin] trial been overlooked? Is it because attention to the validity of therapeutic trials was generally stimulated by the scheme based on random sampling numbers provided by Bradford Hill to Marc Daniels and me for use in the (streptomycin) trial, which subsequently (from 1948) served as a model for randomization in many later randomized controlled trials? Or is it because the results of the patulin trial were negative and those of the streptomycin trial made medical history?"[102] Certainly the methodological details provided in the report of the patulin trial[103] and recent oral testimony suggest[104] that care was taken to make the patulin and placebo groups comparable. The report notes: "Previous experience had convinced us that, in a trial of this nature, it is of great importance that both the medical personnel and the patients be prevented from guessing which of the two treatments is genuine and which spurious. It had further been learnt that two solutions are not sufficient to prevent this. In this present trial therefore, four solutions were used, two of which (R and T) contained patulin and two (Q and S) were simply solutions of the buffer salts used in dispensing patulin."[105]

In a recent interview, D'Arcy Hart said to me: "Joan [Faulkner], Ruth [Hart] and I went to Cardiff to set up the study. Everyone had thought we would use alternation, and we thought we were very clever in setting up a scheme with two patulin groups and two placebo groups using letters to designate each of the four groups, then using rotation to allocate people to the different groups. We thought we were doing something completely new. We wanted to muddle people up. In fact we succeeded in muddling ourselves up! We didn't always remember what the letters stood for! None of us was a statistician, but we felt that the patulin trial was the first decently controlled trial the MRC had done. Some members of the team that had worked on patulin moved on to do the streptomycin trial."[106]

The testimony of D'Arcy Hart and Guy Scadding is consistent with Bradford Hill's response to a more general question, which William Silverman and I put to him when I met him for the first time in 1982. What did he see as the advantages of random allocation over alternation? He made it clear that random allocation was preferable only because it was more likely to prevent advance knowledge of allocations among those involved in recruiting students.[107]

BRADFORD HILL ON ALLOCATION, 1937–55

His 1933 analysis of the MRC trial of serum treatment for lobar pneumonia[108] had introduced Bradford Hill to the problems created by clinicians' departures from allocation schemes based on alternation, and he frequently reiterated the need for strict observance of allocation schemes designed to control bias. None the less, Peter Armitage[109] has suggested that Bradford Hill may have continued to underestimate the danger of bias arising from foreknowledge of allocations. Accordingly I trace the evolution of the relevant text in successive editions of *Principles of Medical Statistics* before and after the streptomycin trial.

In the first edition, published in 1937, the relevant passage is the subsection on 'Allocation to groups' in the section on 'The problems of clinical trials' in the concluding chapter. "By the allocation of the patients to the two groups we want to ensure that these two groups are alike except in treatment. It was pointed out in the first chapter that this might be done, with reasonably large numbers, by a random division of the patients; the first being given treatment A, the second being orthodoxly treated and serving as a control, the third being given treatment A, the fourth serving as a control, and so on, no departure from this rule being allowed. It was also pointed out that this method could be elaborated and the groups made equal in such well defined characteristics as age and sex, and then randomly composed in other respects (and of course, more than one form of treatment could be brought in)."[110]

There was no change in this wording until the fifth edition (1950), where the final sentence reads: "It was also pointed out that this method could be elaborated, *or other 'randomising' methods applied* (emphasis added), and the groups made equal in such well defined characteristics as age and sex, and then randomly composed in other respects."[111]

The preface to the sixth edition (1955) signals a substantial change: "In the first edition of this book, issued in 1937, I wrote my final chapter, entitled 'General Summary and Conclusions', round the problem of clinical trials. The discussion was a broad one, of general principles rather than of detail, but, without much change, it appears to me to have stood up reasonably well to the passage of time. That passage of time has, however, brought clinical trials into prominence and fashion, and I have thought it wise in the present edition to take notice of that development. Accordingly, I have introduced a wholly new chapter (Chapter XX) in which the special problems of clinical trials are set out in detail. For use in clinical trials, and many other purposes, I have added 16 pages of random sampling numbers (some 10,000 in all), together with illustrations of how to use them in practice."[112]

As far as the pages of random sampling numbers are concerned, David Hill has recorded: "When my father produced his own first set of such tables for his book, he did it by using Tippett to take numbers at random from Kendall and Babbington Smith (or vice versa, I do not know which way round it was) but I remember him saying to me 'If anyone wants to sue me for breach of copyright, they will have to demonstrate which particular digits I have copied.' In later editions I produced pseudorandom numbers for him to use, which I would regard as being, in general, just as good as real randomness, provided that the method is a good one."[113]

The subsection on 'The construction of groups' in Bradford Hill's new chapter 20 in 1955 almost certainly reflects the rationale for basing allocation on random numbers in the streptomycin trial.[114] The trial used "a statistical series based on random sampling numbers" to ensure that "the details of the (allocation) series were unknown to any of the investigators or to the coordinator and were contained in a set of sealed envelopes, each bearing on the outside only the name of the hospital and a number."

The next step in the setting up of the trial is the allocation of the patients to be included in the treatment and the non-treatment groups (or to more than two groups if more than one treatment is under test). The aim is to allocate them to these "treatment" and "control" groups in such a way that the two *groups* are initially equivalent in all respects relevant to the inquiry. Individuals, it may be noted, are not necessarily equivalent; it is a group reaction that is under study. In many trials this allocation has been successfully made by putting patients, as they present themselves, alternately into the treatment and control groups. Such a method may, however, be insufficiently random if the admission or non-admission of a case to the trial turns upon a difficult assessment of the patient and if the clinician involved knows whether the patient, if accepted, will pass to the treatment or control group. By such knowledge he may be biased, consciously or unconsciously, in his acceptance or rejection; or through fear of being biased, his judgment may be influenced. The latter can be just as important a source of error as the former but is more often overlooked. For this reason, it is better to avoid the alternating method and to adopt the use of random sampling numbers; in addition, the allocation of the patient to treatment or control should be unknown to the clinician until *after* he has made his decision upon the patient's admission. Thus he can proceed to that decision – admission or rejection – without any fear of bias. One such technique has been for the statistician to provide the clinician with a set of numbered and sealed envelopes. After each patient has been brought into the trial the appropriately numbered envelope is opened (no. 1 for the first patient, no. 2 for the second, and so on) and the group to which the patient is to go, treatment (T) or control (C) is given upon a slip inside. Alternatively a list showing the order to be followed may be prepared in advance, *e.g.* T, T, C, T, C, C, T, T, T, C, etc., and held confidentially, the clinician in charge being instructed after each admission has been made."[115]

Two paragraphs about balanced randomization within blocks follow, before the section concludes: "The prescribed random order must, needless to say, be strictly followed or the whole procedure is valueless and the trial breaks down. Faithfully adhered to, it offers three great advantages: (1) it ensures that our personal feelings, or judgments, applied consciously or unconsciously, have not played any part in building up the various treatment groups; from that aspect, therefore, the groups are unbiased; (2) it removes the very real danger, inherent in any allocation which is based upon personal judgments, that believing our judgments may be biased, we endeavour to allow for that bias and in so doing may 'lean over backwards' and thus introduce a lack of balance from the other direction; (3) having used such a random allocation we cannot be accused by critics of having set up personally biased groups for comparison."[116]

These passages still appeared more than fifteen years later in the ninth edition of the book, with only two sentences added for emphasis at the beginning of the section: "As stated earlier, before admission to a trial *every* patient must be regarded as suitable for *any* of the treatments under study. If this freedom is not present, then equivalent groups cannot be constructed and comparisons are impossible."[117] Nowhere does Bradford Hill allude to randomization as a way of ensuring the validity of tests of statistical significance. His concern continued to be the control of bias, hence his detailed reference to ways of concealing allocation schedules from those involved in recruiting patients for clinical trials.

GRADUAL RECOGNITION OF THE TWO ESSENTIAL COMPONENTS OF UNBIASED ALLOCATION IN CLINICAL TRIALS

The 1948 report of the MRC's streptomycin trial is a landmark in the history of clinical trials because of its clear account of how the researchers had implemented the two essential components of unbiased allocation – an unbiased allocation schedule and prevention of foreknowledge of the allocations among those involved in the recruitment of patients. Empirical research today leaves no room for doubt that both of these steps are important,[118] but surveys of reports of clinical trials make clear that they remain insufficiently appreciated. This unsatisfactory state of affairs has prompted the emergence of an international initiative by researchers, medical journal editors, and others to improve the situation.[119]

Given the confusion among clinical researchers, some historians have made incorrect assumptions about the reason that random allocation was adopted for the MRC clinical trial of streptomycin for pulmonary tuberculosis. First, following Fisher, random allocation rather than alternation has been accorded special status in statistical theory. As I have noted, however, not only are the statistical consequences of random allocation and alternate allocation very similar,[120] but the two methods, and language about them, have intertwined inextricably in the history of clinical trials. Indeed, random allocation has still not replaced alternation, even though schedules based on alternation are substantially more difficult to conceal.

Second, the other element of successful random allocation – concealment of the schedule – may have escaped notice simply because it has had no unambiguous name.[121] Three years after the publication of the sixth edition (1955) of Bradford Hill's book, the statistician David Cox included a section in *The Planning of Experiments* entitled "Randomisation as a device for concealment."[122] However, only the first of his two examples concerns circumstances "where bias may enter the selection of units to take part in the experiment." His second example is concerned with reducing observer biases in assessing outcomes because randomisation may help to 'blind' observers, whether these are patients, professionals, or researchers. "Allocation concealment" has only recently become a more widely accepted term, distinguishing that particular form of "blinding" from other kinds.[123] The latest edition of Last's *Dictionary of Epidemiology*, for example, defines "Allocation concealment": "A method of generating a sequence that ensures random allocation between two or more arms of a study, without revealing this to either study subjects or researchers. The quality of allocation concealment is enhanced by computer-based random allocation and other procedures to make the process impervious to allocation bias. Less satisfactory methods are allocation by alternation or date of birth, case record, day of the week, presenting or enrolment order."[124] Even this definition would have been stronger had the final sentence added: "because these permit foreknowledge of the allocations, and thus the temptation to subvert them."

Although I have not found any evidence that statistical theory influenced the MRC's adoption of random allocation for its trial of streptomycin for pulmonary tuberculosis, it is possible that it may have played a more prominent role elsewhere. One of the earliest clear descriptions of formal randomization in a U.S. clinical trial,[125] for example, reports that a professor of mathematics generated the allocations, and a study published in 1941 used Tippett's random sampling numbers to allocate participants to comparison groups.[126] Furthermore, textbooks (1938 and 1952) written by one of the first medical statisticians active in North America – Donald Mainland[127] – pay explicit tribute to Fisher and are far more 'statistical' than Bradford Hill's *Principles of Medical Statistics.* Future research should look at whether statistical theory was more influential in the evolution of clinical trials outside Fisher's home country than within it.

Further research may also show how Bradford Hill's concern to limit bias when controlled trials begin, and Fisher's desire to quantify the uncertainty left after their completion,[128] merged the 'clinical' and 'statistical' rationales for random allocation and thereby improved the design and analysis of clinical trials during the second half of the twentieth century.

ACKNOWLEDGMENTS

This paper is based on presentations made at the two-day conference "Beating Biases in Therapeutic Research: Historical Perspectives," at the Osler-McGovern Centre, Green College, Oxford, on 4–5 Sept. 2002, which was supported by the UK Cochrane Centre, the Wellcome Unit for the History of Medicine in Oxford, and the Wellcome Trust; and at the three-day conference "La quantification dans les sciences médicales et de la santé: perspective historique et sociologique," at Saint-Julien-en-Beaujolais, France, 24–26 Oct. 2002, which was supported by McGill University, l'Ehess, and the Fondation Mérieux. I am grateful to participants in both these conferences for helpful advice and to

Ben Toth and Alan Yoshioka for copies of their PhD theses. For comments on earlier drafts of this article I am indebted to Doug Altman, Peter Armitage, Luc Berlivet, David Cox, Philip D'Arcy Hart, Richard Doll, David Hill, Michael Kramer, Stephen Lock, Irvine Loudon, Harry Marks, Iain Milne, Keith O'Rourke, William Silverman, Stephen Stigler, Ben Toth, and Ulrich Tröhler. I am especially grateful to Jan Vandenbroucke for his comments on successive drafts and for his studying successive editions of Udny Yule's *Introduction to the Theory of Statistics* and to George Weisz and Annick Opinel for their help and patience in coping with the required format of references.

NOTES

1 R. Doll, "The Role of Data Monitoring Committees," in L. Duley and B. Farrell, eds., *Clinical Trials* (London: BMJ Books, 2002), 97–104.
2 I. Hacking, *The Taming of Chance* (Cambridge: Cambridge University Press, 1990).
3 I. Chalmers, "Comparing Like with Like: Some Historical Milestones in the Evolution of Methods to Create Unbiased Comparison Groups in Therapeutic Experiments," *International Journal of Epidemiology* 30 (2001), 1156–64.
4 T.J. Kaptchuk, "Intentional Ignorance: A History of Blind Assessment and Placebo Controls in Medicine," *Bulletin of the History of Medicine* 72 (1998), 389–433.
5 H.M. Marks, "Trust and Mistrust in the Marketplace: Statistics and Clinical Research, 1945–1960," *History of Science* 38 (2000), 343–55.
6 Medical Research Council (MRC), "Streptomycin Treatment of Pulmonary Tuberculosis: A Medical Research Council Investigation," *British Medical Journal* 2 (1948), 769–82.
7 D. Mainland, "The Rise of Experimental Statistics and the Problems of a Medical Statistician," *Yale Journal of Biology and Medicine* 27 (1954), 5.
8 MRC, "Streptomycin Treatment of Pulmonary Tuberculosis."
9 J. Rosser Matthews, *Quantification and the Quest for Medical Certainty* (Princeton, NJ: Princeton University Press, 1995), 127.
10 H.M. Marks, *The Progress of Experiment: Science and Therapeutic Reform in the United States, 1900–1990*, Cambridge Studies in the History of Medicine (Cambridge: Cambridge University Press, 1997), 132.
11 Ibid., 138.
12 J.-P. Gaudillière, "Beyond One-Case Statistics: Mathematics, Medicine, and the Management of Health and Disease in the Postwar Era," in U. Bottazzini and A.D. Dalmedico, eds., *Changing Images in Mathematics: From the French Revolution to the New Millennium* (London: Routledge, 2001), 283.
13 E. Magnello, "The Introduction of Mathematical Statistics into Medical

Research: The Roles of Karl Pearson, Major Greenwood and Austin Bradford Hill," in E. Magnello and A. Hardy, eds., *The Road to Medical Statistics* (Amsterdam: Rodopi, 2002), 107.

14 Chalmers, "Comparing Like with Like," 1156–64.

15 P. Armitage, cited in ibid., 1157.

16 I. Semmelweis, *Die Aetiologie, der Begriff und die Prophylaxis des Kindbettfiebers* [The Aetiology, Concept, and Prophylaxis of Childbed Fever] (Budapest, 1861); J. Fibiger, "Om Serumbehandling af Difteri" [On Treatment of Diphtheria with Serum], *Hospitalstidende* 6 (1898), 309–25.

17 A. Bradford Hill, *Principles of Medical Statistics,* 1st ed. (London: Lancet, 1937).

18 Armitage, cited in Chalmers, "Comparing Like with Like."

19 See, for example, H.S. Diehl, A.B. Baker and D.W. Cowan, "Cold Vaccines: An Evaluation Based on a Controlled Study," *Journal of the American Medical Association* 111 (1938), 1168–73; I. Sutherland, "Medical Research Council Streptomycin Trial," *Encyclopaedia of Biostatistics* (Chichester: Wiley, 1998), 2559–62.

20 J.F. Box, *R.A. Fisher: The Life of a Scientist* (New York: John Wiley & Sons, 1978), 268– 70.

21 R. Kunz, G. Vist, and A.D. Oxman, "Randomisation to Protect against Selection Bias in Healthcare Trials," *Cochrane Methodology Review* 1 (in The Cochrane Library, Oxford: Update Software, 2003).

22 D.G. Altman and K.F. Schulz, "Statistics Notes: Concealing Treatment Allocation in Randomised Trials," *British Medical Journal* 323 (2001), 446–7; K.F. Schulz, I. Chalmers, R.J. Hayes, and D.G. Altman, "Empirical Evidence of Bias: Dimensions of Methodological Quality Associated with Estimates of Treatment Effects in Controlled Trials," *Journal of the American Medical Association* 273 (1995), 408–12.

23 K.F. Schulz, "Subverting Randomization in Controlled Trials," *Journal of the American Medical Association* 274 (1995), 1456–8.

24 A. Bradford Hill, "Discussion on Dr. Armitage's Paper on 'The Comparison of Survival Curves,'" *Journal of the Royal Statistical Society,* Series A, Part III (1959), 295.

25 MRC, "Streptomycin Treatment of Pulmonary Tuberculosis."

26 J. Lind, *A Treatise of the Scurvy. In Three Parts. Containing an Inquiry into the Nature, Causes and Cure, of that Disease, Together with a Critical and Chronological View of What Has Been Published on the Subject* (Edinburgh: Sands, Murray and Cochran for A. Kincaid and A. Donaldson, 1753).

27 W.A. Silverman and I. Chalmers, "Casting and Drawing Lots: A Time Honoured Way of Dealing with Uncertainty and for Ensuring Fairness," *British Medical Journal* 323 (2001), 1467–8, and "Casting and Drawing Lots," James Lind Library (www.jameslindlibrary.org), Thursday 17 April 2003.

28 C.H. Parry, "Experiments Relative to the Medical Effects of Turkey Rhubarb, and of the English Rhubarbs, No, 1 and No. II Made on Patients of the Pauper Charity," *Letters and Papers of the Bath Society* 3 (1786), 407–22.

29 A.L. Hamilton, *Dissertatio Medica Inauguralis De Synocho Castrensi* (Edinburgh: J. Ballantyne, 1816).

30 Ibid.

31 I. Milne and I. Chalmers, "Tackling Bias in Assessing the Effects of Health Care Interventions: Early Contributions from James Lind, Alexander Lesassier Hamilton and T. Graham Balfour," *Proceedings of the Royal College of Physicians of Edinburgh* 31, Suppl. 9 (2001), 46–8.

32 T.G. Balfour, quoted in *West C. Lectures on the Diseases of Infancy and Childhood* (London: Longman, Brown, Green and Longmans, 1854), 600.

33 I. Chalmers and B. Toth, "Thomas Graham Balfour's 1854 Report of a Clinical Trial of Belladonna Given to Prevent Scarlet Fever," James Lind Library (www.jameslindlibrary.org), 17 April, 2003.

34 W. Fletcher, "Rice and Beri-Beri: Preliminary Report on an Experiment Conducted in the Kuala Lumpur Insane Asylum," *Lancet* 1 (1907), 1776–9; A. Bingel, "Über Behandlung der Diphtherie mit gewöhnlichem Pferdeserum," *Deutsches Archiv für Klinische Medizin* 125 (1918), 284–332; R.A. Johnston and R.S. Siddall, "Is the Usual Method of Preparing Patients for Delivery Beneficial or Necessary?" *American Journal of Obstetrics and Gynecology* (1922), 4645–50.

35 K. Pearson, "Report on Certain Enteric Fever Inoculation Statistics," *British Medical Journal* 3 (1904), 1243–6.

36 See www.jameslindlibrary.org

37 MRC, "Therapeutic Trials Committee, Serum Treatment of Lobar Pneumonia," *British Medical Journal* 1 (1934), 241–5; W.R. Snodgrass and T. Anderson, "Prontosil in the Treatment of Erysipelas: A Controlled Series of 312 Cases [A Report to the Therapeutic Trials Committee of the Medical Research Council]," *British Medical Journal* 2 (1937), 101–4; W.R. Snodgrass and T. Anderson, "Sulphanilamide in the Treatment of Erysipelas: A Controlled Series of 270 Cases," *British Medical Journal* 2 (1937),1156–9; T. Anderson, "Sulphanilamide in the Treatment of Measles," *British Medical Journal* 1 (1939), 716–18.

38 MRC, "Clinical Trial of Patulin in the Common Cold: Report of the Patulin Clinical Trials Committee," *Lancet* 2 (1944), 373–5.

39 P. D'Arcy Hart, "Early Controlled Clinical Trials," *British Medical Journal* (1996), 312.

40 See for example Medical Research Council, "Antibiotic and Chemotherapeutic Agents in the Treatment of Infantile Diarrhoea and Vomiting," *Lancet* 2 (1953), 1164–9; MRC, "Thrombophlebitis Following Intravenous Infusions: Trial of Plastic and Red Rubber Giving-Sets," *Lancet* 1 (1957), 595–7.

41 S. McDonald, M. Westby, and M. Clarke, "Reporting of the Generation and Concealment of the Allocation Schedule in Randomized Trials in the *BMJ* (1948–1997)," Fourth Symposium on Systematic Reviews: Pushing the Boundaries, Oxford, 2–4 July 2002.

42 J.A. Van Helmont, *Oriatrike, or Physick Refined: The Common Errors Therein Refuted and the Whole are Reformed and Rectified* (London: Lodowick-Loyd, 1662), 526.

43 Silverman and Chalmers, "Casting and Drawing Lots" (2001), and "Casting and Drawing Lots" (2003).

44 D. Colebrook, "Irradiation and Health," Medical Research Council Special Report Series, No. 131 (London: HMSO, 1929).

45 J.A. Doull, M. Hardy, J.H. Clark and N.B. Herman, "The Effect of Irradiation with Ultra-violet Light on the Frequency of Attacks of Upper Respiratory Disease (Common Colds)," *American Journal of Hygiene* 13 (1931), 460–77.

46 Ibid.

47 J.B. Amberson, B.T. McMahon, and M. Pinner, "A Clinical Trial of Sanocrysin in Pulmonary Tuberculosis," *American Review of Tuberculosis* 24 (1931), 401–35.

48 G.W. Theobald, "Effect of Calcium and Vitamin A and D on Incidence of Pregnancy Toxaemia," *Lancet* 2 (1937), 1397–9.

49 R. Doll, letter to Iain Chalmers, 28 March 2003.

50 T. Dehue, "Deception, Efficiency, and Random Groups: Psychology and the Gradual Origination of the Random Group Design," *Isis* 88 (1997), 653–73; A. Oakley, "Experimentation and Social Interventions: A Forgotten but Important History," *British Medical Journal* 317 (1998), 1239–42.

51 C.S. Peirce and J. Jastrow, "On Small Differences in Sensation," *Memoirs of the National Academy of Science* 3 (1884), 75–83.

52 E.L. Thorndike and R.S. Woodworth, "The Influence of Improvement in One Mental Function Upon the Efficiency of the Other Functions," *Psychological Review* 8 (1901), 247–61.

53 I. Hacking, "Telepathy: Origins of Randomisation in Experimental Design," *Isis* 79 (1988), 427–51.

54 Ibid., 447.

55 W. McCall, *How to Experiment in Education* (New York: Macmillan, 1923), 42.

56 E.L. Thorndike, G.J. Ruger, and W.A. McCall, "The Effects of Outside Air and Recirculated Air Upon the Intellectual Achievement and Improvement of School Pupils," *School and Society* 3 (1916), 679–84.

57 W.H. Winch, "The Transfer of Improvement in Memory in Schoolchildren," *British Journal of Psychology* (1908), 284–93.

58 D.B. Rubin, "Comment: Neyman (1923) and Causal Inference in Experiments and Observational Studies," *Statistical Science* 5 (1990), 472–80.

59 Student, "On Testing Varieties of Cereals," *Biometrika* 15 (1923), 271–93.

60 J. Splawa-Neyman, "On the Application of Probability Theory to Agricultural Experiments, Essay on Principles," *Statistical Science* 5 (1990), 465–80. This paper appeared originally in Section 9, *Roczniki Nauk Rolniczych* [Annals of Agricultural Science] 10 (1923), 1–51, and was translated and edited by D.M. Dabrowska and T.P. Speed.

61 R.A. Fisher, *Statistical Methods for Research Workers*, 1st ed. (Edinburgh: Oliver and Boyd, 1925); R.A. Fisher, "The Arrangement of Field Experiments," *Journal of the Ministry of Agriculture* 33 (1926), 503–13.

62 Rubin, "Comment: Neyman."

63 Fisher, "The Arrangement of Field Experiments," and R.A. Fisher, *The Design of Experiments* (London: Oliver and Boyd, 1935).

64 A. Bradford Hill, *Principles of Medical Statistics*, 1st ed. (1937).

65 Marks, *The Progress of Experiment*.

66 D. Hill, letter to Iain Chalmers, 15 April 2003.

67 P. Armitage, "Fisher, Bradford Hill and Randomization," *International Journal of Epidemiology* 32 (2003), 925–8; I. Chalmers, "Fisher and Bradford Hill: Theory and Pragmatism?" *International Journal of Epidemiology*, 32 (2003), 922–4.

68 Armitage, "Fisher, Bradford Hill and Randomization"; R. Doll, "Fisher and Bradford Hill: Their Personal Impact," *International Journal of Epidemiology* 32 (2003), 929–31.

69 A. Bradford Hill, *Principles of Medical Statistics*, 1st ed. (1937), 4.

70 A. Bradford Hill, "Memories of the British Streptomycin Trial in Tuberculosis," *Controlled Clinical Trials* 11 (1990), 77–9.

71 J.G. Scadding, "Use of Randomisation in Early Clinical Trials," *British Medical Journal* 318 (1999), 1352.

72 Doll, "Fisher and Bradford Hill: Their Personal Impact."

73 D. Hill, personal communication at meeting on 16 April 2003.

74 A. Bradford Hill, "Some Memories of A.B.H.," manuscript dated January 1988, held in the archive at the London School of Hygiene and Tropical Medicine.

75 A. Yoshioka, "Use of Randomisation in the Medical Research Council's Clinical Trial of Streptomycin in Pulmonary Tuberculosis in the 1940s," *British Medical Journal* 317 (1998), 1220–3.

76 MRC, "Therapeutic Trials Committee."

77 I. Chalmers, "MRC Therapeutic Trials Committee's Report on Serum Treatment of Lobar Pneumonia, British Medical Journal 1934," James Lind Library (www.jameslindlibrary.org), 12 March 2003.

78 B. Toth, "Clinical Trials in British Medicine 1858–1948, with Special Reference to the Development of the Randomised Controlled Trial" (PhD thesis, University of Bristol, 1998).

79 S. Lock, "The Randomised Controlled Trial – a British Invention," in G. Lawrence, ed., *Technologies of Modern Medicine* (London: Science Museum 1994), 81–7.

80 J. Austoker and L. Bryder, eds., *Historical Perspectives on the Role of the MRC* (Oxford: Oxford University Press, 1989), 46–7.
81 Lock, "The Randomised Controlled Trial."
82 A. Bradford Hill, "Serum Treatment of Pneumonia, 22 December 1933," cited in J. Austoker and L. Bryder, eds., *Historical Perspectives on the Role of the MRC* (Oxford: Oxford University Press, 1989), 46–7.
83 Toth, Clinical Trials in British Medicine 1858–1948.
84 MRC, "Therapeutic Trials Committee."
85 J. Vandenbroucke, "A Short Note on the History of the Randomized Controlled Trial," *Journal of Chronic Disease* 40 (1987), 985–7.
86 A. Bradford Hill, letter to Iain Chalmers, 7 Aug. 1988.
87 M. Greenwood and G.U. Yule, "The Statistics of Anti-Typhoid and Anti-Cholera Inoculations, and the Interpretation of Such Statistics in General," *Proceedings of the Royal Society of Medicine* 8 (1915), 113–94.
88 G.U. Yule and M.G. Kendall, *An Introduction to the Theory of Statistics* (London: Charles Griffin, 1937), 337.
89 A. Bradford Hill, letter, 1988.
90 D. Hill, letter, 2003.
91 MRC, "The Prevention of Whooping-Cough by Vaccination," *British Medical Journal* 1 (1951), 1463–71.
92 A.Y. Yoshioka, "Streptomycin, 1946: British Central Administration of Supplies of a New Drug of American Origin with Special Reference to Clinical Trials in Tuberculosis," (PhD thesis, University of London, 1998); A.Y. Yoshioka, "Use of Randomisation in the Medical Research Council's Clinical Trial."
93 M. Daniels, letter to G.S. Wilson, 10 Dec. 1946, FD1/6756, National Archives, Kew, London.
94 Marks, *The Progress of Experiment*, 122.
95 Ibid.
96 Leading article, "The Controlled Therapeutic Trial," *British Medical Journal* 2 (1948), 791–2.
97 Lock, "The Randomised Controlled Trial."
98 S. Lock, e-mail correspondence with Iain Chalmers, 13–21 March 2003.
99 MRC, 1944; J.G. Scadding, "Sulphonamides in Bacillary Dysentery," *Lancet* 2 (1945), 549–53.
100 MRC, 1944.
101 P. D'Arcy Hart, "A Change in Scientific Approach: From Alternation to Randomised Allocation in Clinical Trials in the 1940s," *British Medical Journal* 319 (1999), 572–3; J.G. Scadding, "Use of Randomisation in Early Clinical Trials," *British Medical Journal* 318 (1999), 1352.
102 Hart, "Early Controlled Clinical Trials."
103 MRC, 1944.
104 P. D'Arcy Hart, interview with Iain Chalmers, 2 May 2003.
105 MRC, 1944.

106 Hart, interview, 2003.
107 I. Chalmers, "Why Transition from Alternation to Randomisation in Clinical Trials Was Made," *British Medical Journal* 319 (1999), 1372; Chalmers, "Comparing Like with Like."
108 MRC, 1934.
109 P. Armitage, "Bradford Hill and the Randomized Controlled Trial," *Pharmaceutical Medicine* 6 (1992), 23–37.
110 A. Bradford Hill, *Principles of Medical Statistics*, 1st ed. (1937), 155–60.
111 A. Bradford Hill, *Principles of Medical Statistics*, 5th ed. (London: Lancet, 1950), 235.
112 A. Bradford Hill, *Principles of Medical Statistics*, 6th ed. (London: Lancet, 1955), v.
113 D. Hill, letter, 2003; P. Griffiths and D. Hill, *Applied Statistics Algorithms* (Chichester: Ellis Horwood, 1985), 238–42.
114 MRC, 1948.
115 A. Bradford Hill, *Principles of Medical Statistics*, 6th ed. (1955), v.
116 Ibid., 239–41.
117 A. Bradford Hill, *Principles of Medical Statistics*, 9th ed. (London: Lancet, 1971), 254.
118 Schulz et al., "Empirical Evidence of Bias," 408–12; Kunz et al., "Randomisation to Protect against Selection Bias."
119 D.G. Altman, K.F. Schulz, D. Moher, M. Egger, F. Davidoff, D. Elbourne, P.C. Gøtzsche, and T. Lang, "The Revised CONSORT Statement for Reporting Randomized Trials: Explanation and Elaboration," *Annals of Internal Medicine* 134 (2001), 663–94 and www.consort-statement.org, 19 April 2003.
120 Armitage, cited in Chalmers, "Comparing Like with Like," 1157.
121 Schulz et al., "Empirical Evidence of Bias."
122 D.R. Cox, Planning of Experiments (New York: Wiley, 1958), 79.
123 Schulz et al., "Empirical Evidence of Bias"; K.F. Schulz, I. Chalmers and D. Altman, "The Landscape and Lexicon of Blinding," *Annals of Internal Medicine* 136 (2002), 254–9.
124 J.M. Last, *A Dictionary of Epidemiology*, 4th ed. (Oxford: Oxford University Press, 2001), 4.
125 Doull et al., "The Effect of Irradiation with Ultra-violet Light."
126 J.A. Bell, "Pertussis Prophylaxis with Two Doses of Alum-precipitated Vaccine," *Public Health Reports* 56 (1941), 1535–46.
127 D. Mainland, *The Treatment of Clinical and Laboratory Data* (Edinburgh: Oliver and Boyd, 1938); D. Mainland, *Elementary Medical Statistics* (Philadelphia: Saunders, 1952).
128 H.M. Marks, "Rigorous Uncertainty: Why R.A. Fisher Is Important," *International Journal of Epidemiology* 32 (2003), 932–7.

15

Exigence scientifique et isolement institutionnel : L'essor contrarié de l'épidémiologie française dans la seconde moitié du XXe siècle

LUC BERLIVET

L'évolution du discours et des pratiques de santé publique, dans la seconde moitié du xxe siècle, aura été marquée par un mouvement de systématisation et d'intensification simultanées du recours à l'objectivation statistique. Aux entreprises de description quantifiée de l'état de santé des populations, nées au siècle précédent, vinrent s'ajouter la mobilisation des ressources de la statistique inférentielle au service de la recherche sur l'étiologie des maladies, ainsi que le recours à des méthodologies analogues – développées dans le cadre des essais thérapeutiques dits "randomisés" – afin d'évaluer l'efficacité des actions de prévention et l'organisation des soins[1]. Cette transformation de l'approche étiologique fut très largement le fait des épidémiologistes, groupe professionnel dont les contours restèrent longtemps faiblement objectivés, tant le vocable recouvrait – et recouvre encore parfois – une grande variété de trajectoires, d'affiliations institutionnelles, d'objets de recherche et de pratiques méthodologiques. Les efforts déployés pour élargir leur espace de compétence reconnue ne manquèrent d'ailleurs pas de susciter des résistances, jusque et y compris au sein de cette communauté : en témoignent les propos véhéments d'épidémiologistes britanniques et américains refusant de considérer que la recherche sur les maladies non transmissibles puisse ressortir à la discipline, et appelant ses promoteurs à trouver un autre nom pour désigner leurs pratiques scientifiques[2]... Pour autant, une fois ces objections surmontées, les épidémiologistes en vinrent à occuper une place que leurs prédécesseurs du xixe siècle n'avaient jamais pu guigner[3], affirmant leur présence aussi bien au sein des écoles de santé publique – où ils firent de leur discipline la clef de voûte de l'enseignement et de la quasi-totalité des activités de recherche[4] – que dans les facultés de médecine, les instituts de recherches et les administrations. S'il ne doit pas nous conduire à minorer les développements intervenus précédemment – et particulièrement durant l'entre-deux-guerres, trop longtemps présentée, à tort, comme une période de grand sommeil consécutive à l'obsolescence d'un style de raisonnement inductif, éclipsé par les succès de la microbiologie[5] – ce mouvement historique, au terme duquel la statistique mathématique s'est trouvée légitimée comme la langue vernaculaire que doit maîtriser tout intervenant aux débats pour espérer être écouté, mérite donc que l'on s'y arrête.

Comme bien d'autres disciplines biomédicales, l'épidémiologie a connu un essor proprement mondial, ce qui mine toute tentative (aussi désirable soit-elle) [pour] saisir, en un seul mouvement, ses multiples réalités concrètes et l'extrême variété des usages auxquels elle se prête. Certes, les différences marquées entre les régimes de pratiques privilégiés dans les pays industrialisés et dans les pays en voie de développement apparaissent clairement, qu'elles tiennent au poids relatif des maladies infectieuses et des pathologies non transmissibles, ou aux difficultés, plus ou moins grandes selon les pays, que doivent surmonter les promoteurs d'investigations statistiques. Mais des particularités nationales se laissent également observer à l'intérieur même du groupe, en réalité peu homogène, des pays dits "du Nord". La contribution des chercheurs britanniques et américains au développement de la *modern epidemiology*[6] centrée sur les pathologies chroniques dégénératives – comme les cancers et les maladies cardio-vasculaires – est, elle, bien connue, même si encore peu étudiée, notamment en raison de l'écho qui fut fait aux recherches initiées dans ces deux pays à la fin des années 1940. L'objectivation, dans le cours de ces recherches, d'un lien statistique entre tabagisme et cancer du poumon donna lieu à une controverse fameuse sur la question de savoir si la relation recouvrait un rapport de cause à effet ou si elle masquait au contraire un tiers facteur proprement causal. *A contrario*, les autres traditions nationales en matière d'épidémiologie – entendue aussi bien comme discipline scientifique que comme activité d'expertise auprès des autorités publiques – demeurent largement méconnues. Nous ne savons, par exemple, que fort peu de choses sur ces chercheurs japonais qui, au début des années 1980, conclurent au caractère cancérogène du tabagisme passif[7]. Leurs publications furent pourtant abondamment commentées et contribuèrent grandement à la dramatisation du débat sur les dangers de la "fumée de tabac ambiante". De même, la forte visibilité acquise par les équipes australiennes dans le domaine de l'évaluation des actions de promotion de la santé – l'éducation à la santé en particulier – conduit à s'interroger sur une éventuelle spécificité des liens noués entre statisticiens, épidémiologistes et spécialistes de santé publique dans cette configuration nationale. Les épidémiologistes proposent parfois des explications à ces spécificités d'une nation à l'autre. Ainsi, la qualité des dispositifs publics de recueil de données institués par les pays scandinaves est-elle souvent invoquée pour expliquer les succès académiques des chercheurs nordiques dans le domaine de la santé publique. Au cours d'un séminaire organisé à la London School of Hygiene and Tropical Medicine au printemps 2002, l'orateur, professeur à l'université du Surrey, exprima son émerveillement face à la minutie d'une série de recherches danoises dans un registre délibérément burlesque, où perçait l'envie autant que l'inquiétude : "Au Danemark, vous vous asseyez sur une chaise dans un lieu public et, immédiatement, il y a tout un tas de capteurs qui mesurent un tas de choses, et les données partent directement dans un ordinateur central." Au-delà du caractère caricatural, littéralement grotesque, d'un propos qui profite à plein de la licence comique – puisqu'il s'agissait bien de faire rire les chercheurs et étudiants réunis dans la salle – cet exemple donne à voir comment des différences nationales, différemment perçues par les uns et les autres, peuvent être mobilisées par les épidémiologistes eux-mêmes pour rendre compte des différences manifestes entre les types de recherches privilégiés ici ou là.

Notre objectif sera précisément de contribuer à une meilleure prise en compte des éléments institutionnels[8] dans l'analyse du développement de l'épidémiologie au cours de la seconde moitié du XXe siècle, à partir de l'analyse du cas français. J'entends ici "étude de cas" au sens que donnent à ce terme nombre de sociologues, historiens et politologues ouverts au comparatisme[9] pour dénoter l'analyse d'une configuration nationale dont la singularité est saisie par contraste avec l'évolution d'institutions, de groupes sociaux, de pratiques scientifiques ou culturelles, etc., homologues, dans d'autres pays. De sorte que, même lorsqu'il n'est pas possible de mener à bien une véritable comparaison internationale, demeurent un souci de mise en perspective des situations locales et un refus de borner l'horizon de recherche aux frontières d'un seul État. Dans le cas qui nous occupe, les points de comparaison sont fournis essentiellement par l'histoire de l'épidémiologie britannique et américaine, qui prirent leur essor plus tôt qu'en France et qui, pour cette raison, ont souvent servi de modèle, même lorsque les différences institutionnelles, d'une configuration nationale à l'autre, rendaient illusoire toute tentation d'émulation et contraignaient à des transpositions-adaptations drastiques des programmes de recherche.

Le caractère récent des développements qui nous intéressent a permis de rencontrer les chercheurs et enseignants concernés, si bien qu'une grande part des renseignements sur leurs trajectoires et leurs positions respectives dans la configuration de l'époque sont extraits de vingt-six entretiens – d'une durée moyenne égale à trois heures, environ. Toutefois, nous avons surtout exploité les éléments biographiques et les informations concernant les interrelations entre divers acteurs et les groupes auxquels ils se rattachaient – autant d'éléments importants qui ne laissent pas toujours de traces écrites, mais qu'il est possible d'obtenir par recoupement, en multipliant les entretiens. Nous avons reçu avec beaucoup de circonspection les propos sur "l'état d'esprit" de l'époque, dont on sait combien ils sont travaillés par des reconstructions *a posteriori*.

L'histoire de l'épidémiologie française au siècle dernier ne peut se comprendre si l'on ne saisit pas combien elle fut transformée par l'émergence, au milieu des années 1950, d'un petit groupe défendant une approche des statistiques médicales en rupture affichée avec les traditions – au point, dans un premier temps, de ne pas se définir comme "épidémiologistes" – et qui parvint, dans une certaine mesure, à en effacer jusqu'au souvenir. Cette poignée de chercheurs de l'Institut national d'hygiène n'entretenait aucun lien, initialement, avec l'univers de la santé publique, et leur allégeance allait au contraire au modèle scientifique incarné par les disciplines biomédicales alors en phase d'institutionnalisation dans l'hexagone. Cette "volonté de faire science" (pour reprendre l'expression employée par Isabelle Stengers à propos de la psychanalyse[10]), encouragée par les caractéristiques de l'espace de la recherche médicale française, explique la priorité accordée à un certain type d'épidémiologie au détriment d'autres pratiques statistiques, et le développement tardif – et encore une fois à la marge des institutions dominantes – d'une "épidémiologie d'intervention" portée par un regain d'intérêt pour les pathologies infectieuses de la part des spécialistes de la santé publique et des autorités politiques, à partir du début des années 1980.

DE L'ÉPIDÉMIOLOGIE DESCRIPTIVE À LA STATISTIQUE INFÉRENTIELLE

Le développement, en France, du type d'épidémiologie encore dominant aujourd'hui fut rendu possible par la métamorphose de l'Institut national d'hygiène (INH) amorcée au cours des années 1950. Institué en 1941 par le régime de Vichy, mais avec l'appui de la Fondation Rockefeller, comme infrastructure technico-scientifique au service d'une entreprise de rationalisation de la politique de santé publique, l'INH va évoluer vers un rôle d'agent central du développement de la recherche biomédicale, ce que parachève en quelque sorte sa transformation, en 1964, en un Institut national de la santé et de la recherche médicale (INSERM). Là encore, les modèles se trouvent outre-Manche – la réputation d'excellence scientifique dont jouissent les équipes du Medical Research Council remonte aux années 1920 – et de l'autre côté de l'Atlantique. Dans ce dernier cas, l'homologie apparaît plus clairement encore : le National Cancer Institute, fondé en 1936, et les autres National Institutes of Health (NIH) apparus dans la seconde moitié des années 1940 sont des émanations du Public Health Service fédéral.

Lors de sa création, par une loi du 30 novembre 1941, l'INH est placé sous la direction d'André Chevallier, professeur à la faculté de Marseille et dynamique entrepreneur scientifique qui a su nouer des contacts étroits avec les dirigeants de la Fondation Rockefeller. L'Institut comprend quatre pôles. Une "section de la nutrition" est animée directement par Chevallier, lequel mène, depuis de nombreuses années, une série de recherches sur le rôle des vitamines dans la santé humaine, grâce à des financements de l'organisation philanthropique américaine. Une "section d'hygiène" prend en charge les questions relatives à ce qu'il est traditionnellement convenu d'appeler "l'hygiène des milieux", les adductions d'eau en particulier, mais aussi le domaine en plein développement de la médecine du travail. La troisième section, dite "des maladies sociales", s'intéresse à ces sujets d'angoisse familiers que sont la tuberculose, l'alcoolisme et la syphilis, mais aussi à un nouveau venu : le cancer. Cette section sera l'une des principales productrices et consommatrices de dénombrements statistiques, avec la "section d'épidémiologie", dirigée par Alice Lotte, médecin de formation, dont les travaux sont destinés à éclairer les pouvoirs publics[11]. Leurs études de mortalité et de morbidité s'apparentent plus à ce que les anglo-saxons désignent sous l'expression *vital statistics* qu'aux recherches épidémiologiques des causes de maladies initiées par les chercheurs britanniques de la Statistical Research Unit (SRU) du Medical Research Council ou par les enquêteurs du Public Health Service américain dès l'entre-deux-guerres.

Si cette vision de l'INH comme lieu de production d'un savoir opérationnel en santé publique se voit confirmée à la Libération, l'évolution impulsée par l'élite médicale française va bientôt entraîner une redéfinition des objectifs, des approches et des pratiques scientifiques légitimes et, ce faisant, permettre l'avènement d'un autre type de statistique médicale. Louis Bugnard, nommé en remplacement du trop marqué André Chevallier, amorce cette évolution en travaillant à institutionnaliser le statut de médecin-chercheur et en organisant l'importation de matériels et de produits nécessaires au travail expérimental, toujours avec le soutien d'organisations philanthropiques anglo-saxonnes. Professeur de physique biologique attentif aux expériences étrangères, il s'attache à développer l'usage de produits radioactifs en thérapeutique et, surtout, en biologie cellulaire (sous la forme d'isotopes). Cette priorité donnée à la physique, si elle constitue sans doute la première actualisation en France de ce que l'historiographie appelle classiquement "bio-médecine", ne peut pour autant satisfaire la fraction des jeunes cliniciens désormais rompus aux exigences de la recherche scientifiques. Ceux que l'on qualifie de "néo-cliniciens" entendent plutôt mener des recherches en biochimie, en génétique, en physiologie cellulaire, voire en biologie moléculaire. Avec l'aide d'une structure de financement alimentée par l'Assistance publique parisienne, l'Association Claude-Bernard, ils vont créer des centres de recherche qui préfigurent les premières unités de L'INSERM.

Dans cette nouvelle configuration, les producteurs de statistiques descriptives au service de politiques de santé publique – en réalité embryonnaires, voire hypothétiques – vont se trouver décentrés, tandis qu'une poignée de statisticiens aux caractéristiques sociales fort différentes va tenter de démontrer la parfaite adéquation de leur style de raisonnement probabiliste au nouveau canon scientifique, tout en mettant leurs compétences méthodologiques et mathématiques au service de certains expérimentateurs. La trajectoire de Pierre Denoix, l'un des personnages les plus importants de l'élite médicale et de la recherche biomédicale française de l'après-guerre, éclaire parfaitement ce renouvellement des pratiques statistiques légitimes. Chirurgien et cancérologue, chef de service à l'Institut Gustave-Roussy (IGR), Denoix, qui a développé une activité de recherche dès l'entre-deux-guerres[12], fait office de responsable scientifique de "l'enquête cancer" lancée par l'INH en 1942 et fondée notamment sur la constitution et l'exploitation de 35 000 dossiers – une bonne part en provenance de l'Assistance publique de Paris. Mais c'est ce même Denoix qui en 1954 va introduire à l'IGR et à l'INH, la statistique inférentielle, conçue comme un outil au service de la recherche sur l'étiologie des maladies non transmissibles.

À cette date, plusieurs publications britanniques et américaines avaient déjà mis en cause le tabac dans la survenue du cancer du poumon. L'enquête épidémiologique française, qui vise à reproduire ces résultats sur une autre population, bénéficie du soutien du Service industriel des tabacs et allumettes (le SEITA), à travers le Groupe d'études sur la fumée du tabac[13]. La maîtrise méthodologique de l'étude et son suivi sont d'ailleurs confiés à un ingénieur des tabacs – alors l'un des corps de l'État ouverts aux élèves de l'École polytechnique – Daniel Schwartz, qui abandonne ainsi ses recherches statistiques sur l'incidence des maladies affectant les plants de tabac pour étudier l'effet sur la santé humaine de ladite plante et acclimater en France l'épidémiologie "nouvelle manière". En réalité, cette rencontre apparement providentielle n'est pas entièrement le fait du hasard et le jeune polytechnicien n'est pas totalement étranger au champ de la recherche médicale. Outre son ascendance (il est le fils d'un chirurgien réputé et surtout le neveu de Robert Debré, figure prééminente de l'élite médicale depuis les années 1930, devenu président de l'INH en 1946), Daniel Schwartz a déjà manifesté, au début des années 1950, son inclination pour la recherche scientifique. Ses intérêts le poussent plutôt vers la génétique et il manque de peu de se joindre à un groupe de recherche dirigé par un jeune professeur de génétique médicale, élève de Debré[14]. En 1954, il vient en outre d'accepter de dispenser un enseignement de statistique médicale, à la demande d'un petit groupe de professeurs parisiens conscients de ce que l'opposition traditionnelle des médecins français au style de raisonnement probabiliste les empêche de se familiariser avec les nouvelles pratiques de recherche légitimes.

Si elle constitue donc une sorte de choix par défaut pour l'ingénieur du SEITA, "l'enquête tabac" va néanmoins lui fournir l'occasion de se métamorphoser, avec bonheur, en entrepreneur scientifique. La visibilité conférée par les résultats de l'investigation étiologique[15] justifie la création, au sein d'un IGR désormais dirigé par Denoix, d'une Unité de recherches statistiques placée sous la responsabilité de Schwartz, puis son intégration à l'INH en 1957 – elle devient alors le 21e laboratoire de l'Institut. Et c'est donc dans ce double cadre institutionel de l'IGR et de l'INH, que va s'institutionnaliser le premier pôle de statistique médicale français.

En l'absence de cursus préétabli au sein des facultés de médecine, le recrutement de l'Unité 21 échappe aux modalités classiques de la carrière hospitalo-universitaire. Ainsi, parmi les premiers chercheurs engagés par Daniel Schwartz, on ne compte quère que deux jeunes médecins, Robert Flamant et Claude Rumeau-Rouquette, qui ont découvert l'épidémiologie par hasard, à l'occasion de vacations dans le cadre de "l'enquête tabac". Le premier est surtout intéressé par les possibles applications du calcul probabiliste à la recherche clinique, quand la seconde voit dans l'épidémiologie le moyen de concilier sa formation médicale et un intérêt pour la psychologie sociale, découverte travers l'enseignement de Jean Stoetzel à la faculté des lettres de Bordeaux. Les autres fondateurs de l'Unité 21 (Joseph Lellouch, Philippe Lazar, Pierre Ducimetière et Jacques-Alain Valleron), pour ne citer que les premières recrues, sont tous polytechniciens.

La référence à la recherche statistique dans l'intitulé du centre ne doit pas être entendue comme une simple dénomination de circonstance. Tout d'abord, comme leurs homologues britanniques dans l'entre-deux-guerre et américains à la fin des années 1940, les chercheurs de l'Unité 21 entendent bien promouvoir l'usage du calcul probabiliste dans les divers domaines de la médecine. Ainsi, même si l'épidémiologie prend d'emblée une place essentielle, l'école de Schwartz développe également des méthodologies appliquées à la recherche clinique, autour des essais thérapeutiques notamment[16]. Leur localisation au sein de l'IGR va contraindre ces nouveaux venus à démontrer leur utilité aux yeux de mandarins souvent dubitatifs face aux concepts d'hypothèse nulle et de signification statistique, et peu enclins à s'en remettre à l'expertise de non-médecins, comme en témoigne ce propos du Dr Lacour, ancien chef de service :

> Les médecins étaient assez réticents : "mais enfin, on ne va plus publier sans le label des statisticiens"; or, c'était indispensable. Du jour où l'équipe de Daniel Schwartz est venue, ça nous a donné un label et nos publications étaient reçues dans le monde entier et considérées comme crédibles, alors qu'avant, c'était inconsistant du point de vue scientifique, on comparait des choses qui n'étaient pas comparables. Ça nous a permis de mettre en œuvre des essais thérapeutiques contrôlés, supervisés par l'équipe de Schwartz ... un travail qui était moderne et qui sortait de l'archaïsme de nos vieilles méthodes[17].

Cette résistance des cliniciens, combinée à un complexe de nouveau venu condamné à s'imposer aux yeux d'expérimentateurs déjà installés au cœur de l'institution, explique l'obstination particulière de l'Unité 21 à faire reconnaître la recherche statistique comme une démarche scientifique à part entière, appuyée sur un raisonnement, certes potentiellement déroutant, mais dont la rigueur est gagée sur la rectitude mathématique du calcul des probabilités.

L'insistance avec laquelle le groupe exhibe ces attributs de scientificité, aussi bien dans le domaine des biostatistiques qu'en épidémiologie, dans une configuration qui le contraint terriblement et menace de le marginaliser, rémoigne de sa volonté de se démarquer des formes de statistique descriptive caractéristiques de l'INH des origines, dénigrées comme relevant plus du domaine de la statistique administrative que de la recherche biomédicale. Cette hostilité se traduit notamment par des critiques virulentes à l'adresse de la Division de la recherche médico-sociale, la structure qui au sein de l'Inserm continue le type de recherches lancées par la Section des maladies sociales et la Section d'épidémiologie.

Daniel Schwartz et ses émules ont d'ailleurs soin de marquer la distance entre leur rôle de chercheur travaillant sur des questions lourdes de conséquences pour la santé publique et celui d'activiste, qu'ils refusent délibérément d'endosser. À la différence d'un Ernst Wynder, par exemple, qui choisit de prolonger ses travaux pionniers sur la cancérogénicité du tabac en s'engageant dans des campagnes d'éducation pour la santé et des actions de lobbying, Daniel Schwartz insistera toujours sur la nécessaire distance du chercheur.

FAIRE ÉCOLE : L'ENSEIGNEMENT "HORS LES MURS" DE LA STATISTIQUE INFÉRENTIELLE

Un formidable obstacle à l'institutionnalisation de l'approche défendue par les pionniers de l'Unité 21 tient à la difficulté qu'ils éprouvent à se reproduire socialement. Tandis que leurs homologues britanniques sont fermement implantés à la London School of Hygiene and Tropical Medicine, lieu de formation hégémoniste des médecins de santé publique britannique – mais qui, de surcroît, recrute ses étudiants bien au-delà des frontières du Commonwealth – et que les Américains peuvent compter sur un réseau étendu d'écoles de santé publique, Schwartz ne dispose pas d'un accès à un lieu de formation préexistant. En dépit du fait qu'il jouisse d'une reconnaissance scientifique croissante (il est chef de service à l'IGR, maître de recherche puis, à partir de 1962, directeur de recherche à l'INH) la Faculté de médecine de Paris renâcle à accueillir un polytechnicien sans formation médicale aucune. Il faut attendre 1968 pour que Schwartz soit élu à une chaire, après avoir été professeur associé durant quatre années, et même alors son enseignement reste confiné à la portion congrue.

Dans l'intervalle, il a déjà entrepris de développer, avec la collaboration active des chercheurs de l'Unité 21, une école en marge de la Faculté, expérience qui va se révéler essentielle, non seulement en ce qu'elle permet de recruter des étudiants et de les former, mais parce que l'originalité du mode de formation va contribuer à souder ce groupe en croissance rapide.

Le point de départ de cette expérience originale est ce cours du soir mis en place par Daniel Schwartz à la demande de quelques mandarins et accueilli par l'Institut de statistique de l'Université de Paris (ISUP). Durant la seconde moitié des années 1950, son recrutement s'étend, tandis que le nombre d'options proposées s'accroît. L'enseignement se structure en 1963 avec la création du Centre d'enseignement de la statistique appliquée à la médecine (CESAM), ayant statut d'association régie par la loi de 1901, et dont Philippe Lazar –

chercheur à l'Unité 21 et futur directeur général de l'INSERM – devient le secrétaire général. Un diplôme national est créé, qui comprend des cours, des enseignements dirigés et des devoirs sanctionnés par un examen. Les effectifs vont croître rapidement, passant de soixante étudiants la première année à plusieurs centaines quelques années plus tard, pour atteindre 1 200 en 1985[18], le Centre constituant ainsi un important vecteur de diffusion de l'approche statistique dans le corps médical avant même l'introduction de ces enseignements dans le cursus universitaire. Les membres de l'Unité de recherches statistiques forment le groupe central des enseignants, auquel s'agrègent les jeunes diplômés, certains passant de la position d'enseigné à celle d'enseignant en l'espace de quelques mois. Ceux qui, parmi les personnes interrogées durant notre enquête, participèrent à la création de ces enseignements évoquent volontiers le caractère "pionnier" des débuts. Comme l'explique une épidémiologiste (devenue enseignante au CESAM après avoir obtenu le certificat de bio-mathématique délivré par le Centre) : "C'était semi-militant[19]." L'enjeu de l'entreprise était de hâter l'institutionnalisation d'une nouvelle discipline dans le champ de la recherche biomédicale française. Nombre des plus intéressés et des plus doués vont d'ailleurs faire carrière à l'INSERM, même si l'institution reste dominée par les approches plus expérimentales. De fait, au milieu des années 1970, les effectifs de l'Unité 21 sont devenus quasi-pléthoriques, et s'amorce alors un mouvement d'essaimage qui voit les anciens collaborateurs de Daniel Schwartz partir fonder leurs propres unités sur des thématiques plus précises.

Claude Rumeau, la première, crée l'Unité 149 (Recherches épidémiologiques sur la santé des femmes et des enfants), puis c'est au tour de Joseph Lellouch (Unité 169) et de Philippe Lazar (recherches épidémiologiques et statistiques sur l'environnement et la santé). Au total, près de dix unités vont être fondées par des chercheurs de l'Unité 21, ce qui continue d'assurer à "l'école Schwartz" une place prépondérante en matière d'épidémiologie et de biostatistique.

ÉPIDÉMIOLOGIE ET SANTÉ PUBLIQUE : UNE SINGULARITÉ FRANÇAISE

Cette conception de la statistique médicale et cet éthos du scientifique attaché à marquer la distance qui le sépare des responsables politiques vont se combiner avec les logiques de fonctionnement d'un institut de recherche biomédicale qui récompense ceux qui se consacrent au "fondamental" plutôt qu'à l'appliqué (soulevant d'emblée le problème du départ entre ces différentes pratiques) pour autonomiser les épidémiologistes vis-à-vis des institutions et des professionnels de la santé publique français. Sur ce point fondamental, la singularité française s'avère radicale.

Le groupe réuni autour de Daniel Schwartz met systématiquement l'accent sur l'analyse des liens entre facteurs de risques et survenue d'une pathologie quand les autres types de pratique épidémiologique (en particulier les *vital statistics* et la veille épidémiologique, d'une part, le développement de méthodes d'évaluation des actions publiques de santé, de l'autre) ne trouveront leur place que bien plus tard, et souvent sous l'impulsion de personnalités atypiques.

C'est cette singularité française que va percevoir Philippe Lazar, en 1975, lorsqu'il se joint à l'Université Harvard pour un an, en qualité de professeur invité :

> Un homme comme Brian MacMahon[20], aux États-Unis, ne connaît pas vraiment la statistique et c'est pourtant un grand épidémiologiste. Cela m'a beaucoup appris de constater qu'on peut avoir une approche conceptuelle tout à fait différente. C'est tout juste s'ils parlent de signification statistique. Ce qui les intéresse, ce sont les aspects quantitatifs. Quand ils voient un risque relatif de 3,3, leur premier réflexe c'est de le situer par rapport aux autres RR, avant de se demander s'il est significativement différent de 1. Et s'il y a un risque de 3,5 dans un groupe et un risque de 3,5 dans un autre mais que l'un est sur 1 000 cas et que l'autre sur 10 cas, ils constatent d'abord que c'est toujours 3,5 et ils disent "c'est la même chose". Alors que pour l'école Schwartz, le premier risque est significatif, il y a un phénomène, tandis que l'autre n'est pas significatif, on ne peut rien en dire. La primauté accordée à la signification statistique est la caractéristique de l'équipe de Schwartz, qui a sa noblesse, son sérieux et son grand intérêt, mais qui déforme un petit peu l'esprit par rapport à la culture du risque, du risque relatif et du risque attribuable. La culture de MacMahon, c'est : "Quel est le risque?", "Quel est le risque attribuable?" C'est une forme de culture finalement très différente. L'école de Schwartz est une école qui teste les hypothèses. Les hypothèses sont-elles de nature biologique? On les confronte aux observations et aux expériences et on essaie de répondre à la question : "Est-ce que c'est significatif ou pas?" Et si c'est significatif : "Qu'est ce qu'on peut en penser?" On suit l'hypothèse à la trace, en quelque sorte[21].

La question de l'articulation entre recherche épidémiologique et santé publique fera d'ailleurs l'objet d'une contestation de "l'école de Schwartz" par un groupe de jeunes médecins formés aux statistiques médicales et à l'informatique dans le service de François Grémy, à la Pitié Salpetrière, lui même adossé à l'Unité 88 de l'INSERM. En résumant[22], ces internes (Marcel Goldberg, Roger Salamon, Jacques Chaperon, etc.) professant des opinions de gauche, dénonçaient le faible impact d'une épidémiologie confinée à l'analyse de l'étiologie des maladies non transmissibles sur les politiques de santé et, *in fine*, sur le bien-être des populations. Ils entreprirent donc de promouvoir des approches alternatives, comme la "sanométrie", ou science de l'information statistique utile à la bonne administration des systèmes de santé, inspirée du systémisme caractéristique des années 1970[23]. Une série de handicaps expliquent que cette contestation de l'orthodoxie épidémiologique française fit long feu. D'abord, l'approche défendue par les élèves de Grémy demeurait très théorique, reposant sur l'idée, sans doute quelque peu idéaliste, d'une maîtrise du système de soins par l'information, en dissonance avec l'univers mental des responsables français de la santé publique. Ensuite, des contraintes identiques à celles qu'avaient pu expérimenter Daniel Schwartz et ses collaborateurs pesaient sur un groupe décidé à faire carrière au sein de l'Inserm: la promotion d'une épidémiologie appliquée, même de pointe, pouvait difficilement trouver place dans un institut de recherche biomédicale. Enfin, la polyvalence de cette équipe – engagée aussi bien dans l'informatique médicale, que dans l'analyse des systèmes d'information ou la recherche épidémiologique – a joué contre sa prétention à contester une pratique des statistiques médicales défendue et mise en œuvre par une école exclusivement consacrée à cette activité de recherche.

Outre cette insistance à définir leur discipline comme relevant de la recherche biomédicale, la distance des épidémiologistes français par rapport aux institutions de santé publique s'explique aussi par l'originalité du système de formation hexagonal dans ce domaine. Alors que les écoles de santé publique américaines sont au cœur de la reproduction sociale de ce segment professionnel – leurs *masters* et Ph. D. étant nécessaires à une carrière dans ce secteur – et que les chercheurs de la SRU britannique prirent, dès les années 1930, une part essentielle dans les enseignements du *diploma in public health*, et participèrent ainsi à la formation des futurs *medical officers of health*, les chercheurs de l'Inserm ne tissèrent pas de liens durables avec l'École nationale de la santé publique (ENSP), qui accueille les futurs membres des corps de santé publique français : médecins inspecteurs de santé publique, ingénieurs sanitaires et directeurs d'hôpitaux, en particulier.

Première école française vouée à la santé publique, l'ENSP compte parmi les nombreux produits de l'activité réformatrice qui se fit jour à la Libération dans le domaine sanitaire et social. Suggérée par les organismes de réflexion mis en place par la Résistance, son principe est inscrit dans l'article 13 de l'ordonnance du 19 octobre 1945 réorganisant le ministère de la Santé publique. Elle fut créée comme département de l'Institut national d'hygiène avec pour mission "de compléter la formation scientifique et d'assurer le perfectionnement des médecins, des pharmaciens et des techniciens sanitaires[24]".

Rendue indépendante de l'INH, dotée "de locaux propres, d'enseignants à plein temps et d'un budget autonome[25]" par une loi du 28 juillet 1960, l'ENSP est également décentralisée, ce qui la coupe de l'élite hospitalo-universitaire parisienne. En outre, des considérations politiques conduisent à son installation à Rennes plutôt qu'à Nancy, où la faculté de médecine a pourtant une spécialisation en santé publique depuis la fin du XIXe siècle[26]. Cet isolement va considérablement handicaper les deux médicins chargés, à partir de 1962, de développer l'enseignement de l'épidémiologie et des bio-statistiques au sein de l'École. Yves Biraud et son adjoint Louis Massé présentent la particularité rarissime à cette époque d'être diplômés d'une école de santé publique américaine : le premier a étudié auprès de Wade Hampton Frost à Johns Hopkins dès 1924, obtenant un *master* avant de devenir un expert des statistiques sanitaires et de la santé publique auprès de la SDN puis de l'OMS; quant au second, il est titulaire d'un *master* et d'un Ph. D. de Harvard[27]. Tous deux vont éprouver de terribles difficultés à convaincre une administration de la santé, où l'expertise statistique ne joue pas un rôle prépondèrant de faire de l'information épidémiologique le fondement des choix politiques. À en croire Louis Massé, les différences d'approches demeuraient insurmontables :

> L'épidémiologie ne convenait pas bien aux orientations du ministère ... Un épidémiologiste pose des questions et n'obéit pas. C'est son métier de poser des questions, de dire "il se passe quelque chose là, qu'est-ce qu'on fait?" Le ministère lui, ce qu'il cherche, c'est qu'on lui demande le moins de choses possibles en dehors de sa routine : ce qu'il a fixé comme objectifs aux médecins inspecteurs de la santé, aux pharmaciens, etc. Donc un épidémiologiste gêne, nécessairement.

Pourtant, en dépit de cette double marginalisation, longtemps rédhibitoire, au sein de l'administration de la santé publique et dans l'espace de la recherche en statistique médicale, Yves Biraud et Louis Massé vont finalement exercer une influence notable sur l'évolution de l'épidémiologie française à partir du tournant des années 1980. Le second va ainsi jouer un rôle important dans la genèse d'une pratique épidémiologique alternative à celle qui avait vu le jour dans les unités de l'INSERM, participant activement à une entreprise qui mobilise d'emblée la figure tutélaire du premier. Dans un contexte marqué par une sensibilité croissante des responsables administratifs et ministériels aux enjeux sanitaires mais aussi (et peut-être surtout) politiques des situations de crises – à la suite de l'apparition du sida et de la multiplication des cas d'hépatites – des acteurs hétérogènes et jusqu'alors isolés dans des univers sociaux parallèles vont promouvoir une approche de la statistique médicale qui n'est plus conçue comme une discipline biomédicale mais comme une activité mixte, un outil scientifique plus directement utile à l'administration de la santé des populations humaines.

NAISSANCE D'UNE ÉPIDÉMIOLOGIE APPLIQUÉE : L'INFLUENCE DE LA SANTÉ PUBLIQUE AMÉRICAINE DANS LA FRANCE DES ANNÉES 1980

Qualifiée d'*épidémiologie de terrain*, d'*épidémiologie d'intervention*, voire d'*épidémiologie appliquée*, cette démarche a souvent été présentée par ses promoteurs comme une réaction au 'scientisme' censé caractériser l'approche analytique de leurs homologues de l'INSERM. L'un des effets majeurs de cette initiative sur la santé publique française aura été d'ouvrir, en quelques années à peine, des perspectives de carrière nouvelles aux médecins inspecteurs – en nombre réduit dans un premier temps – intéressés par la mise en œuvre de techniques statistiques. Pourtant, c'est encore une fois à la marge qu'a débuté une entreprise visant explicitement à importer en France une tradition américaine.

Les prolégomènes de cette histoire ont pour cadre l'Institut Pasteur dans les années 1970, lorsque le professeur Henri Mollaret offre à Louis Massé d'y assurer un enseignement de biostatistique. Parallèlement, il fait la connaissance de Charles Mérieux, personnage central de la vaccinologie française, propriétaire des Laboratoires Mérieux, très sensible aux problèmes de santé publique et soucieux de contribuer au développement de cette discipline[28]. Ensemble, ils décident de créer une formation aux techniques et méthodes de l'épidémiologie, baptisée "séminaires Yves Biraud", qui bénéficie du soutien de la Fondation Marcel Mérieux (dirigée par Charles Mérieux) et, au moins dans un premier temps, de la Fondation Rockefeller. Ainsi, un petit groupe de médecins et de spécialistes des maladies infectieuses va prendre l'habitude de se retrouver à Talloires (Haute-Savoie), dans des locaux appartenant à la Tufts University du Massachusetts, pour suivre une formation de quelques jours.

Si les premiers séminaires sont consacrés aux approches et aux outils de base d'une statistique médicale au service de la santé publique[29], les organisateurs confèrent rapidement à leur projet une orientation précise. Il va s'agir d'inventer une "épidémiologie franco-américaine[30]" en prenant modèle sur le fonctionnement des Centers for Disease Control (CDC) – placés sous le contrôle du Department of

Health and Human Services des États-Unis. Cette institution se trouve investie d'une mission de surveillance épidémiologique permanente du territoire américain et a développé des dispositifs socio-techniques à même d'alerter rapidement les autorités fédérales ou locales (ainsi que les professionnels de santé) lorsque survient une épidémie, d'en identifier le foyer et, si possible, la ou les causes[31]. Une telle organisation n'a aucun équivalent dans la France du tournant des années 1980, mais par une démarche pionnière, les promoteurs de l'épidémiologie de terrain espèrent intéresser quelques spécialistes de santé publique à l'approche américaine, de manière à sensibiliser, dans un second temps, l'administration à cette dimension de la sécurité sanitaire.

L'année 1984 marque une étape essentielle à plusieurs égards. Tout d'abord, avec l'appui d'anciens participants aux séminaires Yves Biraud, Louis Massé et Charles Mérieux fondent un Institut pour le développement de l'épidémiologie appliquée (IDEA), hébergé dans les locaux de la Fondation Mérieux à Veyrier-du-Lac (sur les bords du lac d'Annecy), et y organisent des cours annuels d'épidémiologie appliquée. Sans renoncer aux séminaires, ils ont pour ambition avouée de toucher rapidement un public plus large – la première promotion compte 21 stagiaires, beaucoup étant encore issus du cours d'épidémiologie de l'Institut Pasteur. Pour ce faire, l'IDEA s'assure le concours durable de plusieurs intervenants américains, responsables de la formation aux CDC, auxquels viennent s'ajouter des épidémiologistes français et européens, dont une bonne partie a d'ailleurs séjourné à Atlanta ou suivi une formation dans les écoles de santé publique des États-Unis[32]. La même année, un groupe de seize personnes, fidèles des séminaires Yves Biraud restés très actifs au sein du nouvel Institut ou anciens élèves de la première promotion du cours de Veyrier-du-Lac, décident de fonder une association, baptisée EPITER (Association pour le développement d'une EPIdémiologie de TERrain), qui va jouer un rôle important dans l'institutionnalisation de ce nouveau réseau social en fédérant les anciens élèves des séminaires et de l'IDEA[33]. EPITER s'impose ainsi progressivement aux responsables de l'administration française, mais également aux autres épidémiologistes français, comme la représentation légitime[34] d'un usage alternatif des statistiques biomédicales, différent mais complémentaire des pratiques mises en œuvre au sein de l'INSERM[35].

À en croire la définition qu'en donnent ses porte-parole, l'épidémiologie de terrain s'opposerait en effet radicalement à l'épidémiologie théorique, qui serait l'apanage des unités de recherche. Dans son avant-propos au premier manuel d'épidémiologie appliquée[36] (autre signe, quoique plus tardif, de l'institutionnalisation de cette entreprise scientifico-administrative), un haut responsable des CDC très lié à l'IDEA critique ouvertement les orientations prises par la discipline dans sa période moderne, à savoir une focalisation sur les maladies non infectieuses, accompagnée du désir de se voir reconnaître comme une science biomédicale à part entière. À en croire l'auteur, de tels partis pris auraient "eu tendance à éloigner de plus en plus l'épidémiologie de son application quotidienne à la prévention de la morbidité évitable et de la mortalité prématurée." Contre ce qu'il analyse comme une dérive, il s'agirait alors de promouvoir une approche "orientée vers la résolution rapide de problèmes de santé publique[37]". La posture revendiquée par les épidémiologistes appliqués suppose donc l'abandon d'une part de la "distanciation[38]" imposée par Daniel Schwartz et ses continuateurs, au nom d'une recherche d'efficacité impliquant un engagement plus grand dans l'action médico-administrative, notamment lorsqu'il qu'il s'agit d'appréhender des phénomènes de type épidémique.

Reste alors à tenter de comprendre comment une entreprise issue des marges a pu trouver un public de plus en plus nombreux et, forte de ce succès, s'imposer durablement dans l'espace de l'épidémiologie française. La formulation d'une réponse satisfaisante à cette question excéderait de loin le cadre de cet article ; nous nous contenterons donc d'avancer quelques hypothèses et éléments d'explication.

Tout d'abord, l'offre de formation représentée par l'IDEA a suscité l'intérêt des médecins de santé publique – fonctionnaires ou contractuels du service public de santé – qui s'estimaient relativement démunis pour remplir leur fonction de surveillance sanitaire, tant du fait de la faiblesse des moyens à leur disposition que de "l'absence de culture épidémiologique" (l'expression revient très fréquemment dans le discours des acteurs) qui aurait caractérisé l'administration française. De ce point de vue, les cours de l'IDEA leur ont dispensé un savoir spécialisé tout en les confortant dans l'idée que d'autres pratiques étaient envisageables, comme celles qu'avaient imposées leurs homologues américains.

Or, cette forme de mobilisation ascendante a croisé un second mouvement descendant, assez largement indépendant du premier, du moins à l'origine. En effet, dans la première moitié des années 1980, la question récurrente du retard français en santé publique redevient un objet de préoccupation politique et va, une fois n'est pas coutume, déboucher sur des réformes concrètes. Le contexte y est propice : en 1982, deux rapports ont été remis au gouvernement, portant respectivement sur les lacunes du dispositif français d'information sanitaire et sur la faisabilité d'une politique de prévention ambitieuse[39]. En outre, les nombreuses interrogations concernant l'évolution à long terme de l'épidémie de sida commencent à inquiéter les responsables politiques et administratifs – inquiétude qui va croissante à mesure que la maladie devient un problème public. Décision est alors prise de créer de nouvelles institutions spécialisées pour améliorer l'observation de la santé des Français et la surveillance épidémiologique de la population. À partir de 1983, les pouvoirs publics instituent des observatoires régionaux de santé (ORS)[40], chargés de recueillir l'information sanitaire – au besoin au moyen d'enquêtes épidémiologiques *ad hoc* – et de publier des indicateurs statistiques devant permettre de mieux définir les priorités de santé publique locales. Puis en 1992 est institué un Réseau national de santé publique (RNSP) consacré à la surveillance épidémiologique de la population : ses promoteurs le présentent explicitement comme "un CDC à la française[41]". Le nouvel organisme prend la forme d'un groupement d'intérêt public associant le ministère, l'Inserm et l'ENSP. Localisés principalement à l'Hôpital de Saint-Maurice, dans le Val-de-Marne, mais également dans six cellules régionales couvrant l'hexagone, ses agents (une cinquantaine de personnes en 1997) ont reçu pour mission de développer les actions de surveillance, d'alerte et d'investigation dans le domaine des maladies infectieuses et des pollutions environnementales, en coordination avec trois types de partenaires : les services extérieurs du ministère de la Santé (directions départementales de l'action sanitaire et sociale); des réseaux de correspondants constitués d'institutions ou de professionnels de santé (médecins libéraux et hospitaliers, vétérinaires, etc.); enfin, des enseignants et chercheurs en épidémiologie, santé publique et infectiologie, dotés d'une compétence spécifique, mobilisables, ponctuellement, en fonction du type d'épidémie : lystériose, hépatite A, méningites, infection à *Escherichia coli*, etc [42]. Pour se développer, les ORS et le RNSP ont largement fait appel aux anciens élèves de l'IDEA, souvent membres d'EPITER[43] : face à une demande nouvelle, émanant des pouvoirs publics, de personnels formés à l'épidémiologie appliquée, leurs connaissances sont devenues autant de ressources socialement valorisées. Des *outsiders* se sont ainsi retrouvés au centre de l'attention des responsables ministériels.

À cet égard, Jacques Drucker, directeur du RNSP de sa création en 1992 jusqu'en 1999, est l'archétype de ces nouveaux professionnels de santé publique. Qu'on en juge : médecin pédiatre, spécialiste des maladies infectieuses, il a passé trois ans aux États-Unis (1978–1981)[44], obtenant un *master of science in epidemiology* de la Harvard School of Public Health (1981) complété par un stage de trois mois aux CDC – institution à peu près totalement inconnue dans l'hexagone à cette époque. À son retour en France, il est nommé assistant des hôpitaux et chef de clinique assistant au Centre hospitalier universitaire de Tours (1981) et commence, quasi-simultanément, à nouer des liens avec le groupe de Veyrier-du-Lac : il participe aux séminaires Yves Biraud dès 1982 et entre à la direction médicale de l'Institut Mérieux l'année suivante, devenant également conseiller médical de la Fondation Mérieux en 1986. Un an plus tôt, quoique déjà "surdiplômé" en épidémiologie d'intervention, il avait suivi le cours de Veyrier-du-Lac et, depuis lors, il contribue au développement de l'IDEA; il est d'ailleurs l'un des trois coauteurs du manuel de référence[45]. Nommé directeur du RNSP, avec pour mission d'institutionnaliser dans l'espace administratif une surveillance épidémiologique profondément transformée dans ses pratiques, Jacques Drucker est ensuite reconduit, avec le titre de directeur général, à la tête de l'Institut de veille sanitaire qui a succédé au RNSP en 1999. Il occupe parallèlement les fonctions de professeur de santé publique à l'université de Tours depuis 1988, et de chef du service d'information médicale et d'hygiène hospitalière du CHU depuis 1990.

Si l'on élargit maintenant l'analyse au niveau institutionnel, on remarque que l'ENSP constitue un nœud important du réseau social qu'actualise peu à peu cette alliance entre épidémiologistes et administrateurs du système de santé. Les enseignants en épidémiologie ont la possibilité de faire connaître ces initiatives aux futurs fonctionnaires de santé publique (qui passent obligatoirement, à un moment ou un autre, par l'École), ils interviennent à l'IDEA, sont membres d'EPITER et mettent également en place des formations continues en épidémiologie de terrain susceptibles d'intéresser les médecins inspecteurs et les ingénieurs du génie sanitaire attirés par cette pratique administrative relativement nouvelle et en pleine expansion que constitue la "surveillance épidémiologique[46]".

NOTES

1 Jerry Morris, alors directeur de la Social Medicine Research Unit du Medical Research Council britannique, détailla très tôt ces différents types d'usage des méthodologies statistiques, dans son livre *Uses of Epidemiology* (Edinburgh : E. & S. Livingstone, 1957).

2 Ces auteurs s'appuyaient notamment sur l'autorité de l'épidémiologiste américain Wade Hampton Frost, qui, en 1927, avait effectivement défini cette discipline comme la "science des maladies infectieuses" (cf. D.E. Lillienfeld, "Definitions of Epidemiology", *American Journal of Epidemiology*, 107 (1978), 87–90).

3 Pour une présentation des premiers temps de l'épidémiologie, se reporter notamment à Lise Wilkinson "Epidemiology", dans W.F. Bynum

et Roy Porter (dir.), *Companion Encyclopedia of the History of Medicine* (London : Routledge, 1993), II, 1262–82; et à Margaret Pelling, *Cholera, Fever and English Medicine*, 1825–1865 (Oxford : Oxford University Press, 1978).

4 Activités de recherche dont l'objet n'est d'ailleurs plus limité aux seules pathologies mais inclut tout événement, toute pratique susceptible d'influer sur l'état de santé des populations – la pratique sportive, telle ou telle politique publique. Ce mouvement d'élargissement disciplinaire, s'il est ancien, s'est amplifié dans la seconde moitié des années 1970 avec l'intérêt croissant manifesté pour la notion de "promotion de la santé", à la suite, notamment, de la publication en 1974 du Rapport Lalonde, du nom du ministre canadien Marc Lalonde, *Nouvelle Perspective de la santé des canadiens* (Ottawa: Ministère de la Santé nationale et du Bien-être social, 1974).

5 Telle était la thèse avancée, sans guère d'éléments documentaires probants, par Abraham M. Lillienfeld dans Abraham M. Lillienfeld *et al.*, *Time, Places and Persons: Aspects of the History of Epidemiology* (Baltimore : Johns Hopkins University Press, 1980). Cette version est dementie par les travaux de J. Andrew Mendelsohn, "'Typhoid Mary' Strikes Again: The Social and the Scientific in the Making of Modern Public Health," *Isis*, 88 (1995), 268–77, et "From Eradication to Equilibrium: How Epidemics Became Complex after World War I", dans Christopher Lawrence et George Weisz, (dir.), *Greater Than the Parts: Holism in Biomedicine*, 1920–1950 (Oxford : Oxford University Press, 1998), 303–31; et les travaux d'Anne Hardy, "On the Cusp: Epidemiology and Bacteriology at the Local Government Board, 1890–1905", *Medical History*, 42 (1998), 328–46.

6 Kenneth Rothman, *Modern Epidemiology* (Boston : Little Brown, 1986).

7 L'analyse de l'état de santé d'une cohorte de femmes japonaises fit apparaître que celles qui vivaient avec un fumeur étaient plus à risque que les autres. Voir Takeshi Hirayama, "Non-Smoking Wives of Heavy Smokers Have a Higher Risk of Lung Cancer: A Study from Japan", *British Medical Journal*, 282 (1981), 183–5.

8 Les institutions dont il sera question ici sont celles qui construisent l'espace de la recherche biomédicale, de l'enseignement supérieur (les facultés de médecine, mais aussi l'École nationale de santé publique et certains lieux de formation aux statistiques et aux probabilités) et de l'administration de la santé publique, avec le ministère de la Santé et, plus récemment, le Réseau national de santé publique.

9 Voir notamment l'article classique d'Arend Lijphart, "Comparative Politics and the Comparative Method", *American Political Science Review*, 65 (1971), 682–93, ainsi que les contributions réunies dans Robert D. Putnam *et al.*, *Making Democracy Work: Civic Traditions in Modern Italy* (Princeton : Princeton University Press, 1995).

10 Isabelle Stengers, *La Volonté de faire science : À propos de la psychanalyse* (Paris : Éditions Synthélabo/Delagrange, 1993).

11 On peut se reporter aux textes et chronologies mis en ligne par Jean-François Picard sur http://picardp1.ivry.cnrs.fr/. Voir en particulier "De la santé publique à la recherche médicale, de l'INH à l'INSERM". Sur la genèse de l'Institut national d'hygiène, voir Jean-François Picard, "Aux origines de l'INSERM : André Chevallier et l'Institut national d'hygiène", *Sciences sociales et santé,* 21 (2003), 5–26, et William H. Schneider, "War, Philantrhopy, and the National Institute of Hygiene in France", *Minerva,* 41 (2003), 1–23. Sur l'évolution ultérieure de l'institution, voir également Jean-Paul Gaudillière, *Inventer la biomédecine. La France, l'Amérique et la production des savoirs du vivant (1945–1965)* (Paris : La Découverte, 2002).

12 L'IGR, installé à Villejuif, est le principal centre français de recherche sur le cancer. Denoix s'était déjà attaqué au problème de la comparaison des phénomènes pathologiques en participant à l'élaboration d'un système international de classification des cancers. Il élabora également un modèle de dossier médical, toujours dans le but de formaliser les renseignements disponibles sur les patients et, partant, de favoriser la recherche clinique. Voir également Luc Berlivet, *Une santé à risque. L'Action publique de lutte contre l'alcoolisme et le tabagisme en France (1954–2000),* thèse de l'Université Rennes I, 2000, chapitre 1er : "Faire science : transformation de l'épidémiologie et stabilisation d'un style de raisonnement probabiliste".

13 Au même moment, les industriels du tabac britanniques, également inquiets de la mise en cause de leurs produits, vont eux aussi financer les recherches du MRC sur l'étiologie du cancer du poumon, mais sur une toute autre échelle.

14 Entretiens avec Daniel Schwartz janvier 1995, juillet 1995, juin 1996.

15 Daniel Schwartz et Pierre Denoix, "L'Enquête française sur l'étiologie du cancer broncho-pulmonaire : le rôle du tabac", *La Semaine des hôpitaux de Paris,* 33 (1957), 424–37, et D. Schwartz, R. Flamant, J. Lellouch et P. Denoix, "Results of a French Survey on the Role of Tobacco: Particularly Inhalation, in Different Cancer Sites", *Journal of the National Cancer Institute* (1er novembre 1960), 1085–1108. Cette dernière publication, dans une revue scientifique prestigieuse, constitue le premier signe de légitimité scientifique internationale pour la jeune équipe.

16 Cette biostatistique constitue le domaine privilégié de Robert Flamant, mais aussi de Philippe Lazar.

17 Extrait de l'émission radiophonique de France-Culture "Profil perdu" du 31 octobre 1991. Robert Flamant fut l'un des acteurs essentiel de cette évolution. S'il parvint finalement à convaincre ses pairs et devint directeur de l'IGR, il a raconté dans son autobiographie (*Malade ou cobaye? Plaidoyer pour les essais thérapeutiques* (Paris : Albin Michel, 1994),

24–5) les moqueries de ses collègues : "Lorsque j'étais interne en médecine et que je commençais à travailler dans la petite équipe de Daniel Schwartz ... mes collègues des autres disciplines avaient écrit sur les murs de la salle de garde, entre autres déclarations remarquées, la phrase suivante : 'La statistique est au statisticien ce que le bec de gaz est à l'ivrogne; elle le soutient plus qu'elle ne l'éclaire.' S'embarquer dans la statistique en médecine était, en 1955, une véritable aventure!" Sa trajectoire ascendante ne doit d'ailleurs pas faire oublier que les critiques et refus ont perduré dans bien d'autres lieux du champ médical. Les essais thérapeutiques ont été violemment combattus, à la fois sur le principe du tirage aléatoire des groupes, parfois qualifié de "non éthique", et sur la nécessité d'un protocole qui retire au médecin sa liberté de prescription.

18 Le CESAM s'est rapidement doté d'un enseignement par correspondance, si bien que ce chiffre inclut également de nombreuses inscriptions hors de France.

19 Entretien avec Francine Kauffmann, directrice de recherches à l'Inserm, 1er juin 1995, Villejuif.

20 Épidémiologiste de réputation mondiale, MacMahon a dirigé pendant longtemps le département d'épidémiologie de la Harvard School of Public Health. Il a participé au travail de formalisation disciplinaire en écrivant des manuels qui sont toujours très utilisés, notamment dans le monde anglo-saxon.

21 Entretien avec Ph. Lazar mai 1995, Paris.

22 Il est impossible de détailler ici l'histoire des relations de rivalité entre ces groupes.

23 Voir leur long article-manifeste publié en deux parties : M. Goldberg, W. Dab, J. Chaperon, R. Fuhrer et F. Grémy, "Indicateurs de santé et 'sanométrie' : les aspects conceptuels de recherches récentes sur la mesure de l'état de santé d'une population", *Revue d'épidémiologie et de santé publique*, 27 (1979), 51–68 et 133–52.

24 Louis Massé, "L'École Nationale de la Santé Publique à Paris", dans *Histoire de l'enseignement à l'École Nationale de la Santé Publique*, Cahiers de L'ENSP, 10 (janvier 1987), 13. Il s'agissait, autrement dit, de doter le ministère de la Santé d'une véritable école d'application, capable de former les cadres de cette administration.

25 *Ibid.*, 16.

26 L'excellence nancéienne dans ce domaine est d'ailleurs publiquement marquée par la nomination de Jacques Parisot, doyen de la faculté de médecine, à la présidence du comité scientifique et pédagogique de l'ENSP (*ibid.*, 17).

27 Louis Massé, ami autant que collaborateur d'Yves Biraud, a publié une notice biographique de ce dernier dans les actes du *Neuvième séminaire*

Yves Biraud (Lyon : Fondation Marcel Mérieux, 1987), 193–4. Ces renseignements ont été complétés au cours de plusieurs entretiens avec Louis Massé en juin 1995 et mai 1998.

28 À en croire Louis Massé (entretien), tous deux se sont rapidement découvert une préoccupation commune pour les problèmes sanitaires du tiers-monde. Ils partagent également un point de vue très négatif sur les carences de l'administration française en matière de santé publique en regard de ses homologues américaines ou d'Europe du Nord.

29 Louis Massé, *Origine et évolution des séminaires Yves Biraud*, s.d., multigraphié, 4, à la p. 3. Entre 1979 et 1983, les séminaires réunirent un total de 149 participants. Outre des universitaires et des chercheurs en épidémiologie (français et américains, pour la plupart), on compte parmi eux des anciens élèves de l'ENSP (des médecins inspecteurs de la santé, notamment) qui s'étaient découvert un intérêt pour l'épidémiologie lors de leur formation à Rennes, ainsi que des spécialistes des maladies infectieuses que leur travail conduisait à faire largement appel aux biostatistiques.

30 Préface de Charles Mérieux à F. Dabis, J. Drucker et A. Moren, *Épidémiologie d'intervention*, (Paris : Arnette, 1992).

31 Les six CDC disposent de plusieurs moyens pour rendre publiques les informations qu'ils recueillent quotidiennement, dont le très fameux *Morbidity and Mortality Weekly Report* (*MMWR*). Le rôle joué par le centre d'Atlanta dans le processus d'alerte ayant abouti à l'objectivation de l'épidémie de sida est devenu quasi-légendaire; sur ce point, voir notamment l'étude très complète de Gerald M. Oppenheimer, "Causes, Cases and Cohorts: The Role of Epidemiology in the Historical Construction of AIDS", dans Elizabeth Fee et Daniel M. Fox (dir.), *AIDS: The Making of a Chronic Disease* (Berkeley : University of California Press, 1992), 49–83 (not. 52–6); le terme nosographique "AIDS" apparaît pour la première fois dans un article du *MMWR* en septembre 1982. Pour une présentation synthétique du développement des CDC (à partir de 1946) et de leurs modes de fonctionnement, voir également François Dabis, "Les *Centers for Disease Control* : mythe et réalité", *Le concours médical* (21 mai 1988), 1711–9, et Jean-Claude Desenclos, "Les *Centers for Disease Control and Prevention* : historique, fonctions actuelles et originalité", *Revue française des affaires sociales*, 51, 3–4 (1997), 49–61.

32 Les éléments d'information présentés ici ont été recueillis au cours d'entretiens avec Louis Massé, ainsi qu'avec trois autres professeurs d'épidémiologie de l'ENSP ayant participé au développement de l'IDEA et d'EPITER : Robert Freund, qui a effectué un voyage d'étude au CDC d'Atlanta en juin-juillet 1986; Bernard Junod, titulaire d'un *master of public health* et d'un *master of science in epidemiology* de la School of Public Health de Harvard et ancien stagiaire du CDC; et Laurent Chambaud, titulaire

d'une maîtrise en santé publique de l'Université de Montréal et ancien stagiaire du CDC. Ces trois derniers entretiens ont été réalisés à Rennes, dans les locaux de l'ENSP, respectivement les 5 juillet, 13 juillet et 6 septembre 1993. D'autres enseignants en épidémiologie de l'ENSP ont également participé au développement de l'IDEA (en tant qu'élèves ou formateurs) et fait le "voyage d'Atlanta" : c'est notamment le cas de Rémi Demillac.

33 La création de l'association (loi 1901) est officialisée en février 1985. Cf. Anne Mosnier-Mantel *et al.*, *L'Histoire d'Epiter*, document multigraphié, 1999, 9 p.

34 Selon les chiffres aimablement transmis par le bureau de l'association, en novembre 1998 EPITER comptait 456 membres; 90 % d'entre eux ont suivi au moins un cours de l'IDEA ou sont intervenus dans cette formation; 85 % de ses membres sont docteurs en médecine. Au total, 553 personnes ont suivi le cours de l'IDEA entre 1984 et 1998 (avec une crête à 80 élèves en 1990), auxquels il faut ajouter les participants aux séminaires Yves Biraud. (Cf. EPITER, Annuaire 1998/9, Hôpital national de Saint-Maurice, novembre 1998, document multigraphié, 45 p.)

35 Ce qui ne signifie pas que les chercheurs de l'Inserm soient totalement absents de ce mouvement. F. Dabis, de l'Unité 330 (Bordeaux), est même l'un des trois auteurs du manuel de référence dans ce domaine : cf. F. Dabis, J. Drucker et A. Moren, *Épidémiologie d'intervention* (Paris : Arnette, 1992). D'autres chercheurs appartenant à plusieurs unités participent également à cette entreprise.

36 Michael B. Gregg, avant-propos à F. Dabis, J. Drucker et A. Moren, *Épidémiologie d'intervention.*

37 Idem. Ancien directeur-adjoint de l'Epidemiology Program Office et rédacteur en chef du *MMWR*, Michael Gregg a eu l'occasion de développer son point de vue dans plusieurs publications françaises : "Le pouvoir de l'épidémiologie dans la pratique de la santé publique," *Bulletin épidémiologique Hebdomadaire*, 14 (10 avril 1989), 53–5, et "Entretien avec le Docteur Michael Gregg", *Afrique médecine et santé*, 45 (mai 1990), 23–8.

38 Au sens que donne Norbert Elias à ce terme dans *Engagement et Distanciation* (Paris : Fayard, 1993).

39 Ces documents sont connus sous les noms de Rapport Taïeb et Rapport du groupe Grémy-Pissaro.

40 Même s'ils s'inscrivent presque toujours dans le cadre territorial de la région administrative française, les observatoires sont des institutions autonomes par rapport aux services déconcentrés du ministère de la Santé. Leur mise en place effective va s'étaler sur plusieurs années, en fonction (notamment) des compétences disponibles localement : en 1998, on comptait 26 ORS, regroupés dans une Fédération nationale des Observatoires régionaux de santé. Leur importance politique s'est

trouvée renforcée avec l'institution, dans le cadre du plan Juppé de maîtrise des dépenses de santé, des Conférences régionales, puis nationale, de santé (art. 1 de l'ordonnance du 24 avril 1996). Chargées de définir les priorités de santé publique, tant au niveau national que régional, ces conférences restent tributaires des informations chiffrées fournies par les observatoires locaux.

41 Cf., par exemple, J. Drucker, "Des CDC d'Atlanta à l'Institut de veille sanitaire en passant par le Réseau national de santé publique : l'essor de l'épidémiologie d'intervention en France", *Revue française des affaires sociales*, 51, 3–4 (1997), 63–9.

42 Les éléments concernant le RNSP sont repris de l'article mentionné à la note précédente, ainsi que du texte rédigé (respectivement) par son directeur et son secrétaire général : Jacques Drucker et Patrice Barberousse, "Le Réseau national de santé publique", *Gestions hospitalières* (mai 1997), 338–40.

43 Sur ce point, la consultation des annuaires de l'association s'avère très éclairante : en 1998–99, 33,7 % des 456 membres ressortissaient à la catégorie professionnelle "administration de la santé" (de loin la plus représentée), la plupart d'entre eux étant chargés d'un travail de veille sanitaire, soit au sein des organismes spécialisés (RNSP, ORS, etc.), soit dans un des services extérieurs du ministère (inspecteurs des DDASS et DRAS, etc.). À ce premier groupe viennent s'ajouter les universitaires et chercheurs (11 %), ainsi que les personnels contractuels travaillant directement pour l'administration (une part non négligeable des effectifs des ORS et du RNSP entrent dans cette catégorie), ou dans des associations auxquelles les pouvoirs publics font régulièrement appel (10,7 %).

44 Cf. Pascale Deschandol, "Le Réseau national de santé publique : un petit CDC aux grandes ambitions. Entretien avec Jacques Drucker", *Décision Santé*, 52 (15 décembre 1993), 9–11. Les éléments biographiques contenus dans ce document ont été complétés à partir de la biographie officielle diffusée par l'INVS (*Biographie du Directeur général de l'Institut de veille sanitaire*, document multigraphié, s.d., 2 p.).

45 F. Dabis, J. Drucker et A. Moren, *Épidémiologie d'intervention*.

46 Pour une tentative de formalisation de ce régime de pratiques administratives et d'exploration prospective de ses usages potentiels, on peut se reporter à William Dab, *La Décision en santé publique. Surveillance épidémiologique, urgences et crises* (Rennes : Éd. de l'ENSP, 1993). L'auteur est enseignant à l'ENSP et a contribué très régulièrement aux travaux du RNSP.

16

L'infléchissement du travail politique autour des essais contrôlés : L'épidémie de sida à la fin du XXe siècle

NICOLAS DODIER

Plusieurs chapitres de ce recueil portent sur le raisonnement statistique et la quantification dans l'évaluation des thérapeutiques, couvrant une large période qui va du XVIIIe siècle au début du XXe. J'aimerais prolonger cette interrogation par une réflexion sur le nouveau contexte qui prévaut à la fin du XXe siècle, et qui amorce sans doute les évolutions que nous vivons aujourd'hui. Une caractéristique essentielle du monde médical depuis le milieu des années 1950 est la victoire progressive des essais contrôlés comme méthode d'évaluation scientifique canonique des médicaments[1]. Méthode au fondement de la *médecine des preuves,* l'essai contrôlé s'est imposé dans les pays occidentaux, puis au niveau de la médecine transnationale, comme référence légale universelle pour l'homologation des médicaments. L'objet de ce chapitre est d'examiner plus précisément comment les différents acteurs du monde médical se sont emparés de cette nouvelle donne. Il est évident que l'essor des essais contrôlés a redistribué d'une façon très sensible l'agencement des pouvoirs dans le monde médical, mais la situation ainsi créée est loin d'être statique. Un nouvel espace s'est ouvert pour le *travail politique,* entendu ici comme l'ensemble des interventions par lesquelles les acteurs défendent ou contestent la légitimité des pouvoirs existants et s'attachent, le cas échéant, à en établir de nouveaux.

Je me focaliserai sur l'épidémie de sida, qui constitue à la fin du XXe siècle un moment particulièrement intense de controverses publiques autour des essais contrôlés. Le travail politique autour du sida est aujourd'hui largement repris, discuté ou critiqué dans d'autres domaines de la médecine. Dans ces conditions, et avant d'envisager des considérations plus globales, il peut être utile de faire la lumière sur cet exemple.

Ce chapitre s'appuie sur une enquête collective couvrant l'ensemble de la mobilisation qui a accompagné en France le développement et la mise à disposition des traitements du sida[2]. Nous avons étudié cette mobilisation depuis le début de l'épidémie en 1981 jusqu'à la fin de l'année 1999, lorsque certains militants du sida ont rejoint les manifestations de Seattle contre la réunion de l'Organisation mondiale du commerce, moment exemplaire car il marque l'inscription de cette pathologie dans de nouvelles causes internationales. Nous avons constitué et travaillé avec plusieurs séries de données : un corpus d'environ 3 000 articles de la presse générale ou médicale, que nous avons complété par 1 500 dépêches de l'Agence France-Presse; plusieurs centaines d'articles de la presse spécialisée en France sur le sida[3]; les répertoires des essais thérapeutiques en France, publiés par l'association Arcat-sida; une soixantaine d'entretiens auprès de médecins et méthodologistes; des observations de réunions associatives; des articles émanant de la presse associative ainsi que des entretiens avec des militants associatifs[4]. Nous nous sommes concentrés sur le cas français[5], tout en restant attentifs à la manière dont cette mobilisation s'est construite en rapport étroit avec ce qui se passait outre-Atlantique. Le positionnement des acteurs vis-à-vis des États-Unis est en effet, dans le domaine biomédical, un élément récurrent du travail politique conduit en France[6].

Les réglementations associées aux essais contrôlés définissent un certain nombre de *places*. Un essai est financé par un *promoteur*, privé ou public. Il est placé sous la responsabilité d'un *investigateur principal*, généralement un médecin. D'autres médecins sont de simples *participants* à l'essai : ce sont eux qui recrutent les malades et qui leur dispensent les traitements. Des statisticiens sont présents comme *méthodologistes*. Chacune de ces places fait aujourd'hui l'objet, dans chaque pays, d'une réglementation à laquelle s'ajoutent l'ensemble des règles propres à chaque essai. Mais chacune de ces places a été investie, dans l'histoire du sida, par des *générations* d'acteurs très contrastées. Et c'est sur ce point que je mettrai ici l'accent. On doit comprendre la notion de génération dans un sens large, lié évidemment à des questions d'âge mais nullement réductible à l'appartenance à une classe d'âge. Une génération peut être definie comme l'ensemble des acteurs qui ont tiré des leçons semblables des mêmes épisodes marquants. Nous verrons que l'appartenance à une génération influence de façon très sensible la manière dont chaque acteur aborde les questions éthiques et scientifiques complexes soulevées par les essais contrôlés. Je me concentrerai ici sur le jeu qui s'est instauré, au carrefour de différentes générations, entre les médecins, les laboratoires pharmaceutiques, les responsables des agences publiques et les militants associatifs[7].

On peut distinguer deux temps dans le travail politique autour des essais contrôlés du sida. Pendant la première décennie, ces essais sont promus par des institutions médicales et scientifiques *enclavées*, au sens où elles cherchent à se protéger au maximum de l'immixtion d'acteurs qui leur sont extérieurs (cliniciens, médias, associations de malades). La mobilisation des institutions médicales et scientifiques autour du sida est en France un processus long, difficile, émaillé de nombreuses controverses. Et le principe même des essais contrôlés a constitué à cet égard un point d'achoppement crucial. On peut néanmoins affirmer qu'à la fin des années 1980, la plupart des acteurs se sont ralliés au principe des essais contrôlés. Mais ce ralliement ne clôt pas les controverses, il les déplace. Un nouvel espace de polémiques s'ouvre à partir des années 1990. Il est typique d'un monde médical que l'on qualifiera, par contraste, de *désenclavé*. L'ouverture des institutions médico-scientifiques sur l'extérieur est devenue pour elles, beaucoup plus qu'auparavant, une source de légitimité. De nouvelles formes de mobilisation et de contestation apparaissent, à l'intérieur même du jeu d'acteurs défini par la médecine des preuves, au niveau national, puis international. C'est la dynamique plus précise de ce mouvement que je souhaiterais maintenant examiner. Mais il convient, avant d'aborder l'exemple du sida, de revenir brièvement sur la situation dans laquelle se trouve le monde médical en France vis-à-vis des essais contrôlés au moment où éclate l'épidémie.

LA MÉDECINE DES PREUVES EN FRANCE À L'ORÉE DES ANNÉES 1980

Le statut des essais contrôlés reste, au début des années 1980, très contrasté. Certains segments du monde médical français sont déjà très marqués par la montée de la médecine des preuves. La lutte en faveur des essais contrôlés interfère, en France, avec une critique particulièrement vigoureuse de la *tradition clinique*, auparavant dominante dans la médecine et caractérisée par la grande légitimité accordée au clinicien concernant la dimension à la fois éthique et cognitive de ses interventions auprès de ses malades[8]. Une spécificité de la France est l'implantation très forte de cette tradition clinique dans le monde hospitalier[9]. Une nouvelle génération de médecins hospitaliers commence dans les années 1950 à s'attaquer à cette tradition[10]. Il s'agit d'un segment marginal, même s'il est très actif, et bien connecté aux instances politiques. Ce segment s'appuie dans un premier temps sur le développement des organismes publics de recherche (Centre national de la recherche scientifique, Institut national de la santé et de la recherche médicale (Inserm)). Il n'investira les essais contrôlés que progressivement, dans des conditions qu'il reste à préciser sur le plan historique[11]. Des témoignages concernant cette volonté d'émancipation vis-à-vis de la tradition clinique apparaissent très clairement dans les entretiens que nous avons réalisés auprès des médecins qui ont occupé des positions de responsabilité dans les institutions médico-scientifiques du sida, notamment à l'Agence nationale de recherches sur le sida (ANRS), créée en 1989. Ces médecins ont été formés par un petit cercle de médecins prestigieux, tous membres du petit milieu qui a commencé, dans les années 1950, la lutte contre la tradition clinique hospitalière. Ils en sont restés les héritiers directs.

La montée de la médecine des preuves aux États-Unis a été décrite de façon très approfondie par Harry Marks[12]. Sans doute parce que notre enquête concerne une époque postérieure à celle sur laquelle a principalement travaillé Harry Marks, la médecine des preuves à laquelle nous avons affaire est beaucoup plus en symbiose, aujourd'hui, avec l'industrie pharmaceutique. Ce que montre l'ouvrage de Marks c'est, pour l'essentiel, comment le gouvernement américain, lié à un ample mouvement de réforme du monde médical, cherche, depuis le début du XXe siècle, à établir un point d'appui solide pour évaluer scientifiquement les médicaments mis sur le marché par les laboratoires pharmaceutiques. L'État, en effet, ne fait pas confiance aux médecins cliniciens pour former un jugement scientifique étayé sur les nouveaux médicaments. À partir des années 1950, il trouve dans les essais contrôlés l'outil qu'il recherchait. Le pas supplémentaire, dont nous héritons aujourd'hui, c'est l'assimilation, par les laboratoires pharmaceutiques, de cette imposition des essais contrôlés comme base réglementée de l'évaluation scientifique. Le capitalisme pharmaceutique s'est coulé dans ce moule. De telle sorte que, lorsque le sida apparaît, et cela jouera un rôle essentiel dans le travail politique, les grands laboratoires sont déjà devenus les garants, aux yeux d'un certain nombre d'acteurs, de la mise en œuvre professionnelle, compétente, d'une recherche thérapeutique à la fois éthique et scientifique.

Cela dit, au début des années 1980, les essais contrôlés n'ont pas encore étendu leur influence sur tous les secteurs de la médecine française. D'une part, certains segments concernés par le sida, telle l'infectiologie, n'en font pas un usage systématique. De nombreuses évaluations reposent sur des protocoles non randomisés, sans comparaison entre plusieurs groupes (essais à un seul bras). Par ailleurs, l'encadrement légal et réglementaire de l'expérimentation médicale est loin d'être consolidé. Certes, l'autorisation de mise sur le marché date de 1972, mais de nombreux commentateurs parlent encore, dans les années 1980, d'un vide juridique autour des tests de molécules, tout en reconnaissant la difficulté de légiférer en la matière[13]. De nombreuses contradictions sont notées entre le droit de la médecine et la mise en œuvre d'essais contrôlés *versus* placebo. Il faudra attendre la loi Huriet-Sérusclat en 1987 pour que la France soit dotée d'un droit spécifique en matière d'expérimentation médicale. Et ce n'est qu'en 1993 qu'est créée l'Agence du médicament, instance en change de l'homologation des nouveaux traitements.

L'ENCLAVEMENT DE LA MÉDECINE DES PREUVES

L'espace de la mobilisation collective autour des traitements du sida lors de la première décennie de l'épidémie en France se structure autour de deux générations de médecins. Les premiers à se mobiliser contre le nouveau syndrome forment une génération de "jeunes médecins" peu familiarisés avec les essais contrôlés. Ces médecins, qui sont pour une grande part encore en formation, soignent les malades et expérimentent des traitements selon des méthodes diverses, sans suivre une méthodologie standard réglementée. Des associations de défense des malades commencent à émerger peu après (Vaincre le sida en 1983, Aides en 1984). Ces associations sont très proches de ces jeunes médecins, même si elles mobilisent leurs militants dans des milieux plus larges, liés notamment à l'homosexualité. Elles tendent globalement à déléguer à ces médecins la réflexion sur l'éthique des essais thérapeutiques[14]. On assiste un peu plus tard, dans les années 1986–1988, à l'arrivée d'une deuxième génération de médecins du sida, très différente de la première. Ils viennent de l'hématologie, de la médecine interne ou de l'immunologie clinique. Ils défendent fermement, contrairement aux premiers, le principe des essais contrôlés. Ce sont en quelque sorte les nouveaux mandarins des institutions médico-scientifiques, liés non plus à la tradition clinique mais à la médecine des preuves. Souvent directeurs d'unités de recherche à l'Inserm, c'est à eux qu'est confiée, en collaboration avec des statisticiens qui ont travaillé dans leurs unités, la responsabilité des institutions spécialisées dans le sida, et notamment l'ANRS.

Une alliance de fait s'instaure alors entre ces médecins, bien établis dans les agences d'État, et les grands laboratoires pharmaceutiques face aux acteurs qui n'adhèrent pas au principe des essais contrôlés. La symbiose entre médecine et industrie pharmaceutique dans le cadre d'un monde de spécialistes des essais contrôlés apparaît clairement. La méfiance vis-à-vis des autres acteurs est renforcée par le contexte d'urgence sanitaire propre au sida. Au nom de celle-ci, des pressions fortes s'exercent sur les scientifiques. Les responsables de l'ANRS regardent en retour les cliniciens, les associations de malades, et les médias avec beaucoup de méfiance. Et les actions engagées outre-Atlantique par les activistes américains, dont les médias français commencent à se faire l'écho, les inquiètent plus particulièrement. Cette montée d'une nouvelle génération de médecins, son raidissement vis-à-vis de tout ce qui est extérieur aux institutions scientifiques, suscite en retour une radicalisation des médecins de première génération. Ces derniers s'en prennent vigoureusement aux nouvelles institutions du sida, d'autant plus que certains n'admettent pas d'en avoir été écartés. Cette opposition initiale est renforcée par la critique globale des institutions que certains jeunes médecins, ou certains militants associatifs, ont héritée des mouvements des années 1970. Pour ces médecins, la lenteur des institutions médicales et scientifiques à réagir face au sida est caractéristique de leur conservatisme et de leur incapacité à être en prise, rapidement, sur des questions sanitaires émergentes. Cette radicalisation de l'opposition suscite en retour un *enclavement* d'autant plus important des institutions. Les premiers essais que l'ANRS met alors en place, et dont elle veut faire les emblèmes de sa politique (en particulier les essais Concorde, Alpha, puis Delta), sont conçus selon des protocoles particulièrement stricts. L'Agence favorise ainsi des essais longs, portant sur des milliers de patients, randomisés, en double aveugle, contre placebo, fondés sur des critères cliniques (apparition d'infections opportunistes, décès) plutôt que sur des marqueurs biologiques (CD4, puis charge virale). Ces protocoles confirment que les jugements cliniques, autant que les avis des malades, n'ont pas droit de cité, du point de vue de l'Agence, dans la recherche médicale : ce ne sont que des opinions externes, des biais dont il convient d'autant plus de se prémunir que les pressions sont fortes pour les intégrer à la démarch scientifique.

LA SUBVERSION DES INSTITUTIONS MÉDICALES ET SCIENTIFIQUES

À cette tension caractéristique de la fin des années 1980 succède le basculement du début des années 1990. La majeure partie des médecins, des associations françaises de lutte contre le sida et des médias grand public se rallient aux essais contrôlés. Pourquoi n'en reste-t-on pas là? Pourquoi un nouvel espace de mobilisation se crée-t-il alors, autour du *désenclavement de la médecine des preuves*? Cette dynamique s'enclenche autour des demandes de transparence adressées à l'État par les associations de lutte contre le sida et par le milieu gay concernant les essais de molécules – en particulier lors de l'arrivée en France en 1990 de la ddI, deuxième antiviral à faire preuve après l'AZT d'une certaine efficacité, au vu des essais de phase 1 ou 2. L'Agence nationale de recherches sur le sida répond à ces demandes par l'instauration d'un rapport *pédagogique*. Cette pédagogie prend la forme de réunions d'information sur les protocoles d'essais à l'intention des associations. Les responsables de l'Agence se considèrent également investis d'une mission pédagogique vis-à-vis de la première génération des médecins du sida. Ils cherchent à mieux les former aux essais contrôlés, notamment en les faisant participer aux grands essais de l'Agence. L'essai Concorde, qui mobilise en France des centaines de services hospitaliers, est ainsi, pour beaucoup de médecins, une véritable initiation à la machinerie complexe de l'essai contrôlé. On observe alors, et c'est un point essentiel de la dynamique politique autour des essais, un processus de *subversion* de ce rapport pédagogique. Les nouveaux acteurs qui se saisissent des essais contrôlés vont en faire un autre usage que celui qui était initialement défini par les responsables de l'Agence. Cette subversion ne présente pas le même visage selon que l'on se place du côté des associations, ou du côté des jeunes médecins du sida. Mais elle est tout aussi frappante.

Côté associations, la subversion résulte de deux types d'apprentissage. D'une part, certaines associations, parmi les plus engagées dans les essais contrôlés, viennent aux réunions d'information organisées par l'ANRS avec une option *épistémique* qui leur est personnelle, et qui s'avère très différente de celle qui est véhiculée par l'Agence. Cette posture est développée par les associations de *deuxième génération*, celles qui sont apparues en France au début des années 1990 (Act-Up Paris, Actions-Traitements)[15]. Si les militants membres de ces associations assistent aux réunions d'information, ils ne considèrent pas l'Agence comme étant détentrice d'un avis de référence en matière d'essais. Un tel avis, de leur point de vue, n'existe pas. Pour ces militants, les réunions organisées par l'Agence constituent l'une de leurs sources d'information sur les nouveaux médicaments, mais une source parmi d'autres. Les militants vont puiser à bien d'autres sources : les congrès scientifiques, la presse associative américaine, les revues scientifiques internationales, les discussions informelles avec divers médecins, les témoignages de malades sur les traitements. En tant que malades ou séropositifs, ces militants théorisent cette posture comme processus "d'autoformation"[16].

Une fois ces réunions mises en place, une autre forme d'apprentissage fait son œuvre, qui concerne cette fois-ci l'ensemble des militants associatifs, toutes générations d'associations confondues, regroupés dans le collectif TRT-5 qui organise les rencontres avec l'ANRS, ou avec les laboratoires[17]. Les militants qui participent aux réunions prennent en effet conscience, progressivement, du caractère négociable des protocoles d'essais. De réunions "d'informations", ces rencontres se transforment d'ailleurs en réunions dites "de concertation". Les négociations portent par exemple sur le nombre de malades inclus dans l'essai, sur les critères d'inclusion, sur la longueur de l'essai, sur les critères susceptibles de justifier une sortie de l'essai, sur la fréquence des examens biologiques. Ces militants, dont certains siègent en réunion en tant que séropositifs, découvrent en même temps que les protocoles issus des négociations avec les chercheurs ne sont pas moins scientifiques que les autres. Certains protocoles négociés sont même parfois plus performants car plus réalistes, et donc plus fiables. Cette confrontation des militants à une pratique concrète de la science change l'image qu'ils se font de celle-ci.

Une fois ralliés aux essais contrôlés, les médecins de la première génération du sida vont également subvertir l'usage qui en est prôné par les institutions scientifiques. Ils imaginent d'une manière générale des protocoles plus souples que ceux élaborés par l'Agence. Cette souplesse signifie par exemple des essais plus courts, sur la base de marqueurs biologiques plutôt que de marqueurs cliniques, avec une marge de manœuvre plus grande du clinicien pour changer le traitement du patient. D'une manière générale, leurs protocoles laissent plus de place à l'expérience clinique et au jugement des cliniciens. Ces médecins justifient cette souplesse des protocoles par l'urgence sanitaire. Dans un tel contexte, le jugement clinique retrouve selon eux une nouvelle légitimité au sein des protocoles d'essais contrôlés. On peut s'appuyer, de leur point de vue, sur le jugement clinique pour être plus rapide dans l'évaluation. Les essais souples s'avèrent ainsi plus en prise sur la dernière actualité de la recherche thérapeutique. Cette revalorisation de la clinique n'est donc pas un retour à la tradition. On peut l'appeler *clinique de veille*, nouvelle forme d'appui sur l'expérience clinique, à l'intérieur même d'une médecine des preuves confrontée à la rapidité de l'évolution des connaissances en matière thérapeutique.

Dans ce nouvel espace de mobilisation, les essais contrôlés deviennent un *objet-frontière* dans un monde médical lui-même désenclavé. Tout en étant commun à l'ensemble des protagonistes de la médecine officielle, l'essai contrôlé est susceptible d'une certaine malléabilité. C'est un outil partagé par des médecins qui développent par ailleurs des philosophies d'essais différentes. Autour de cet outil se mobilisent des acteurs (jeunes médecins du sida, militants associatifs) dont le rapport aux institutions scientifiques n'est pas un simple rapport d'affiliation. Ces acteurs adhèrent à un outil, qui constitue une base de négociations, mais pas à l'ensemble des conceptions de l'éthique et de la scientificité promues par l'institution médico-scientifique.

LES NOUVELLES PERSPECTIVES DU TRAVAIL POLITIQUE

Cette subversion des institutions médicales et scientifiques a eu deux conséquences importantes : elle a contribué à durcir la lutte contre les marges de la médecine instituée; elle a relancé la critique des laboratoires pharmaceutiques.

L'ouverture d'un espace de négociation entre chercheurs et associations n'a pas eu pour effet d'augmenter la tolérance vis-à-vis des marges de la médecine officielle. Bien au contraire. Avec le ralliement d'une partie des médecins du sida et des associations aux essais contrôlés, un nouveau milieu s'est formé, propice à la négociation des essais contrôlés. Mais ce milieu est borné par de nouvelles frontières. Les quelques médecins hospitaliers qui dorénavant critiquent les essais contrôlés se retrouvent marginalisés. Ces médecins ont eux-mêmes tendance à globaliser le type d'acteur auquel ils sont confrontés. Ils envisagent le monde qui s'est construit autour des essais comme un véritable "système", entité qui englobe selon eux l'État, les nouveaux mandarins de la médecine et le capitalisme pharmaceutique international. Ces médecins essayent de se situer en dehors de ce système. Ils sont déçus par le mouvement associatif. Ils en attendaient une ligne d'action plus critique vis-à-vis du système. Cette marginalisation touche également les associations de malades qui refusent le principe des essais contrôlés. L'association Positifs est ainsi écartée du collectif interassociatif TRT-5.

Les associations de lutte contre le sida ralliées aux essais contrôlés, y compris les associations de malades (Act-Up, Actions Traitements), changent par ailleurs sensiblement de politique vis-à-vis du charlatanisme et des médecines parallèles. Jusqu'à la fin des années 1980, ces associations sont tentées par une politique de recherche de médicaments tous azimuts. Elles se montrent ainsi plutôt tolérantes envers certaines pistes de recherche non estampillées par les institutions officielles. Mais à partir des années 1991–1992, à l'occasion de plusieurs affaires sensibles[18], les mêmes associations se convertissent très nettement à la lutte contre tous les acteurs, médecins ou non, qui n'en passeraient pas par les essais contrôlés. Un front élargi d'acteurs, qui inclut les grandes associations de malades, se construit dès lors contre les médecines parallèles lorsque celles-ci proposent des traitements alternatifs à ceux qui sont homologués par les essais contrôlés. Les médecines parallèles sont cantonnées dans des rôles de médecines d'appoint, tout juste bonnes à proposer des compléments.

On observe par ailleurs, à partir du milieu des années 1990, l'émergence d'une nouvelle critique des laboratoires pharmaceutiques, dans un cadre que l'on pourrait qualifier de *réformiste,* c'est-à-dire respectueux du principe des essais contrôlés. Maîtrisant désormais les méthodes réglementées de l'évaluation scientifique, les associations sont en mesure de critiquer de façon plus étayée les stratégies des laboratoires pharmaceutiques. Elles prennent la parole sur des problèmes jusqu'à présent laissés de côté : la gestion des stocks de molécules, l'allocation des molécules entre les différents pays, les délais et les conditions d'approvisionnement des hôpitaux dans le cadre d'autorisations "temporaires" désormais clairement réglementées. Si ces associations occupent le devant de la scène, c'est aussi parce que les médecins prennent peu la parole pour critiquer les laboratoires pharmaceutiques. Les médecins du sida, quelle que soit leur génération, sont en effet fortement liés à l'industrie, ne serait-ce que pour accéder aux nouvelles molécules expérimentées. Les seuls médecins qui s'en prennent au capitalisme pharmaceutique sont ceux qu'a marginalisés leur hostilité globale aux essais contrôlés. Ils se retrouvent suspects dans leur travail, du fait même de leur distance vis-à-vis d'une industrie pharmaceutique considérée comme garante de l'éthique et de la scientificité. Ils sont vus comme des artisans qui veulent s'abstraire de la rigueur des essais.

Dans un contexte où, en dehors de quelques personnages isolés, les médecins ne constituent plus un contrepoint critique aux stratégies des laboratoires pharmaceutiques, les associations de défense des malades relancent le débat. Cette prise de parole émergente concerne en premier lieu les protocoles d'essais, comme le montre la controverse autour de l'essai Saquinavir organisé par le laboratoire Roche en 1994. Elle s'étend ensuite aux conditions de mise sur le marché des molécules. À partir de la crise des antiprotéases en 1996, crise provoquée par le décalage entre le caractère très prometteur des nouvelles molécules et la quantité infime de produits mise à disposition par les firmes concernées, cette prise de parole porte plus directement sur la dimension internationale des stratégies des laboratoires. C'est en effet lors de cette crise que les associations françaises prennent conscience du fait que les laboratoires approvisionnent d'abord le marché américain.

Cette prise de conscience de la stratégie différenciée des firmes sur les différents marchés nationaux va favoriser l'alliance avec les organisations non gouvernementales qui relèvent de la médecine humanitaire. La nouvelle convergence porte sur la mise à disposition des médicaments dans les pays du Sud. Jusqu'au milieu des années 1990, celle-ci est pensée pour l'essentiel, concernant le sida, selon les catégories de la philanthropie internationale et de l'aide au développement. Mais l'ONG Médecins sans frontières propose un abord nouveau de la santé dans les pays du Sud, avec sa campagne pour l'accès aux médicaments essentiels, au début de l'année 1999. Le problème des brevets devient crucial. Les controverses se déplacent vers un chaînon encore non problématisé du dispositif juridique sur lequel s'appuient les essais contrôlés : les conditions d'appropriation des molécules par les laboratoires pharmaceutiques. Act-Up se joint quelques mois plus tard à l'action des ONG et trouve dans la question des brevets un nouveau levier d'action sur les pratiques des laboratoires pharmaceutiques. Les alliances s'étendent plus loin. Au-delà de la médecine humanitaire, on observe en effet une convergence entre des associations de lutte contre le sida et les mouvements qui s'opposent d'une manière générale à la libéralisation des règles du commerce international. Les controverses sur les brevets de médicaments contre le sida vont jalonner, à partir de 1999, les réunions internationales de l'OMC, de l'OMS, ainsi que les sommets entre États (G7 ou G8).

SPÉCIFICITÉ D'UN CAS ET FÉDÉRATION DE CAUSES

L'accession des essais contrôlés au rang de méthode standard soutenue par l'État ne ferme donc pas le jeu politique, elle ouvre plutôt un espace pour de nouvelles formes de contestation qui ne pouvaient pas exister dans le cadre de la tradition clinique. On assiste à un déplacement important du jeu des acteurs à l'intérieur de la médecine des preuves, que l'on peut résumer de la façon suivante. Pendant la montée de la médecine des preuves, l'essai contrôlé est pour l'essentiel une arme de l'État pour modérer et encadrer le capitalisme pharmaceutique. Lorsque la médecine des preuves est officiellement établie, l'essai contrôlé change de statut. Il devient une arme de l'État et des firmes pharmaceutiques contre l'ensemble des acteurs qui ne sont pas des spécialistes attitrés de cette médecine des preuves : les cliniciens, les médias, les malades qui font pression pour avoir des médicaments. Avec l'avènement d'une médecine des preuves désenclavée, l'essai contrôlé acquiert encore un nouveau statut. Il est devenu une arme commune aux firmes, aux médecins cliniciens, aux associations, aux médias, ou à la plupart d'entre eux, contre les nouveaux "marginaux" de la médecine : les médecins ou les malades qui restent radicaux dans leur critique du système des essais. Mais l'essai contrôlé est en même temps un point d'appui des associations pour une critique étayée de l'État et des firmes pharmaceutiques. Une fois enclenchée, cette critique s'étend ensuite aux conditions d'appropriation des médicaments. Elle cherche à infléchir la médecine transnationale.

Cet infléchissement du travail politique s'appuie sur des ressorts de la mobilisation propres au sida. Le rapport aux institutions y joue tout d'abord un rôle crucial. La lutte contre le sida a drainé une première génération de médecins déjà engagés, avant l'épidémie, dans une critique globale des institutions. Ceux-ci ont converti cette critique globale en une subversion des institutions médicales et scientifiques du sida qui les a conduits vers une critique plus étayée des nouveaux mandarins de la médecine, menée de l'intérieur même de la médecine des preuves. Un autre ressort de la mobilisation propre au sida est l'intensité du travail produit sur la notion de stigmate. On ne comprend pas la manière dont les acteurs se sont mobilisés autour d'une cause sanitaire comme le sida si l'on ne saisit pas comment ils ont articulé cette cause avec la lutte contre la stigmatisation des groupes concernés par cette pathologie, les malades ou les séropositifs, bien sûr, mais également les homosexuels, les toxicomanes, les immigrés. Cette lutte contre le stigmate, de la part des acteurs qui font partie du monde du sida, est beaucoup plus forte que dans d'autres pathologies. Il n'est pas simple, en même temps, d'en saisir toutes les dimensions. Ses implications sur le travail politique autour des essais contrôlés ont été en effet très contrastées. On peut distinguer trois dimensions.

La lutte contre la stigmatisation a joué tout d'abord dans le sens d'un affaiblissement de la tradition clinique. Car les illustres représentants de cette tradition, lorsqu'ils ont voulu s'engager sur le sida, étaient loin de satisfaire aux exigences de cette cause. Ils faisaient souvent figure de réactionnaires insupportables.

Cette exigence de non-stigmatisation a joué par ailleurs dans le sens d'un raidissement de la médecine des preuves. Dès les premières années de l'épidémie, la cause *moderne-libérale* est devenue le ciment commun du monde du sida. *Libérale* au sens où l'on souhaitent éviter de stigmatiser de toute une série de conduites. *Moderne* au sens où l'on considérait en outre les pratiques de stigmatisation comme “irrationnelles” et où l'on croyait en la science pour faire valoir un rapport “éclairé” au stigmate[19]. Maintenir les institutions scientifiques à l'abri des pressions extérieures, faire parler les scientifiques d'une seule voix, semblait aux responsables de ces institutions une manière de prévenir les dérives stigmatisatrices liées à l'irrationalité et à la panique, et de contrer le recours à des solutions “autoritaires” dans un contexte où, de surcroît, l'extrême droite commençait à s'emparer de la question de l'épidémie[20].

La lutte contre la stigmatisation a joué enfin, mais seulement dans un deuxième temps, dans le sens du désenclavement du monde médical. La volonté, chez les associations de deuxième génération, de dépasser la “tolérance” vis-à-vis des personnes stigmatisées, forme euphémisée de la lutte contre le stigmate, a conduit ces militants à se déclarer ouvertement malades, ou homosexuels, et à agir comme tels. C'est ainsi que les militants d'Act-Up ont revendiqué, y compris vis-à-vis des essais, une fierté homosexuelle. Celle-ci n'est pas étrangère à la mise en avant de “l'auto-formation” et à la subversion des institutions. Alors que la cause libérale a joué dans un premier temps dans le sens d'un raidissement de la médecine des preuves, il faut bien comprendre qu'elle a ensuite joué, en se radicalisant, en faveur de la subversion des institutions propres à cette médecine.

Ces spécificités de la lutte contre le sida ont eu tendance, pendant longtemps, à isoler cette cause. Le sida paraissait une pathologie singulière, une exception. En fin de période, à partir de 1996, certains acteurs tentent de désingulariser le travail politique conduit autour du sida. Ils vont chercher des alliances au-delà de la maladie, d'autant plus que la mobilisation autour de de celle-ci traverse une crise profonde[21]. D'où une nouvelle dimension du travail politique, qui va consister à former *de nouvelles fédérations de causes*, dans lesquelles la cause du sida n'est plus qu'une cause parmi d'autres. Ce mouvement de désingularisation du sida comme cause s'oriente alors selon deux vecteurs principaux.

Le premier concerne ce qui aujourd'hui s'organise, de manière encore floue, autour de la notion de “démocratie sanitaire”. Le cas du sida est pris alors comme exemple d'une démocratisation possible de la science biomédicale, au sens où les associations de lutte contre le sida participent directement à la production des connaissances médico-scientifiques.

Par ailleurs, le sida devient l'un des domaines en pointe pour la réévaluation des règles régissant le commerce international, en particulier le droit de propriété intellectuelle. La cause du sida s'inscrit dans l'ensemble des causes défendues par les mouvements altermondialistes. Dans les deux cas, c'est la capacité des acteurs qui n'en étaient pas les spécialistes à se rapprocher d'une manière critique des essais contrôlés qui a ouvert ces nouvelles perspectives de mobilisation.

NOTES

1 On appelle “essai contrôlé” une méthode qui consiste à répartir les malades en plusieurs groupes et à comparer les traitements dispensés dans chacun de ces groupes. Généralement, on considère comme véritablement contrôlé un essai *randomisé*, dans lequel l'affectation d'un malade à l'un des groupes résulte d'un tirage au sort. Les essais contrôlés effectuent dans la mesure du possible des comparaisons *versus* placebo et recourent au *double aveugle*, technique qui permet de maintenir le médecin clinicien et le malade, pendant toute la durée de l'expérimentation, dans l'ignorance du traitement dispensé.

2 Le programme a été conduit en collaboration, notamment, avec Janine Barbot, Andrei Mogoutov et Sophia Rosman. Il a reçu des financements de l'Agence nationale de recherches sur le sida, de l'association Ensemble contre le sida, et de la mission Recherche-expérimentation du ministère de la Santé.

3 Deux journaux ont été systématiquement analysés : *Le Journal du sida* et *Transcriptase*.

4 Le travail sur les associations a fait l'objet de l'ouvrage de J. Barbot, *Les Malades en mouvements : La médecine et la science à l'épreuve du sida* (Paris : Balland, 2002). Un certain nombre d'arguments présentés dans ce chapitre sont développés dans N. Dodier, *Leçons politiques de l'épidémie de sida* (Paris : Éditions de l'EHESS, 2003).

5 L'histoire de la mobilisation associative autour des essais thérapeutiques aux États-Unis dans le cadre du sida, pour les années 1981–1995, est bien documentée par Steven Epstein, *La Grande Révolte des malades : Histoire du sida*, tome 2 (Paris : Seuil, 2001); édition originale en anglais : 1996.

6 J.-P. Gaudillière, *Inventer la biomédecine : La France, l'Amérique et la production des savoirs du vivant* (1945–1965) (Paris : La Découverte, 2002); L. Murard dans ce volume.

7 J'ai tenté dans mon livre (Dodier, *Leçons politiques de l'épidémie de sida*) de donner une vision plus ample de cette histoire, en incluant également les médias et le mouvement gay.

8 Dodier, Médecine, science et capitalisme.

9 G. Weisz, *The Medical Mandarins: The French Academy of Medicine in the Nineteenth and Early Twentieth Centuries* (Oxford : Oxford University Press, 1995).

10 H. Jamous, *Sociologie de la décision: La Réforme des études médicales et des structures hospitalières* (Paris : Éditions du CNRS, 1969).

11 Sur le cas de la cancérologie, voir I. Löwy, *Between Bench and Bedside: Science, Healing and Interleukin-2 in a Cancer Ward* (Cambridge et Londres :

Harvard University Press, 1996). On trouvera dans la thèse de Luc Berlivet, *Une santé à risques : L'Action publique de lutte contre l'alcoolisme et le tabagisme en France (1954–1999)* (thèse pour le doctorat de science politique, Université de Rennes, 2000) des éléments sur l'histoire de l'épidémiologie en France qui interfèrent fortement avec le développement des essais contrôlés.

12 H. Marks, *La Médecine des preuves : Histoire et anthropologie des essais cliniques (1900–1990)* (Synthélabo : Les Empêcheurs de penser en rond, 1999); édition originale en anglais : 1997.

13 A. Fagot-Largeault, *L'Homme bio-éthique : Pour une déontologie de la recherche sur le vivant* (Paris : Maloine, 1985).

14 C'est une grande différence avec les États-Unis. Les premiers activistes américains engagés dans la lutte contre le sida sont très liés au mouvement gay, ils se construisent rapidement des positions personnelles sur la recherche médicale (Epstein, *La Grande Révolte des malades*). En France, le mouvement gay réagit tout d'abord avec beaucoup de méfiance à l'égard de l'alerte à l'épidémie lancée par les jeunes médecins hospitaliers. Les premières associations de lutte contre le sida, même si leurs militants viennent en grande partie du milieu gay, affichent une distance par rapport aux collectifs construits autour de la cause homosexuelle et s'en remettent aux jeunes spécialistes du sida pour faire avancer la recherche.

15 Act-Up Paris est créé en 1989, avec des références fortes au modèle d'Act-Up New York. Une autre association, Positifs, est créée la même année. Elle se veut une association de malades sans lien avec le milieu gay. Actions-Traitements rassemble en 1991 des malades initialement engagés dans un groupe de travail de Positifs consacré aux traitements. Alors que les militants de Positifs refuseront toujours les essais contrôlés, ce n'est pas le cas d'Actions-Traitements.

16 D. Lestrade, *Act Up: Une histoire* (Paris : Denoël, 2000).

17 Barbot, *Les Malades en mouvements.*

18 Il s'agit essentiellement en 1991 de l'affaire Miesch, du nom d'un médecin généraliste à la retraite qui propose l'Aviral, cocktail de médicaments supposé guérir du sida, et en 1992 de l'affaire Song Wa, du nom d'une femme originaire de Hong Kong qui propose des traitements basés sur la pharmacopée chinoise.

19 Voir M. Pollak, *Les Homosexuels et le sida : Sociologie d'une épidémie* (Paris : Métailié, 1988) sur l'instauration d'un régime *moderne* d'épidémie.

20 Cette inquiétude devant l'exploitation que l'extrême droite pouvait faire du sida est très nette en France à la fin des années 1980.

21 Début 1996, l'arrivée des trithérapies à base d'antiprotéases correspond au développement de traitements plus efficaces qui conduisent à une

baisse sensible de la mortalité liée au sida. Les années 1997–1998 sont marquées par une baisse très nette de la mobilisation collective quels que soient les indicateurs considérés : militantisme dans les associations, participation aux manifestations, montant des dons, financements publics. Des associations disparaissent (Vaincre le sida) ou se restructurent (Arcat-sida, Aides).

PART FIVE

Afterthoughts

17

From Clinical Counting to Evidence-Based Medicine

GEORGE WEISZ

Several years ago, I gave a talk in Gérard Jorland's seminar on the quantification debates that stirred the Parisian medical world during the 1830s. During question period, one of my listeners asked whether the "numerical method" advocated by P.C.A. Louis was in fact evidence-based medicine (EBM). The query struck me as historically naïve; but both advocates and opponents of EBM have since made this very same connection; the latter use it to emphasize the historical legitimacy of their enterprise, while the former argue that there is nothing particularly original about EBM – old French wine with a new Canadian label.[1] The more interesting question is whether parallels and differences between nineteenth-century debates and today's can tell us something about long-standing medical efforts to quantify.

To that end, this essay looks at quantification in the nineteenth and early twentieth centuries and then considers the rise of objectification as a social movement as manifest in the recent intense interest in evidence-based medicine.

QUANTIFICATION IN THE NINETEENTH AND EARLY TWENTIETH CENTURIES

Quantification in medicine is part of the growing trust in numbers that has gradually affected all aspects of social life during the past centuries.[2] More narrowly, it is part of a process of objectification in clinical medicine that has been going on since at least the eighteenth century[3] It has been most evident in diagnosis, which has come to depend less and less on patients' accounts or physicians' subjective judgment and more and more on objective signs that, in theory at least, transcend subjectivity and compel agreement among qualified observers. Among the first and most compelling of these signs are the anatomic lesions that defined the scientific medicine of the Paris School during the first half of the nineteenth century.[4] These are so forceful precisely because we can see them (and, as we know, "seeing is believing"). Once observable only in post-mortem dissections, lesions can now appear as images in living patients produced by CAT-scans, MRIs, or x-rays or, at the cellular level, by microscopes of various sorts. Frequently when we cannot see lesions directly, laboratory tests – counting something produced by the body – serve as a proxy. Or mechanical means measuring specific functions serve similar ends, defining variations outside specific numeric parameters as disease. When no external sign of this nature manifests itself, doctors frequently dismiss illness as psychological in nature. Quantification in this context seems to be one of many techniques of objectification; it is, however, particularly central and ubiquitous because numbers seem especially "objective" and are applicable to so many domains.

The diagnosis of illness had by the early twentieth century become highly objectified; however, the same was not true of therapeutics. Doctors and patients – as always – defined success subjectively. If a new therapy came along, doctors used it and decided, on the basis of patients' experiences and colleagues' reports, whether it was effective or not. Quantification, we know, had surfaced in the eighteenth century – to evaluate smallpox vaccination and as the basis of Lind's famous scurvy experiment. It was the subject of philosophical controversy in France, and medical reformers in Britain made it the cornerstone for a new program of clinical medicine that was quite visible by the beginning of the nineteenth century.[5] Louis presented it as a methodological innovation and research program in 1830s' Paris, provoking much controversy. Scholars have written much about these debates, and Ann La Berge discusses them in this volume.[6] I therefore do not explore this debate except to observe that nineteenth-century criticisms of clinical quantification were essentially of two kinds:[7] it was not effective, and it limited the freedom of doctors.

First, quantification did not work. Objections were both practical and theoretical. Among the latter was Risueño d'Amador's philosophical critique of quantification based on his vitalistic convictions. Many critics argued that it was impossible to transfer data about groups or populations to individual cases. Isolated individuals such as Jules Gavarret in France emphasized the mathematical limitations involved in counting via averages and means. Many defended clinical experience, informed by pathological and physiological knowledge, as a more valid form of knowledge than mere counting. Decades later, Claude Bernard presented his philosophical objections to "observational" knowledge, which he contrasted to the certain results of laboratory experimentation.

But even without such theoretical underpinnings, scepticism was widespread because results of quantification were frequently unconvincing. Disease categories being counted were too imprecise – if they in fact existed at all – to take account of individual variability among people and cases of a given disease. Therapies moreover were never applied in exactly the same way. Different observers thus quite regularly came up with very different if not contradictory results. There was no response to such objections except to say that correctly made observation under proper conditions could yield consistent results and that individual variability did not affect efficacy in the aggregate.

Second, decisions based on counting threatened both the therapeutic freedom and the judgment of the doctor. At a time when physicians took pride in their ability to make subtle distinctions among patients, diseases, and therapies on the basis of their understanding of pathology and physiology, and also to weigh and judge large numbers of factors and the consequences of various choices, it was easy to imagine that quantifiers were looking for the one best way that would promote profession-wide conformity and destroy traditional medical intelligence.

This threat of course did not materialize, largely because the critics were right about the limitations of counting. Simple counting of therapeutic results by individual doctors *was* inadequate in many and perhaps most situations for producing conclusive results. The standard historiographical argument is that this technical inadequacy prompted doctors largely to abandon quantification. According to this view, first popularized by Major Greenwood, clinicians rejected quantification, which the new public-health movement of the mid-nineteenth century took over and that became eventually the basis of epidemiology.[8] Clinical rejection of statistics, according to this view, did not dissipate until the twentieth-century development of new techniques made possible a more effective program of quantified therapeutic evaluation, based on advanced mathematical statistics. However, I have argued elsewhere that this view is at best partially true. Far from disappearing, counting came to be standard for many doctors after 1850. They could easily incorporate it in practice routines, and it came to serve as an extension of practical medical judgment. Counting alone might bring about consensus in a few cases where results were particularly striking – such as averting certain death; but often in such cases, quantifying results merely formalized direct experience and perception. Most often, clinical statistics were one element among many in medical discussions. The weight that they received depended on who was presenting them and what other kinds of evidence were available.[9]

As it became routine, quantification lost its normative and programmatic character. Few individuals followed Louis in arguing that it would transform medical practice. Counting in fact had rather low epistemological status in the latter half of the nineteenth century. A doctor did not achieve a reputation for being scientific by presenting clinical results in quantified form. The mark of science in the late nineteenth and early twentieth centuries was the laboratory, which had produced astonishing successes and demanded skills that most doctors lacked. To the extent that doctors worried about threats to traditional clinical judgment, they feared laboratory tests or new forms of imaging such as the x-ray when these received a definitive role in diagnosing diseases, superseding clinical judgment.[10] Even in the case of a highly technological procedure such as electrotherapy, some observers insisted that the doctor's senses should determine the amount of electricity to be applied to the patient rather than relying on precision instruments of measurement.[11] Eventually clinicians accommodated themselves to those innovations that proved more consistently reliable than clinical observation and experience; doctors dealt with the resulting tensions by adopting some variant of the cliché that medicine is both science AND art.

By the end of the nineteenth century, counting results no longer seemed a threat to clinical judgment. Any physician who kept records could do it. It was highly individualized and did not require the enormous infrastructures that were necessary for compiling public-health statistics. If enough people reached the same conclusion, a collective change in practice might occur. Clinical counting could take various forms. One strategy was the retrospective audit of results,[12] comparing, for instance, two hospitals or wards with different practices. (This was a very old technique, used in French debates on tracheotomy of the 1840s.)[13] A variation was to compare results in the same institution before and after a particular innovation. (Lister's results on amputation before and after antiseptic method, or Semmelweis, discussed by Jorland in this volume.) The work of Karl Pearson transformed clinical counting but only slowly and gradually. Quantification took many forms. The famous debate between Pearson and Sir Almroth Wright was not really about the role of statistics in clinical medicine. Rather, it concerned two competing scientific models for quantification in clinical medical research – one based on statistics, and the other on quantified laboratory procedures that left some room for the researcher's subjective judgment.[14]

The new statistical procedures developed by Pearson and pupils such as Major Greenwood gained in influence because, during the first half of the twentieth century, distrust of subjective experience continued to grow.[15] Part of this followed expansion of the pharmaceutical industry and the glut of therapeutic products on the market. The old reliance on practitioners' experience was visibly unequal to the task of evaluating and choosing from among so many products. And it did not help that many people thought producers of pharmaceuticals or apparatuses to be venal. Medical researchers gradually came to understand that effective counting requires sophisticated techniques, large infrastructures, and rigorous regulation of conditions. The development of new statistical techniques such as randomization and the chi-square test was certainly necessary to the development of randomized clinical trials (RCTs). But equally vital were new forms of social organization and regulation. We know that these forms of regulated testing emerged in Britain during the interwar years and in the United States, on an even larger scale, after 1945.[16]

Since the 1960s, RCTs have assumed canonical significance everywhere in the Western world – they are the gold standard. They do not always resolve controversies or convince everyone, as sociologists of science have repeatedly documented,[17] but unsuccessful test results usually keep new drugs off the market. The acceptance of RCTs has reawakened fears that mechanistic formulae are displacing individualized medical judgment. More seriously, to the extent that RCTs appear to provide reliable information about efficacy, it seems logical to seek to eliminate wide variations in medical practice that seem to deviate from correct clinical procedure. This pressure comes not only from third-party payers who have an interest in cutting costs by eliminating ineffective treatments, but even more from within the medical profession; it is a logical consequence of the quest for objectification that has energized and transformed medical research during the past two centuries.

Marc Berg has provided an interesting analysis of how the barriers to "objective knowledge" were understood in the years following 1945. His work suggests that perceptions have changed continually. Starting in the postwar years with the notions that external, structural forces impeded the correct application of science to practice, professional rhetoric increasingly came to blame misunderstanding by individual physicians, making the problem essentially a "cognitive" deficiency.[18] It begins to make sense then to seek to displace judgment from individual physicians and to argue that algorithms or expert systems can do a better job than individual doctors in diagnosing and choosing therapies. In response, doctors argue that physical examination and judgment will always be indispensable, no matter how smart the computer or the algorithm.[19]

RCTs are not a panacea and have thus become the starting point for an entire infrastructure of practices that aim to clarify frequently confusing and contradictory test results – Cochrane collaborations, consensus conferences, meta-analyses, etc. – and that try to monitor or shape doctors' actual behavior – medical audits, practice guidelines, courses in medical schools in evaluating clinical research. In the context of efforts by governments and private insurance providers to slow rising health costs, these emerging practices have again raised the old fear that reliance on numbers threatens individual clinical judgment. This brings me back to the ubiquitous notion of evidence-based medicine that somehow exemplifies all these different concerns and pressures.

EVIDENCE-BASED MEDICINE: OBJECTIFICATION AS A SOCIAL MOVEMENT

In preparation for the conference on which we based this volume, I did a search on PubMed web site for articles that contained the term "evidence-based medicine" in their title. Since this is a book about quantification, it seems appropriate to inundate the reader with some numbers. I found 1,255 articles published before 1 October 2002. Using just "evidence-based" resulted in over 3,400 listings; a broader search including keywords and NLM categories produced about 9,000. This torrent of publications started in 1992 with an article in the *Journal of the American Medical Association* (*JAMA*) by a group based at McMaster University in Hamilton, Ontario.[20] In 1995 there were 55 articles with "evidence-based medicine" in the title; in 1997, 110; and in 2001, 256. The vast majority of papers published before October 2002 are in English (958), with German a distant second (89) and French third (45). The three journals with the most titles are British, the *British Medical Journal* (*BMJ*), *Lancet*, and what is now called the *Emergency Medicine Journal*; these make up 16 per cent of the entire sample and over 20 per cent of the papers published since 1998. *JAMA*, dominant in the early years, is now in fourth place.

This of course raises interesting questions about the apparent taste in Britain for evidence-based medicine (EBM) that may shed light on the emergence of clinical trials there early in the twentieth century. (I would suggest as possible reasons the long history of statisticians on staff in British public health institutions and the managerial, indeed accounting, ethos in the National Health Service where "audit commissions" seek to standardize all aspects of medical training and practice.) In recent years, medical journals in almost every country, and representing every specialty, have published some articles on this topic. The *New York Times Magazine* "Year in Review" included EBM among the most influential ideas of 2001.[21]

Articles are of various sorts. A large group has to do with educating doctors to use on-line evidence. A variation attempts, in true evidence-based fashion, to test the effectiveness of such educational programs. Another category, exemplified by reports from the Cochrane collaboration but extending far beyond it, evaluates the literature on various medical problems in order to generate recommendations for practice. A large group of articles makes rhetorical statements in favour of EBM in one field or another. Early papers in this genre were highly polemical. The very first, published in *JAMA* in 1992, was a call to medical arms robed in the language of Kuhnian philosophy of science. EBM was replacing an old paradigm based on a variety of bad things – intuition, unsystematic, and pathophysiologic rationale as sufficient grounds for clinical decision making; the New Paradigm emphasized examination of evidence from clinical research ... and the application of formal rules of evidence evaluating the clinical literature.[22] One was the Way of the Past; the other, The Way of the Future. (Which would you choose?)

Since then this language has substantially moderated. The most prolific advocate of EBM, David Sackett, together with a number of co-authors, published an editorial in the BMJ in 1996 that exemplified this growing moderation: EBM "means integrating clinical expertise with the best available external evidence ... neither alone is enough."[23] This changing tone, with its constant insistence that EBM complements rather than replaces traditional clinical virtues, is a result of EBM's critical reception from many sectors of the profession.

The literature certainly includes many critiques of the concepts behind EBM; frequently the authors are Europeans, but there are considerable numbers of North Americans. Unlike the situation in 1830s' Paris, these critics seem to be swimming against an immensely powerful tide. They have political allies that were not available to their predecessors – a public-health left, for instance, which sees EBM as part of the reductionist trend that obfuscates social causes of disease, and a popular movement that supports alternative medicine. None the less, the concept's power is such that each of these two domains has generated its own EBM claims – evidence-based public health or evidence-based alternative medicine.[24] The overall thrust of the critics' arguments is not unfamiliar to the historian of nineteenth-century medicine and testifies to the enduring tensions inherent in all efforts to "objectify" medicine. First, critics argue that EBM does not work in many cases – where good evidence is lacking; where variations in skill are very marked, as in surgery or psychodynamic therapy; where the numbers of cases are small and not susceptible to RTCs or, on the contrary, where very large numbers produce great variability in the nature of the condition being tested.[25] RTCs are "bedeviled by low inclusion rates and potentially important recruitment biases. 'Real world' trials often do not give the same results as these highly artificial controlled clinical studies ... There is a bias in the hypotheses tested in large clinical trials, as the costs involved are usually covered by commercially interested companies."[26] The contradictory results yielded by different trials are striking reminders that they do not "work" very well. That is why consensus conferences and meta-analyses are necessary to adjudicate such discrepancies. One recent critic has argued that evidence-based medicine is in fact opinion-based and suggests that there are parallels here with the emperor's new clothes. Most of the time, results are inconclusive and reflect the opinions of experts on how to interpret them. Meta-analysis is particularly untrustworthy and gives the impression of trying to wring statistical significance out of a morass of small effects.[27] Not only does it occult hidden variations in procedure, but it underrepresents trials with negative results, which are frequently never published.[28]

The original popularizers of EBM cast this method, rather naïvely, as a new "paradigm." They have thus been fair game for epistemologically sophisticated critics who have pointed out the EBM is at best a set of practices with almost no features of a classical Kuhnian paradigm. It is suggested that the insistence that information from the medical literature should have precedence even when it contradicts the dominant pathophysiological paradigm goes directly against Kuhn's understanding of paradigms and is in reality profoundly anti-scientific. If the clinical trial always takes precedence over medical theory, "why not conduct double-blind, controlled, randomized clinical trials of the effectiveness of Voodoo, followed by a meta-analysis?" It is, moreover, self-contradictory to demand a change in practices when there is not the slightest evidence of the kind that EBM regularly demands to demonstrate that such practices provide better outcomes. The only possible justification is one of theoretical plausibility, a form of argument that EBM advocates regularly label as "unsubstantiated claims."[29]

Other critics have used philosophical theories of science in an even more scathing way. One of these examines the claims of EBM in term of Popperian standards of verifiability and points out that what it calls evidence consists of many levels of subjective interpretation of empirical data. "Unfortunately there are no rules of logic that can guarantee a truthful interpretation. There is no *evidence* in the sense of proofs; there are assertions which are held to be true by some people, by many people, or by practically everyone and which might be false, regardless of how many believers line up to support them."[30]

The nineteenth-century argument that individual clinical expertise retains its legitimacy continues to be advanced.[31] Repeated even more frequently is the old proposition that quantitative knowledge applies to collectivities and thus cannot apply to individuals.[32] It is not that such knowledge is totally inapplicable – we now can speak in terms of probabilities – but specific results do not apply to real individual people because trials tend to enrol patients who are younger and healthier and in general of lower risk than real-world patients.[33] (A fascinating political dimension to this critique involves identity groups of various sorts apparently excluded from testing, and that has led to radically transformed regulations for recruiting test subjects.)[34] But we return to conclusions remarkably similar to those of Louis's opponents in the 1830s. Patients are individuals, and need individual treatment.[35] As in the previous century, proponents of pathophysiological reasoning and laboratory experimentation in medicine are among those most threatened by the new trust in numbers.[36]

Second, the old fear resurfaces that clinical authority will shift from doctors. For many people, particularly policy types, this is not a threat but an occasion for beneficial change. EBM provides managers with information that allows them to question the judgment and autonomy of physicians. The techniques that produce data typically require many sorts of non-medical expertise (notably statistical); this breaks the lockhold that the medical profession traditionally has had over judging medicine ... Now armed with more and better information about medical practices, payers and purchasers can deny payment for medical services that they deem medically unnecessary or ineffective.[37]

This of course revives an old nightmare for doctors – that others will make medical decisions on their behalf. Critics consistently use the term "orthodoxy" in speaking about EBM;[38] words such as "rigid," "politically correct," and "knee jerk–like" are frequent qualifiers of EBM in this literature. The fear is that EBM will dictate practices, not just in the obvious sense that those who pay health costs will impose practice guidelines to save money, but more subtly by defining out of existence what cannot be measured by RCTs (environmental or psychosocial factors) or what is uninteresting to those who pay for tests – usually pharmaceutical companies – (conditions and therapies from which no one is going to make much money and, more generally, prevention as opposed to cure). From his Popperian perspective, Eyal

Shahar sees EBM as using logically meaningless terms such as "systematic" and "evidence" in order to impose "a new type of authoritarianism" that makes some interpreters of the evidence dominant. "What is behind the title if not other doctors who claim to know better? Who claim that what they call *evidence* is more valid than another doctor's interpretation of empirical experience?"[39] As is often the case, sociologists follow the protagonists in emphasizing that political and social factors underlie EBM. Some seek to analyse it a "social movement";[40] similarly, the rise of a new stratum of professional "experts" producing guidelines fits with Freidson's "stratification theory".[41]

Other critics worry less about power than about the "dumbing down" of the medical profession, as doctors lose their ability to judge and discriminate and understand disease mechanisms.[42] In response, spokesmen for EBM such as Sackett insist that it is not "cookbook" medicine but depends on individual clinical expertise. "External clinical evidence can inform, but can never replace, individual clinical expertise." To fears that the hidden agenda is cutting costs, Sackett replies, "this may raise rather than lower the cost of their care."[43]

Not all the arguments against EBM are traditional. The medical field, for one thing, now includes a large number of occupational groups, many of which do not share the values of doctors. A variety of other forms of expertise are struggling to make themselves heard. Research in health administration, for instance, emphasizes that clinical effectiveness is only one criterion of decision-making, others include "cost-effectiveness" and "patient and public preferences." Some observers argue for a much more complex form of administrative decision-making to take account of these different imperatives.[44] Allan Maynard sees EBM as concerned just with what is effective for the patient, whereas the economist or public-health physician looks at the interests of society as a whole – "the population-health ethic."[45] Ours is a far more cynical, relativistic culture than was 1830s' Paris; the idea that evidence alone drives practice has become unconvincing to some. Some critics maintain, for instance, that EBM reflects specific ideological investments – in curative medicine rather than prevention. EBM is bound to fail in shaping practice, others say, because it does not recognize the complex nature of medical decision-making.

One such article coming out of the health-management domain applies Aristotle's analysis of rhetoric to argue that *logos*, in this case evidence, is only one element in the arts of persuasion, which also include *pathos*, the power to stir the emotions, and *ethos*, the authority of the speaker. "Perhaps the most obvious lesson we can take away from the rhetorical triangle is that scientific evidence is but *one* component of persuasion. Health care innovation adoption is not only a function of the argument, but also of the credibility of the proponents and the values, experience, and interests of potential adopters. Innovations are more like to be adopted when a convincing argument (logos) is presented by credible research proponents (ethos) who stir the interests, needs, and emotions of adopting practitioners (pathos)."[46]

The authors add: "in this pluralistic situation there is no such thing as '*the* evidence.' Instead, there are several competing bodies of evidence that are subject to multiple interpretations by different stakeholders."

In the face of this onslaught, prominent leaders of EBM have not just moderated their rhetoric but conceded to the critics on many points. R. Brian Haynes of McMaster University, a major figure in the movement, has admitted that no direct evidence exists to show that practice based on the principles of EBM is in any way superior to that based on clinicians' experience. He agrees that "the research methods of medical science are pluralistic and expanding, driven by attempts to address a broader range of questions" and that "evidence from research can be no more than one component of any clinical decision." He admits that it is difficult to argue for EBM's superiority when results of methodologically similar trials frequently disagree with one another and when findings of observational studies frequently agree with supposedly more potent RCTs. Among EBM's greatest failings is its inability to distinguish between doing the greatest good for the individual patient and doing the greatest good for all patients, collectively.[47]

Stripped of its preachy tone and moral fervour, and presented in this new and distinctly ecumenical mode, EBM does not mean very much. As critics have noted, admitting the validity of many different forms of knowledge without prescribing a strategy for evaluating them and resolving conflicting conclusions hardly amounts to a new paradigm and may not be distinguishable from traditional practice.[48] (In any case, the majority of more hardline EBMers do not shrink from claiming a strict evidentiary hierarchy.) None the less, pronouncements to the effect that EBM has been a failure seem wildly premature. Not only do they ignore the time required for even the most successful innovations to take root, they understand success as the unrealistic expectation that most physicians will suddenly change their ways and practice the "best" medicine. The reality is likely to be much more modest. I suspect that EBM will continue to gain in popularity, at least as a slogan and as a claim and, not incidentally, as an ever-expanding multitude of procedures, instruments, and guidelines. Certainly my own distinctly non-evidence-based impression of the literature is that criticism is becoming less frequent as the movement gradually loses its threatening edge (even as it becomes more powerful). It may even someday become – like simple clinical counting in the nineteenth century – a routine part of medical practice. It may or may not lead to better clinical decisions, as more and more medical students receive indoctrination in its principles. (This is certainly the case at McGill University, where I teach.) Certainly the widespread availability of practice guidelines has reduced the economic implications of spending hours at a computer instead of seeing billable patients. There is no reason to assume that the underdetermination of medical practice by solid evidence or expert opinion will not continue, given the complexity of so much "real-life" medical practice. Whatever form EBM comes to assume, it will not go away. It is perhaps a slogan as much as a concrete program (let alone a paradigm), but it serves a wide variety of functions.

First, it is clearly plays a rhetorical role in defending medical authority from a variety of contemporary threats. This is of course the function that sociologists of science and of the professions tend to emphasize.[49] EBM identifies medicine as scientific and distinguishes it from various forms of alternative healing, the heartless cost-cutting of insurance providers, and the irrational whims of patients. This collective authority may limit somewhat the clinical autonomy of individual clinicians (and concentrate authority in the hands of clinical elites), but this may be unavoidable. And one of its side-effects is to make doctors feel that they are coping with an ever-expanding volume of medical literature that they would otherwise never master.

Second, within the hierarchy of clinical research, EBM particularly valorizes patient-centred clinical research – a form of science that has never achieved the success or status of the laboratory sciences. It thus places clinical research on a more nearly equal footing. If it does not have the epistemological status of the laboratory experiment, it at least has the immediate relevance of rigorous applied research that defines effective practice, not to mention statistical techniques that few people can fully comprehend. It joins to medicine's existing status the new status and power of the computer while allowing doctors – and especially the men among them – to play with computers as a routine part of their work.

Third, EBM is such a protean concept that anyone can appropriate it. Politicians and health administrators can invoke it to argue for cost-cutting and for limiting the autonomy of doctors; simultaneously, doctors can use it to defend clinical practices and judgment against economic pressures to cut costs. Everyone from public-health professionals, through nurses, to alternative practitioners can associate himself or herself with both the term and the scientific rigour that it supposedly embodies.

It is thus possible that EBM will lose its ideological and programmatic edge and become just one routine part of practice, among many others, in much the way that clinical counting did in the nineteenth century. However, several important variables have changed since the nineteenth century. Chief of these is the sheer size of the medical enterprise. Medicine has become so institutionalized, bureaucratized, and central to social concerns that one cannot dismiss the possibility that the increasing numbers of practice guidelines will eventually become rigidly enforced criteria of practice. Courts may come to use practice guidelines as standards in litigation judgments.[50] It is equally possible that insurers, both public and private, will use them to determine which procedures to reimburse and which not. There is little evidence that this process has begun, in North America at least, but this does not mean that it will not occur in the future.[51]

A less likely alternative to EBM receives frequent mention in leading medical journals. Even those clinicians who most fervently support EBM understand that there is a major gap between evidence about populations and evidence about individuals. The former may provide us with the best existing "objective" data about the latter, but "average responses" cannot replace knowledge of the individual. This latter form of knowledge has traditionally been subjective and thus unreliable. If knowledge of the individual could become truly "objective," there would be no need to rely on "averages." This is precisely the promise that genotyping seems to offer: "objective" genetic data, some people think or hope, may allow clinicians to individualize therapy in a way now possible only through trial and error.[52] Such claims or hopes reveal a great deal about the tensions within the EBM movement and clinical medicine in general. There is, I would argue, fundamental incommensurability between forms of collective objectification and the aims of the clinician at the bedside, however loudly he or she clamours for EBM. Therapy based on genotyping – "objectified" individuality in therapy – would allow clinicians to have their cake and eat it too. However, this is at present a distant hope rather than an immediate prospect. In the interim we have EBM. Available to everyone, and meaning relatively little, EBM will probably remain a popular catchphrase, at least until something better comes along.

NOTES

1 P.K. Rangachari, "Evidence-Based Medicine: Old French Wine with a New Canadian Label," *Journal of the Royal Society of Medicine* 90 (1997), 280–4. A more positive spin on this connection appears in Han P. Van-

denbroucke, "Evidence-Based Medicine and 'Médecine d'Observation,'" *Journal of Clinical Epidemiology* 49 (1996), 1335–8.

2 Theodore Porter, *Trust in Numbers: The Pursuit of Objectivity in Science and Public Life* (Princeton, NJ: Princeton University Press, 1995).

3 By using this term I mean to suggest the various efforts made to achieve what Lorraine Daston has called "aperspectival objectivity" by externalizing subjective judgment. Lorraine Daston, "Objectivity and the Escape from Perspective," *Social Studies of Science* 22 (1992), 597–618. On quantification and objectivity, see Theodore M. Porter, "Quantification and the Accounting Ideal in Science," ibid., 633–52.

4 The classic study of Paris medicine during the first half of the nineteenth century is Erwin Ackerknecht, *Medicine at the Paris Hospital, 1794–1848* (Baltimore, Md.: Johns Hopkins Press, 1967). A more theoretical analysis of its intellectual origins is Michel Foucault, *The Birth of the Clinic: An Archaeology of Medical Perception*, trans. A.M. Sheridan Smith (London: Tavistock, 1973). The most recent comprehensive re-evaluation is Caroline Hannaway and Ann La Berge, eds., *Constructing Paris Medicine,* Clio Medica 50 (Amsterdam: Rodopi, 1998).

5 On these matters, see the essays in this volume by Marks, Rusnock, and Tröhler.

6 Ann La Berge in this volume.

7 I draw on my own account of this debate in George Weisz, *The Medical Mandarins: The French Academy of Medicine in the 19th and Early 20th Centuries* (Oxford: Oxford University Press, 1995), 159–88.

8 Major Greenwood, "Louis and the Numerical Method," in *The Medical Dictator,* first pub. 1936 (London: British Medical Association, 1986).

9 I describe a number of examples in Weisz, *The Medical Mandarins,* 159–88.

10 For one example, Bernike Pasveer, "Depiction in Medicine as a Two-Way Affair: X-Ray Pictures and Pulmonary Tuberculosis in the Early 20th Century," in Ilana Loewy, ed., *Medicine and Change: Historical and Sociological Studies of Medical Innovation* (London: John Libby, 1993), 85–106.

11 John Senior, "Metrological Awakenings: Rationalizing the Body Electric in Nineteenth-Century Medicine," in Eileen Magnello and Anne Hardy, eds., *The Road to Medical Statistics,* Clio Medica 67 (Amsterdam: Rodopi, 2002), 77–94.

12 The term is in John R. Hampton, "Evidence-Based Medicine, Opinion-Based Medicine, and Real-World Medicine," *Perspectives in Biology and Medicine* 45 (2002), 554.

13 Weisz, *The Medical Mandarins.*

14 J. Rosser Matthews, "Almroth Wright, Vaccine Therapy and British Biometrics: Disciplinary Expertise versus Statistical Objectivity," in Eileen Magnello and Anne Hardy, eds., *The Road to Medical Statistics,* Clio Medica 67 (Amsterdam: Rodopi, 2002), 125–48.

15 Harry Marks, "Trust and Mistrust in the Marketplace: Statistics and Clinical Research, 1945–1960," *History of Science* 38 (2000), 343–55.

16 This perception may be based on simple ignorance. We do not really know what was going on in other countries, because research is lacking.

17 Among many works in this vein, see Harry Marks, *The Progress of Experiment: Science and Therapeutic Reform in the United States, 1900–1990* (Cambridge: Cambridge University Press, 1997); Steven Epstein, *Impure Science: AIDS, Activism and the Politics of Knowledge* (Berkeley: University of California Press, 1996); David S. Jones, "Visions of a Cure: Visualization, Clinical Trials, and Controversies in Cardiac Therapeutics, 1968–1998," *Isis* 91 (2000), 504–41; Nicolas Dodier and Janine Barbot, "Le temps des tensions épistémiques. Le développement des essais thérapheutiques dans le cadre du sida (1982–1996)," *Revue française de sociologie* 41 (2000), 79–118.

18 Marc Berg, "Turning a Practice into a Science: Reconceptualizing Postwar Medical Practice," *Social Studies of Science* 25 (1995), 437–76.

19 Anthony L. Komaroff, "Algorithms and the 'Art' of Medicine," *American Journal of Public Health* 72 (1982), 10–12; Robyn M. Dawes, David Faust, and Paul E. Meehl, "Clinical versus Actuarial Judgment," *Science* 243 (1989), 1668–74; Collin K.L. Phoon, "Must Doctors Still Examine Patients?" *Perspectives in Biology and Medicine* 43 (2000), 548–61.

20 The movement began long before the appearance of this term in 1992. For some background, see Steven Timmermans and Marc Berg, *The Gold Standard: The Challenge of Evidence-Based Medicine and Standardization in Health Care* (Philadelphia: Temple University Press, 2003), 13–15.

21 J. Hitt, "Evidence-Based Medicine," *New York Times Magazine*, 2001.

22 Evidence-Based Medicine Working Group, "Evidence-Based Medicine: A New Approach to Teaching the Practice of Medicine," *Journal of the American Medical Association* 258 (1992), 67.

23 David L. Sackett et al. "Editorial: Evidence Based Medicine: What It Is and What It Isn't," *British Medical Journal* 312 (1996), 71–2.

24 R.F. Heller and J. Page, "A Population Perspective to Evidence Based Medicine: 'Evidence for Population Health,'" *Journal of Epidemiology and Community Health* 56 (2002), 45–7.

25 On this last point, Douglas Black, "The Limitations of Evidence," *Perspectives in Biology and Medicine* 42 (1998), 4. Also see A.R. Feinstein and R.I. Horowitz, "Problems in the 'Evidence' of 'Evidence-Based Medicine,'" *American Journal of Medicine* 103 (1997), 529–35.

26 D.S. Celermajer, "Evidence-Based Medicine: How Good Is the Evidence?" *Medical Journal of Australia* 174 (2001), 293–5; quote from abstract.

27 Hampton, "Evidence-Based Medicine," 550, 561.

28 Black, "The Limitations of Evidence," 4.

29 Joaquim S. Couto, "Evidence-Based Medicine: A Kuhnian Perspective of a Transvestite Non-Theory," *Journal of Evaluation in Clinical Practice* 4 (1998), 271.

30 Eyal Shahar, "A Popperian Perspective of the Term 'Evidence-Based Medicine,'" *Journal of Evaluation in Clinical Practice* 3 (1997), 110.
31 D.D.R. Williams and Jane Garner, "The Case against 'The Evidence': A Different Perspective on Evidence-Based Medicine," *British Journal of Psych* 180 (2002), 8–12.
32 S.J. Tanenbaum, "What Physicians Know," *New England Journal of Medicine* 329 (1993), 1268–9; N.W. Goodman, "Who Will Challenge Evidence-Based Medicine?," *Journal of the Royal College of Physicians of London* 33 (1999), 249–51.
33 Hampton, "Evidence-Based Medicine," 563.
34 Stephen Epstein is writing a book on test recruitment. Among his articles, see "Bodily Differences and Collective Identities: The Politics of Gender and Race in Biomedical Research in the United States," *Body and Society* 10 (2004), 183–203.
35 Hampton, "Evidence-Based Medicine," 565.
36 Burton E. Sobel and Mark A. Levine, "Medical Education, Evidence-Based Medicine, and the Disqualification of Physician-Scientists," *Experimental Biological Medicine* (Maywood) 226 (2001), 716.
37 Marc Rodwin, "Commentary: The Politics of Evidence-Based Medicine," *Journal of Health Politics, Policy and Law* 26 (2001), 440–1.
38 David Graham Smith, "Evidence-Based Medicine: Challenging the Orthodoxy," *Journal of the Royal Society of Medicine* 91 Suppl. 35 (1998), 7–11; Williams and Garner, "The Case against 'The Evidence'"; Goodman, "Who Will Challenge Evidence-Based Medicine?"
39 Shahar, "A Popperian Perspective," 115.
40 Catherine Pope, "Resisting Evidence: The Study of Evidence-Based Medicine as a Contemporary Social Movement," *Health: An Interdisciplinary Journal for the Social Study of Health, Illness and Medicine* 7 (2003), 267–82.
41 Sue Dopson et al., "Evidence-Based Medicine and the Implementation Gap," *Health: An Interdisciplinary Journal for the Social Study of Health, Illness and Medicine* 7 (2003), 311–30, especially 323.
42 Sobel and Levine, "Medical Education," 713–6.
43 Sackett et al., "Editorial: Evidence Based Medicine."
44 J. Dowie, "'Evidence-Based', 'Cost-Effective' and 'Preference-Driven' Medicine: Decision Analysis Based Medical Decision Making the Prerequisite," *Journal of Health Services Research Policy* 1 (1996), 104–13.
45 Alan Maynard, "Evidence-Based Medicine: An Incomplete Method for Informing Treatment Choices," *Lancet* 349 (1997), 126–8.
46 Andrew H. Van de Ven and Margaret S. Schomaker, "Commentary: The Rhetoric of Evidence-Based Medicine," *Health Care Management Review* 27 (2002), 90.
47 R. Brian Haynes, "What Kind of Evidence Is It That Evidence-Based Medicine Advocates Want Health Care Providers and Consumers to Pay

Attention to?" BMC *Health Services Research* 2 (2002). The copy that I consulted on the internet is paginated 1 to 7 but warns on the bottom not to use this numbering for citation purposes. I have been unable to find any other pagination. The quotes in the text are from pages 2, 4, 5, and 6, respectively, of the internet version.

48 Geoffrey R. Norman, "Examining the Assumptions for Evidence-Based Medicine," *Journal of Evaluation in Clinical Practice* 5 (1999), 141.

49 Keith Denny, "Evidence-Based Medicine and Medical Authority," *Journal of Medical Humanities* 20 (1999), 247–63.

50 This has not yet occurred, according to A.J. Rosoff, "Evidence-Based Medicine and the Law: The Courts Confront Clinical Practice Guidelines," *Journal of Health Political Policy Law* 26 (2001), 327–68.

51 In Germany, sickness insurance funds have implemented mandatory guidelines. G. Ollenschlager et al, 'The German Guidelines Clearing House (GGC) – Rationale, Aims and Results," *Procedures of the Royal College of Physicians Edinburgh* 31 Suppl. 9 (2001), 59–64.

52 To cite just some very recent examples: David M. Herrington and Timothy D. Howard, "From Presumed Benefit to Potential Harm – Hormone Therapy and Heart Disease," *New England Journal of Medicine* 349 (2003), 519–21; S. Fredericks, D. Holt, and I. MacPhee, "The Pharmacogenetics of Immunosuppression for Organ Transplantation: A Route to Individualization of Drug Administration," *American Journal of Pharmacogenomics* 3 (2003), 291–301; Eliot Marshall, "First Check My Genome, Doctor," *Science* 302 (2003), 589.

18

Medical Quantification: Science, Regulation, and the State

THEODORE M. PORTER

B.J.I. Risueño d'Amador spoke for many doctors in 1836 when he told the Académie Royale de Médecine in Paris that statistics is profoundly anti-medical. An ancient tradition of medical practice, backed up by extensive theorizing, insisted on the subtle skills of medical practice and the individuation of patients and conditions. The anti-statistical animus was often expressed as a moral claim about treating the sick. If a course of therapy is indicated by the preponderance of the numbers, wrote Risueño, this still means that it will work only for some, and a physician who chooses remedies based on statistics will in effect condemn some patients to death. But medical individualism was also, perhaps even more, about the professional standing of doctors, who did not want their art to be reduced to something formulaic and indiscriminate. Through long experience, at first under the guidance of a master, the physician should acquire a refined and subtle judgment. Although in retrospect it is easy to doubt the efficacy of many of the therapies proffered by these doctors, they prided themselves on their capacity to adapt treatments to the particular temperaments and conditions of their patients. Often they claimed a kind of intuition or feel – "medical tact" – that eluded formal rationality.

But medicine was never a pure relation of doctor to patient. The medical involvement of states and insurance organizations helped to open up medicine to new kinds of science and to an increasingly systematic reliance on quantification.

STATE AND STATISTICS

The Greek heritage claimed by the European medical tradition provided also a basis for regarding patients collectively. Medicine was a kind of social science – a "science de l'homme" – that classified disease according to customs and temperaments. The Hippocratic text on "Airs, Waters, and Places" explained how sickness was related to geography and climate. This was put forth in the guise of instructions for doctors working at a new location, to inform them of what diseases to expect there. But these environmental doctrines came increasingly to be valued as the basis for public-health measures. In the seventeenth century, when states began to collect numbers about causes of death, organized medicine was able to draw on familiar causes and categories to explain the results.

John Graunt's treatise of 1662 on the London bills of mortality provided a model for how to present the new statistics and judge their significance. Natural history, too, was becoming increasingly quantitative in the era of the Royal Society and the Académie des Sciences, and medical writers in the eighteenth century began using these numbers to associate environments with their characteristic diseases. Networks of doctors formed to assemble in quantitative form their collective experience and to assess the effectiveness of medical interventions. They sought particularly to determine the effectiveness of inoculation against smallpox – a controversial issue that aroused great interest and provoked public controversy through much of the eighteenth century, which was debated by mathematicians such as Daniel Bernoulli and Jean D'Alembert.[1]

Significantly, in this last discussion, Bernoulli deployed numbers and calculations to defend the rationality of inoculation from the standpoint of the state, while d'Alembert doubted if the tendency of mortality tables could outweigh the tender caution of a father or mother faced with a choice that might lead to the immediate death of a beloved child. Not for nothing did this aspect of health come in the nineteenth century to bear the name of statistics (i.e., state-istics), the descriptive science of the state. This was not merely a vehicle for the guidance of public interventions and the expansion of state power. Statistics became also a tool of liberalism, a way of informing the people about the condition of society and about the effectiveness of their governments.

The broad area of public health, including endemic as well as epidemic disease, was widely regarded in the period of early industrialization as an index of social danger and of progress. Under the name of *hygiène publique*, it was extended also to diseases of the social body, including crime, pauperism, and ignorance. For many nineteenth-century liberals, the remedy for such ills might as often require the retreat of the state – for example, from the attempt to tax and to regulate commerce – as the expansion of its role in regard, for instance, to schools and sanitation. Nineteenth-century reformers often supposed that private initiative and employer paternalism were the more effective and appropriate means to clean up urban slums or to provide insurance against unexpected illness or death. The expansion of medical statistics in the eighteenth and nineteenth centuries, then, is not simply synonymous with the growth of the state. It was, however, closely linked to public action and social reform.[2]

Statistical medicine fit neatly into the statistical movements that became so active in Europe and North America beginning in the 1820s. Along with these efforts to redefine the role of the state, statistics entailed also a new form of knowledge. German academic statisticians of the later nineteenth century developed an appropriate terminology for the new reality – "mass phenomena" (Massenerscheinungen) – which required a method of "mass observation." In this stance, however, they were followers of the Belgian Adolphe Quetelet and his English popularizer Henry Thomas Buckle, who emphasized the astonishing collective regularity of phenomena, such as crime and suicide, that seemed very far from orderly at the level of individuals. Epidemics were not stable in the same way, since they interrupted the normal patterns of disease and death. For statisticians such as William Farr, however, they had their own distinctive pattern of increase and decay, and their effects were not so great as to destroy the regularities of death by age as summarized in a life table, on which insurance companies depended. This faith in a collective order of society, a special form of human science, underlay the first influential form of medical quantification.[3]

SCIENCE AND MEASUREMENT

Even if medicine was often regarded as more art than science, it was taught already in the medieval universities, in part through instruction in such medical sciences as anatomy and pathology. Personal experience within a kind of apprenticeship, however, seemed generally more vital for the physician in training. Doctoring was about skill and judgment as well as formal learning, and the medical sciences, far from ineluctably dissolving this art into them, were in many ways subordinate to medicine as a profession. Medical knowledge meant skill in interpreting signs, rather than, as modern doctrines of evidence-based medicine would have it, processing information. Strictly codified or objective facts and laws had only a modest place in orthodox medicine up to the period of the Enlightenment.

The claims of medical science began to gain in effectiveness and influence in the late eighteenth century. The hospital – now increasingly a centre of research and of care for the seriously ill, rather than a charitable institution for poor invalids – became a major site of scientific medicine and also, as in Paris, a place to study disease as a mass phenomenon. Until about 1850, however, medical science in established institutions did not often aspire to explanation in terms of general laws, and the biological vitalism of the late eighteenth century remained pervasive. Such doctrines were nicely compatible with the faith of many practitioners in the ineffable medical touch. Physicians associated them with doubts regarding numbers and measures, and sometimes also about medical instruments. A fever was much more than a thermometer reading, just as the pulse did not reduce to a heart rate.

Still, it would be a mistake to suppose that medicine was singularly resistant to quantification, or that early efforts to incorporate measurement into medicine were at bottom an attempt to reject medical traditions and absorb the extraneous ideals of astronomy or physics. The role of measurement in most of science was quite limited until the late eighteenth century. Physics took part in the massive expansion of quantification after about 1750, but it was not notably in the forefront. Land surveys, accounts, and population statistics had at least as great a role in the new quantitative enthusiasm as did experimental physics.[4] Public-health statistics were part of the same movement. The numerical method of P.C.A. Louis, against which Risueño d'Amador inveighed, involved statistics on the scale of a great Paris hospital, yet depended on experiment and not on censuses or surveys.

It would be more accurate to say that medicine participated in the quantification of science, rather than that it imitated or resisted an ideal of exact science that was external to it. Even the noted opponent of statistical medicine Claude Bernard was a pioneer of a new movement of experimental precision in physiology, and such ambitions were increasingly characteristic of nineteenth-century science. Bernard, however, was anything but a spokesman for the medical profession. His great campaign was precisely to narrow the tacit domain of medical art and to replace it with science. The proper site for making medical knowledge, according to him, was not the hospital but the laboratory, and he was an unflagging champion of what he called experimental determinism. The point was not to detect loose correlations but to comprehend causes, in an effort to explain what happens not most of the time, but every time.[5]

The campaign for a scientific medicine accelerated in the late nineteenth century and continued throughout the twentieth. Its core was then and to a large degree remains the laboratory sciences, beginning with physiology and bacteriology. In the biomedical laboratory, as in the chemistry laboratory since Lavoisier, measurement was a normal part of competent practice. But this had more to do with procedures than with results, for the understanding of physiological processes was rarely precise in a quantitative sense. The new physiology did not put much emphasis on variability. Major Greenwood, trained in biometrics by Karl Pearson in the first decade of the twentieth century, assisted with laboratory experiments as well as therapeutic ones. He was still complaining in the 1940s of medical experimentalists who put their faith in an *experimentum crucis* rather than performing enough trials on diverse individuals to comprehend the range of variation. They even imagined that they could understand epidemics by investigating mechanisms of infection in the individual, while he saw the epidemic as a phenomenon of populations, whose effects could not be predicted without exact quantification.[6]

INSURANCE AND REGULATION

The private practice of medicine was still less favourable to measurement activities than the physiology laboratory. The enormously increased reliance on instrument readings in clinical settings over the course of the twentieth century reflects an ever-closer relationship between practising physicians and medical laboratories. The emergence of a fundamental role for science in medical education is an important part of that story. There was also an institutional and cultural dynamic at work, which indeed helped to shape the science. Medical instruments and laboratories developed in a way that could accommodate the needs and expectations of their customers.

As ever, the hospital defined an intermediate case between individual consultations and public-health actions, and certain measurements, such as bodily temperature readings, began to penetrate there in the mid-nineteenth century. But insurance companies and the state – or in some cases state-provided insurance – played a crucial role in the quantification of medical practice. The thermometer as a measure of fever, for example, was particularly in demand where it was required to provide objective evidence of sickness, and hence of the need for medical treatment, which a third party, a medical insurer, then paid. Objectivity, in the sense of neutral indicators or measures that could supposedly not lie no matter what interests were at stake, plays an essential role in this story.[7]

Since the late nineteenth century, insurance institutions have been central to the movement towards a more collectivized form of medicine. For a time, life insurance was as important in this respect as health or medical insurance. In the United States in the early twentieth century, life-insurance examinations provided as much as 12 per cent of the income of doctors. Young physicians, just starting out, were particularly dependent on such work while they tried to build up a base of patients. In part because they needed to attract and hold new patients, they rarely were willing to assess unfavourably the health of an applicant for life insurance. This would incur the wrath of the applicants, and also of the salesmen who stood to reap a generous commission if the insurance policy should be issued. These insurance agents, whose persistence and resourcefulness became legendary, were indispensable for companies selling policies to individuals. Few people apply on their on initiative for life insurance, and those who do are automatically suspect as likely to be bad risks. One key to the success of insurance institutions, according to the actuaries and other professionals who run them, is to avoid the "adverse selection" that came from admitting a substandard population of policy-holders. The medical directors of early-twentieth-century life insurance companies, who were responsible for accepting applications and determining a proper rate for new customers, found it extremely difficult to get an honest and informed evaluation of the health of applicants.

Faced with so difficult a problem of trust, medical directors came increasingly to favour objective criteria, such as the relationship of height and weight, and they developed tables based on their own experience for linking such measures to mortality rates. In the early twentieth century, insurance companies collected the evidence linking elevated blood pressure ("hypertension") to health risks, and they were early advocates of electrocardiograms and x-rays for prognostic purposes. "Modern" medical practitioners, they thought, should have such equipment in their offices, and in this way they helped to define such instruments as a basic feature of modern medicine.[8]

Most of the "basic" medical sciences of the twentieth century, right up to the present, have not been particularly quantitative ones. This is especially true of molecular biology, which for about three decades now has been regarded by many as virtually synonymous with another modernism, "modern" biology. Systematic quantification and rigorous statistical testing have been more prominent in applied aspects of medicine, especially in the design and analysis of therapeutic trials. Such methods are often powerful and effective, and many, including the randomized clinical trial, have a compelling theoretical rationale.

Yet instrument readings, laboratory tests, and controlled trials have succeeded in medicine by taking part in a sweeping cultural transformation, one that is not merely internal to medicine, but includes its relations to state bureaucracies, insurers, and the law. The randomized clinical trial, however persuasive its inherent logic, owes its immense authority to its role in government efforts to regulate the pharmaceutical trade – and with it, to the extent possible – the practices of physicians.[9] Doctors order lab tests because they may provide valuable information for a diagnosis, but also to give evidence to insurance companies of the need for treatment and to reduce the exposure of doctors to legal claims. In the modern medical climate, at least in the United States, medical judgment that seems to go against statistical evidence is automatically suspect and leaves the practitioner vulnerable to charges of malpractice. The relationship of patient to doctor, once relatively unconstrained, is now bound up with myriad systems of regulation and oversight and intricate problems of trust and authority. The modern role of science in medicine, and particularly the role of measurement and quantification, are part of this new moral order, which has reined in the discretion of a once-free profession. In an important sense, the private practice of medicine has been made public. If the expanding role of quantification in medicine is part of the history of science, it is also one of the forms of knowledge that mesh most effectively with the prevailing contemporary forms of administration and government.

In this brave new world, measurement and statistics have become a part of the work of medicine. Since the early eighteenth century, probability mathematicians have argued that theirs was the proper logic for this world, a place of uncertainty and imperfect knowledge. But converting the uncertainties that pervade life into numbers is quite impossible in a state of nature, without elaborate infrastructures for generating and compiling data, and such reasoning does not conform very well to untutored modes of understanding. For a long time statistics threatened also the professional interests of doctors. The modern politics of health, backed up by a remarkable flourishing of quantitative expertise, has generated the data and the modes of calculation that really have made statistics central to medical practice. Epistemology, I would suggest, is becoming a subfield of administration, and this is nowhere more significant, or more consequential, than in medicine.

NOTES

1 Andrea Rusnock, *Vital Accounts: Quantifying Health and Population in Eighteenth-Century England and France* (Cambridge: Cambridge University Press, 2002).

2 William Coleman, *Death Is a Social Disease: Public Health and Political Economy in Early Industrial France* (Madison: University of Wisconsin Press, 1982); François Ewald, *L'Etat providence* (Paris: Bernard Grasset, 1986).

3 Theodore M. Porter, *The Rise of Statistical Thinking, 1820–1900* (Princeton, NJ: Princeton University Press, 1986); Ian Hacking, *The Taming of Chance* (Cambridge: Cambridge University Press, 1990).

4 Tore Frängsmyr, J.L. Heilbron, and Robin Rider, eds., *The Quantifying Spirit in the Eighteenth Century* (Berkeley: University of California Press, 1990).

5 J. Rosser Matthews, *Quantification and the Quest for Medical Certainty* (Princeton, NJ: Princeton University Press, 1995).

6 Major Greenwood, *Authority in Medicine: Old and New* (Cambridge: Cambridge University Press, 1943), 16; Greenwood, *Medical Statistics from Graunt to Farr* (Cambridge: Cambridge University Press, 1948); also Theodore M. Porter, *Karl {Pearson: The Scientific Life in a Statistical Age* (Princeton, NJ: Princeton University Press, 2004).

7 Volker Hess, *Der wohltemperierte Mensch: Wissenschaft und Alltag des Fiebermessens* (Frankfurt: Campus, 2000); John Harley Warner, *The Therapeutic Perspective: Medical Practice, Knowledge, and Identity in America, 1820–1885* (Cambridge, Mass.: Harvard University Press, 1986); Theodore M. Porter, *Trust in Numbers: The Pursuit of Objectivity in Science and Public Life* (Princeton, NJ: Princeton University Press, 1995).

8 Theodore M. Porter, "Life Insurance, Medical Testing, and the Management of Mortality," in Lorraine Daston, ed., *Biographies of Scientific Objects* (Chicago: University of Chicago Press, 2000), 226–46.

9 Harry M. Marks, *The Progress of Experiment: Science and Therapeutic Reform in the United States, 1900—1990* (Cambridge: Cambridge University Press, 1997).

Index

The index uses French, in a sans-serif font, for topics in French-language papers, except for proper names. Cross-references provide a guide to topics covered in both languages. Where authors have used terms that are identical or very close (for example, government and gouvernement), the index cites the English term. Some terms appear in both languages.

Abramowski, Edward, 153–4
Academy of Medicine (Paris), 3, 9, 45, 89–104; medical statistics at, 93–6, 394
Academy of Sciences (Paris), 3, 395
accouchements, 218–20, 221–3
Actions-Traitements, 365, 367
Act-Up, 365, 367, 371
Adams, Robert, 37
aetiology, 226, 335, 340
Affymetrix, 199n64
Agence du médicament, 363
Agence nationale de recherches sur le sida (ANRS), 362, 363, 364, 365–6
agriculture, 282–3, 316, 317
Aides (association), 363
AIDS. *See* sida
Airborne Instruments Limited, 179–80
Aldersgate Dispensary, 40, 41
Alembert, Jean Le Rond d', 53–9, 395
alimentation. *Voir* diet
Allen, Frederik Madison, 129–30, 133, 135, 136, 140
allocation (in clinical trials): alternation in, 311–14, 316–18, 320, 321–2, 324–7; bias in, 309–13, 320, 323, 325, 326–7; evolution of, 313–15; Hill on, 323–6; knowledge of, 312–13, 326–7; by rotation, 322–3; schedules for, 311–12. *See also* randomization
Amberson, J.B., et al., 314–15
American Association of the History of Medicine, 310
American Cancer Society, 177, 179
American Child Health Association, 279
American Management Association, 275
American Public Health Association (APHA), 268–71, 274–5, 289; appraisal forms, 267, 271–5, 277–8, 280, 292; Committee on Administrative Practice (CAP), 271, 274–5, 279–80, 281, 288, 289; Committee on Municipal Health Department Practice, 270–1; *Health Practice Indices,* 288; information collected by, 267–8, 288
American Society for the Control of Cancer, 228
American Society of Cytology, 181
American Telephone and Telegraph Company, 275
American War of Independence, 27
Andral, Gabriel, 92, 101
angina pectoris, 44
l'Angleterre. *Voir* Britain
ANRS. *Voir* Agence nationale de recherches sur le sida
antibiotics, 230. *See also* streptomycin
antibodies. *See* immunophenotyping
antigens, 178, 183
APHA. *See* American Public Health Association

Arcat-sida, 360
Armitage, Peter, 312, 323
Armstrong's Dispensary for the Infant Poor, 41
Arneth, Franz Hecktor, 208–12
arthritis, 34
l'Asie, 291
Assistance publique parisienne, 340
Association Claude-Bernard, 340
Association for Molecular Pathology, 191
assurance, 270, 271–2, 274–5. *Voir aussi* insurance industry
asthma, 41, 257
Atlas Human Hematology Array, 190–1
Atwater, Reginald M., 289
Austoker, Joan, 319
Australia, 336–7
autopsies, 214–15, 216–17
Aykroyd, W.R., 282
AZT (azidothymidine), 365

Bacon, Francis, 19–20, 24, 37, 42
bacteriology, 236, 398
Badinter, Elisabeth, 58
Baglivi, Giorgio, 20
Bailar, John, 234
Baillie, Matthew, 43
Balfour, Thomas Graham, 313
Banque mondiale, 292
Banting, Frederick, 131–2
Bardsley, Samuel Argent, 41
Basel Institute of Pathology, 189
Bateman, Thomas, 31–2, 36
Belgium, 147–8, 149–50, 154, 156–8, 160
Belvedere Isolation Hospital, 320
Berg, Marc, 381
Berkson, Joseph, 232, 235, 236, 240
Bernard, Claude, 103, 127–8, 140, 379–80
Bernoulli, Daniel, 52–5, 58, 395
Bertillon, Jacques, 281
Best, Charles, 131–2
Bethlehem Asylum ("Bedlam"), 35, 41
Bhore Report (1944), 291
bias, 28; in allocation, 309–13, 320, 323, 325, 326–7. *See also* clinical trials
Billings, John S., 276, 280
bills of mortality, 70–4, 77, 257; Black and, 39, 40; Graunt and, 66–7, 252, 395
Binet, Albert, 156–7
biochips, 187–92
biology: molecular, 399; and pathology, 183, 185–6, 189, 193; quantification in, 146, 182
biometricians, 310
biostatisticians: and cohort studies, 234–5; epidemiologists and, 226–7, 228, 233, 237–8; in public health, 270
Biraud, Yves, 347
Birmingham Hospital, 22
Bishop, E.L., 287
Blache, Vidal de la, 287
Black, William, 35, 37–41, 44, 67; *Arithmetical and Medical Analysis,* 39, 70; *Historical Sketch,* 37–9; on infant mortality, 70–1, 74, 75, 77, 79
bladder stones, 29–31, 34, 41, 43. *See also* lithotomy
Blane, Gilbert, 27, 37
blood: circulation of, 40; sugar in, 128, 133
bloodletting, 206, 313, 314; as treatment, 31, 33, 90, 92
Blum, Emile, 156, 157
Bouchut, Eugène, 206
Boudreau, Frank, 276, 288
Bouillaud, Jean-Baptiste, 96, 205, 206
Brackel (Westphalia), 221–2
Braun, Lilly, 117
breastfeeding, 65–6
Brian, Eric, 51, 58
Britain: cancer research in, 184–5; child care in, 80–1; class distinctions in, 25, 41–2; commerce in, 6; contagion theory in, 215; evidence-based medicine in, 382–3; hospitals in, 42, 43–4, 207–8, 213; infant mortality in, 65–82, 260; inoculation in, 52; and League of Nations, 285; medical statistics in, 4, 19–24; nosography in, 33–7; public health in, 251–63, 292, 343; quantification in, 4, 22, 66–7; research in, 19–24, 42–3, 184–5
British Lying-In Hospital, 80
British Medical Journal (*BMJ*), 321–2, 382
Broussais, François, 90, 128
Bruce, Stanley M., 282–3, 285
Bryder, L., 319
Buckle, Henry Thomas, 396
Bugnard, Louis, 339–40
Bureau international du travail, 291
Burnet, E., 282

Buyse, Raymond, 149

Campbell, W.B., 131–2, 136
Canada, 288
cancer: age and, 230, 231; biomedical measurement in, 173–94; breast, 229; causes of, 236; cervical, 176–7, 179–82, 234; clinical trials for, 235–6, 237–8; deaths from, 227–8; diagnosis of, 184–5, 188–92, 228, 230, 231; epidemiology of, 227–9, 239–40; gender and, 230, 231; genetics and, 186, 191; larynx, 233; lung, 226–40, 336, 340–1; pathology of, 173–94; patient attitude and, 131; prostate, 178; race and, 228–9, 231; research on, 184–5, 232–4, 237–9, 336, 339, 340; staging of, 178; treatment of, 206. *See also* leukemia; lymphoma
Cancer Genome Anatomy Project (CGAP), 187
Canguilhem, Georges, 173
CAP. *See under* American Public Health Association
carcinoma. *See* cancer
Castelnau, Henri de, 212–31
Cauchy, A.L., 91
cells, 184–6
censuses, 257, 258
Centers for Disease Control (CDC), 348–9
Centre d'enseignement de la statistique applique à la médecine (CESAM), 343–4
Centre national de la recherche scientifique, 362
Chadwick, Edwin, 276
Chaperon, Jacques, 345–6
Chapin, Charles V., 269, 270–1
Charité Hospital (Berlin), 112
Chatelier, Henry le, 154–5
Cheselden, William, 29
Chevallier, André, 339
Cheyne, John, 36–7
childbirth, 218–20, 221–3
child labour, 79–80
children: care of, 65–6, 80–1; in cities, 67, 75, 77–9, 157, 260; foundling, 80–1; measurement of, 156–60. *See also* infant mortality; pedology
China, 292
chlorure de chaux (chloride of lime), 210–13
cholera, 261
Chomel, A.F., 96
Chrisman, O., 156
cinchona (Peruvian bark), 31, 33, 40
cities, 102; and children's health, 67, 75, 77–9, 157, 260; public health services in, 269–70
City Manager Movement, 269, 270
Civiale, J., 91
Clark, John, 28, 40, 41
class. *See* social status
Clifton, Francis, 19–21
clinical accounting, 380
clinical medicine: in France, 97–8; and molecular genetics, 191–2; quantification in, 4, 43; research in, 23; screening techniques in, 177; and social change, 112–15
clinical trials, 4, 11; and AIDS, 362–3, 364, 366; for cancer, 235–6, 237–8; and diabetes, 135–9; documentation of, 28, 29–30, 135–6; in 18th and 19th centuries, 22–3, 27–8, 29–32, 98; social change and, 381; and social class, 320; statistical theory and, 310, 327. *See also* allocation; controlled trials; essais cliniques; placebos; randomization
Clontech, 190–1
Clowes, Henry A., 132, 133–4
Cochrane collaboration, 383
Collip, Bertram, 131–2
Colombier, Jean, 21
commerce, 6, 140, 371. *See also* globalisation
Commission spéciale des indices sanitaires (1938), 289
Committee for Diagnostic Morphometry. *See* International Society of Diagnostic Quantitative Pathology
Committee for Diagnostic Quantitative Pathology. *See* International Society of Diagnostic Quantitative Pathology
Commonwealth Fund, 280, 288
complementary medicine. *See* medicine, alternative
Concerted Action Automated Analytical Cytology (CAAAC), 182
Condorcet, Marquis de, 58–9, 93
Conférence mondiale économique et monétaire (1932), 282
Connaught Laboratories, 132–3

Conseil supérieur de la statistique, 291
controlled trials, 309–27; control groups in, 320; criticism of, 384; development of, 381–2; government and, 400; selection for, 22–3, 232–4, 236, 385; statistical theory and, 310. *See also* allocation; clinical trials; randomization
Coover, John Edgar, 315
Cornfield, Jerome, 227, 231, 233, 238, 239–40
Coudray, Madame du, 66
Cournot, A.A., 3
Cox, David, 326
Crofton, John, 318
la Croix-Rouge, 281
croup, 205–6
Cruveilhier, Louis, 207, 220
Cullen, M.J., 253, 259
Cumming, Hugh S., 285
CYDAC, 180
Cytoanalyzer, 179–80
cytology, 179–82

Daniels, Marc, 321, 322
Danyau, Dr, 212, 216–17, 221–2
D'Arcy Hart, Philip, 314, 322–3
Daston, Lorraine, 51, 53, 55
data: analysis of, 26–8; genetic, 389; presentation of, 135–6; qualitative, 135. *See also* statistics
ddI (dideoxyinosine), 365
décès: causes, 281; par diabète sucré, 134; par fièvre puerpérale, 207–8; statistiques de, 211, 218. *Voir aussi* statistics, vital
Decroly, Ovide, 157
de Haen, Anton, 110–12
demographics, 39, 276
Denis, Hector, 147, 149, 161
Denmark, 285, 337
Denoix, Pierre, 340
Depaul, Dr, 207, 212, 215–16, 218–20, 222
Depression. *See* Great Depression
désinfection, 210–13
determinism, 160, 397
diabète, 127–41; complications, 130, 137; comportement des patients, 130; essais cliniques, 135–9; quantification, 128–31; régime alimentaire, 128, 129–30, 136–7, 140; traitement, 130–1, 136–7, 138–9; travaux expérimentaux, 129–30, 132–3, 134, 137, 139
Diabetes Control and Complications Trial Research Group, 137–9
diagnosis: of cancer, 184–5, 188–92, 228, 230, 231; instrumentation and, 98, 380; and mortality statistics, 257–8; objectification of, 378, 380. *See also* screening
diarrhée infantile, 274
Dictionary of Epidemiology (Last), 327
Diderot, Denis, 57
diet: diabetes and, 128, 129–30, 136–7, 140; and health, 282–4; vegetarian, 149
digitalis, 22–3
diphtérie, 273
disease: analysis of, 35, 127–9; case-to-population ratios in, 257–8; causes of, 236; in children, 67; climate and, 32, 33, 34, 37, 75–7, 395; nomenclature of, 257; poverty and, 291; probability of, 236; specificity of, 99, 379; standardization and, 120; theory and, 32, 215, 236; transmission of, 214–15, 236–7; views of, 32, 44, 98–9, 252. *See also* maladies; nosography
disinfectants, 210–13
dispensaries, 26–7, 40, 41, 42
dissections, 209–11, 213
DNA microarrays, 187–92
Dobson, Matthew, 34, 41
doctors: and evidence-based medicine, 385–6, 388; government and, 388, 400; and health insurance, 120; in hospitals, 43; and patients, 94, 97–8, 113–15, 119; and statistical approach, 344, 394; status of, 25, 41–2, 98, 385–6, 394; student, 208–10, 213; and thermometer use, 119–20; and vital statistics, 257–8. *See also* médecins; surgeons
Doll, Richard, 232, 315, 318
données, 135–6, 208
Dorn, Harold, 227, 228–30, 232, 233–4, 240
Double, François-Joseph, 91–2, 98, 99–100, 101
Doull, John, 314
dropsy (oedema), 22–3, 24, 41
Drucker, Jacques, 351–2
drugs. *See* therapeutics

Dublin, Louis I., 270, 271, 273, 274, 275, 281
Dubois, Dr, 216, 217, 221–2
Ducimetière, Pierre, 341
Duffin, Jacalyn, 98
Duncan, Andrew, Sr, 41

École clinique de Paris, 89–104
École nationale de la santé publique (ENSP), 346–7, 351, 352
economics, 278–80, 282–3, 290. *See also* commerce
Edinburgh, 213–15
Edinburgh Infirmary, 24
Edinburgh Maternity Hospital, 213
Edmonds, Thomas, 259
education: experiments in, 316, 317; for mentally handicapped, 161; reform of, 159–60; and social status, 153–6, 160; for workers, 153, 154, 160
Eli Lilly and Co., 132–3, 135, 140
Emergency Medicine Journal, 382
empiricism, 26–37, 41–2; versus rationalism, 19–21, 24–7, 43–4. *See also* observation
l'Encyclopédie (ed. Diderot), 56, 57
l'Encyclopédie scientifique (ed. Toulouse), 161–2
energy (human), 147, 152, 154
Enfants malades (hospital), 206
England. *See* Britain
ENSP. *Voir* École nationale de la santé publique
environment, 74–80, 252, 339, 351
epidemics, 396, 398; influenza, 257–8; lung cancer as, 229–31; sickness tables of, 253–5
épidémiologie: appliquée, 348–52; enseignement, 347, 348, 349; en France, 10, 338, 345–52; *vs.* microbiologie, 336; et la santé publique, 335–6, 337, 344–8; et la Société des Nations, 268, 276; et les statistiques, 336, 338, 345. *Voir aussi* epidemiologists; epidemiology; recherches
epidemiologists (épidémiologistes), 11–12, 335–7, 339, 342, 343; and aetiologic approach, 335; and biostatisticians, 226–7, 228, 233, 237–8
epidemiology, 4, 10, 226–40; of cancer, 227–9, 239–40; in France, 10, 338, 345–52; promotion of, 237–8; rise of, 173, 379. *See also* épidémiologie
EPITER (Association pour le développement d'une épidémiologie de terrain), 349, 351, 352
Equitable Insurance Company, 274
ergonomics, 152
essais cliniques: controverses, 140; et le diabète, 135–9; et les hôpitaux, 361; dans l'industrie pharmaceutique, 362; résultats, 135–6, 139; et le sida, 362–3, 364, 366. *Voir aussi* clinical trials
essais contrôlés, 359–71; acteurs, 265, 360; essai Concorde, 365; opposition, 367; protocoles, 366, 368; rêglementations, 360; essai Saquinavir, 368; et le sida, 362–3, 364, 366; soutien, 364, 367–8. *Voir aussi* clinical trials; médecine des preuves
les États-Unis: et la coopération internationale, 285, 288–9, 292; et la formation en santé publique, 346, 349; et la médecine des preuves, 362; et le sida, 360, 364; statistiques de la santé, 266–97; survols de la santé publique, 271, 276–81, 286, 288. *Voir aussi* United States
étiologie, 335, 340
étudiants en médicine, 208–10, 213
eugenics, 157
Europe, 283, 284–5; eastern, 283, 284–5, 286–7; health surveys in, 277–8, 286–7; Pap tests in, 181–2; public health in, 281–7, 288; rural health in, 291–3; United States and, 288–9
European Association for Analytical Cellular Pathology (ESACP), 183
evidence-based medicine, 382–9; in Britain, 382–3; criticism of, 383–7; development of, 387–8; doctors and, 385–6, 388; literature about, 382–3; as paradigm, 383, 384; and public health, 383; as social movement, 386; in United States, 362. *See also* médecine des preuves
experiments, 43, 397; and causal inference, 234–7; design of, 237–8, 315–16; in diabetes, 129–30, 132–3, 134, 137, 139; in education, 316, 317; morality and, 158; in physiology, 397; standardization in, 133. *See also* observation; research

l'Extrême-Orient, 291
Eyler, John, 255, 263

Faculté de médicine (Paris), 343; Clinique de la, 218, 219, 220, 223
Falconer, William, 34
Falk, Isidore, 277, 279–82, 285, 287, 288, 291
Farr, William, 251–63, 271, 274; statistical laws of, 253–7, 263, 279, 396
fascisme, 282, 284
fatigue, 151–6
Faulkner, Joan, 322–3
feminism, 148, 151, 154
Ferriar, John, 23–4, 41
Feudtner, Chris, 130, 131
fever, 31–2, 34, 36; classification of, 40; measurement of, 109; puerperal, 102, 207–23; treatment of, 41, 119; typhoid, 269
fièvre puerpérale, 102, 207–23; son caractère contagieux, 213–14, 215, 221–2; moyens prophylactiques contre son apparition, 210–13, 214, 215–16
fièvre typhoïde, 269
fire insurance, 271–2
Fisher, Irving, 269
Fisher, R.A., 235, 239, 240, 310, 320–1; and randomization, 312, 316, 317, 326, 327
Flamant, Robert, 341
Fletcher, A.A., 131–2, 136
Fondation Marcel Mérieux, 348, 352
Fordyce, George, 21
Foucault, Jean Bernard Léon, 109–10
Foucault, Michel, 162
Foundling Hospital, 80
Fowler, Thomas, 33
Fox, Renée, 140–1
France: AIDS in, 360; child care in, 80–1; contagion theories in, 215, 222; epidemiology in, 12, 338, 345–52; hospitals in, 98, 99, 206, 218–20, 222; infant mortality in, 65–82; inoculation in, 52–9; medical statistics in, 89–104; medicine in, 97–8, 222; public health in, 338–9, 348–52; quantification in, 3–4, 6–7, 67–70, 378–9; research in, 21, 99, 342
Frankel, Lee K., 270
Frederick II of Prussia, 57
Frost, Wade H., 273
Gaudillière, Jean-Paul, 310
Gavarret, Jules, 378
gender, 77, 161, 230, 231
GeneChip, 199n64
General Dispensary for Poor Married Women (London), 37, 74
General Register Office (GRO) (Britain), 253, 279
genetics: and cancer, 186, 191; data on, 389; molecular, 175, 187–92
geography, 32, 75, 258, 259–61, 395
géomédecine, 286–7
George III of Britain, 35
Germany, 117, 119, 278, 292; hospitals in, 110–11, 112–15
germ theory, 236
Gilliam, Alexander, 227, 229–31, 233–4, 236, 240
globalisation, 288–92, 371
glycémie, 129, 134, 135, 138
glycosurie, 128, 129, 131
Goldberg, Marcel, 345–6
Golub, Todd, 188, 192
government (gouvernement): and child welfare, 66; and doctors, 388, 400; versus individual, 55–9, 101–2; and medicine, 101, 388, 394–400; and public health, 346–7, 350–1; and quantification, 55–9, 101–2, 398, 400; and technical standards, 117–18
Grant, John B., 266, 286, 290
Graunt, John, 42, 66–7, 70–5, 252, 253, 395
Great Depression, 275–6, 277–8, 281–2
Greaves, Melvin, 184–6
Greenhouse, Samuel, 231
Greenwood, Major, 285, 310, 379, 381; and controlled trials, 314, 320, 398
Gregory, John, 28, 32
Grémy, François, 345
Groupe d'études sur la fumée du tabac, 340
Grzegorzewska, Maria, 150, 154, 161
Guéneau de Mussy, François, 97
Guérard, Dr, 207, 223
Guy, William, 252, 255–6
Guy's Hospital, 29–30
Guyton de Morveau, Louis Bernard, 210–11

Hacking, Ian, 256, 315
Haenszel, William, 231, 239–40

Halley, Edmund, 52, 252–3
Hamilton, Alexander, 313
Hammond, E. Cuyler, 238, 239
Hardwicke Fever Hospital, 36–7
Hart, Ruth, 322–3
Harvey, Joy, 99
Haygarth, John, 33–4, 82
Haynes, R. Brian, 387
Hazemann, Robert-Henri, 272, 273, 285, 286, 288, 291
health, 128; diet and, 282–4; surveys of, 271, 276–81, 286–7, 288. *See also* hygiène; public health; santé
health administration, 386, 388
health insurance, 120–1
Heberden, William, the elder, 44
Heberden, William, the younger, 67, 77
hematopoiesis, 184–6
Henry, Charles, 152
Hersch, L., 276
Hill, Austin Bradford, 232, 240, 310, 311, 315, 316–21; on allocation, 323–6; *Principles of Medical Statistics,* 312, 316, 320, 323–6, 327
Hill, David, 320–1, 324
Hilleboe, Herman, 237
Himsworth, Harold, 314
Hippocratic tradition, 39, 44, 91, 93, 97–103, 395
Hoffman, Frederick, 228
Hoffman–La Roche Limited, 368
Holmes, Frederic, 128
Home, Francis, 24
homosexuels, 363, 365, 371
Hôpital des Enfants malades (Paris), 206
Hôpital Lariboisière (Paris), 218, 222
Hôpital Saint-Antoine (Paris), 218
Hôpital Saint-Louis (Paris), 218, 220
hôpitaux, 206, 213, 218–23, 361. *Voir aussi* hospitals
hospitals: in Austria, 208–9; in Britain, 42, 43–4, 207–8, 213; in 18th century, 21, 23, 26–7, 397; feeding patients in, 114; in France, 98, 99, 206, 218–20, 222; in Germany, 110–11, 112–15; maternity, 80–1, 207–9, 213, 218–20, 221–2; in 19th century, 31–2, 99, 110, 398; research in, 21, 23, 133, 232, 361; social change in, 112–15; teaching role of, 222. *See also specific hospitals*
Hungary, 284, 289, 290, 297
Hunter, John, 42, 43
Huriet-Sérusclat, loi de, 363
hygiene, 215. *See also* fever, puerperal; fièvre puerpérale
hygiène: écoles d', 286, 288; des milieux, 339; rurale, 271, 275, 280, 281, 283–94
hyperglycémie, 128, 129, 137–9
hypoglycémie, 132, 134. *Voir aussi* insuline

Imbert, Armand, 154–5
immunology, 184, 191
immunophenotyping, 175, 183–7
Imperial Cancer Research Fund (ICRF), 184–5
Imperial Physical-Technical Institute (Germany), 117, 119
India, 291, 292
indices: experiments with, 285; international system of, 275–8; League of Nations and, 284–5, 288–90, 291, 292; of life expectancy, 59; of poverty, 286; of public health, 271–3, 296; of rural health, 289–90; tropical applications of, 291; usefulness of, 272–3, 287
industrialization, 102
industrie pharmaceutique, 362, 363, 368–9. *Voir aussi* pharmaceutical industry
infant mortality, 260; explanations for, 74–80; in France, 65–82; methods of calculating, 66–74; social status and, 79–80; tobacco and, 236. *See also* children
infirmières, 272
influenza, 36, 257–8
inoculation, 37, 40, 51–9, 66, 81–2, 395
insanity, 35, 41
Institut de statistique de l'Université de Paris (ISUP), 343
Institut de veille sanitaire, 352
Institut d'hygiène de Budapest, 289
Institut für Konjunkturforschung, 278
Institut Gustave-Roussy (IGR), 340, 341, 342
institutions, subversion des, 364–7, 370–1
Institut national de la santé et de la recherche médicale (Inserm), 339, 344, 346, 349, 351, 362; Division de la recherche médico-sociale, 342; et le sida, 363; Unité 88, 345–6; unités de

recherches épidémiologiques, 344; Unité de recherches statistiques (Unité 21), 341–4, 345
Institut national d'hygiène (INH), 338–40. *Voir aussi* École nationale de la santé publique (ENSP)
Institut Pasteur, 348, 349
Institut pour le développement de l'épidémiologie appliquée (IDEA), 349–50, 352
Institut régional d'hygiène de Nancy, 286
instruments, medical, 7, 98, 100, 103–4, 152; computerized, 174, 179–82; and diagnosis, 98, 380; doctors and, 380, 397, 398; insurance industry and, 399; physiological, 150, 151, 157, 159; and public health, 266–97
insuline, 129, 131–6
insurance industry: and medicine, 389, 394–400; and objective measurement, 398–9, 400; and public health, 270, 274–5; statisticians in, 228. *See also* health insurance
interleukin, 131
International Academy of Cytology, 182
International Faculty of Pedology, 149–50, 154, 158, 162
International Labor Organization, 291
International Society of Diagnostic Quantitative Pathology (ISDQP), 173, 174, 182–3
Ipsen, Johannes, 239

Jameson, William, 285
Japan, 336
Jesuits, 57–8
Jewson, N.D., 43
Johan, Bela, 284, 290
Jorland, Gérard, 102
Joslin, Elliot P., 130–1, 133, 134
Joteyko, Jozefa, 145–63; career of, 146–51; on fatigue, 151–6
Journal of Metabolic Research, 135–6
Journal of the American Medical Association (*JAMA*), 382, 383
Jurin, James, 39–40

Kamentsky, L.A., 180, 181
Kaptchuk, T.J., 309
W.K. Kellogg Foundation, 275
Kingsbury, John, 275
Kipiani, Varia, 149
Kraus, Arthur, 234
Kreager, Phillip, 6
kystes ovariens, 206

Laboratoires Mérieux, 348
laboratoires pharmaceutiques, 366, 368–9
laboratories, 29–30, 157, 397–8
labour movement, 120. *See also* workers
labour (work), 79–80, 153, 154–5, 291
Lachmund, Jens, 116–17
La Condamine, Charles de, 52
Laennec, René, 98
Lahy, Jean Maurice, 154–5
Lancet, 382
Lander, Eric, 188
Laplace, P.S., 91, 93, 96
Latour, Bruno, 136
Latvia, 285
law of large numbers (Poisson), 91, 92, 95
Lazar, Philippe, 341, 343–4, 345
League of Nations. *See* Société des Nations
Lebert, Hermann, 98
Le Bon, Gustave, 163
Le Bras, Hervé, 56
Leipzig Hospital, 114
Lellouch, Joseph, 341, 344
Lettsom, John Coakley, 37, 40
leukemia, 184–6, 229, 231
Levin, Morton, 234, 240
Levret, André, 34, 35
liberalism, 102, 395
Lichter, Peter, 189
life expectancy, 59
life insurance. *See* insurance industry
life tables, 253
Lilienfeld, Abraham M., 238, 239, 240
Lilly, J.K., 132. *See also* Eli Lilly and Co.
Lind, James, 27, 28, 40, 313
Lister, Joseph, 380
lithotomy, 29–30, 91
Lock, Stephen, 319, 322
London Fever Hospital, 31–2
London School of Hygiene and Tropical Medicine, 343
Lordat, Jacques, 100
Lotka, Alfred, 274
Lotte, Alice, 339
Louis, Pierre C.A., 3, 37, 90, 216, 378;

numerical method of, 3–4, 96–7, 205, 397
Louis XV of France, 57
Löwy, Ilana, 131
lumbago, 33
lymphoma, 189–90, 229

MacMahon, Brian, 239, 345
Madsen, Thorvald, 283–4
Magnello, Eileen, 310
Mainland, Donald, 310, 327
maladies, 127–9; cardio-vasculaires, 336; infectieuses, 351. *Voir aussi* disease
Malgaigne, Joseph François, 206, 218
Manchester Infirmary, 23, 214
Manitoba Health Plan (1945), 291
Mantel, Nathan, 231, 239–40
Marcet, Alexander, 29–30
Marey, Jules Etienne, 152
Marks, Harry, 4, 309, 310, 362
Massachusetts General Hospital, 130
Massachusetts Institute of Technology. *See* MIT Center for Genome Research
Massé, Louis, 347–8, 349
Maternité de Paris (hospital), 218, 219, 220
Matthews, J. Rosser, 102, 310
Maynard, Allan, 386
Mazower, Mark, 282
McCall, William, 316
McCulloch, J.R., 253
McDougall, Frank L., 282, 283, 288
McGill University, 388
measurement: biomedical, 173–94; of children, 156–60; objectifying, 113–15; physiological, 150, 151–6; quantification as, 174; role of, 117–19, 397; social status and, 117–21; statistics and, 279; of time, 155; of weight, 115. *See also* microscopes; thermometers
médecine: affaiblissement, 370; humanitaire, 368–9; keynésienne, 283; parallèle (complémentaire), 367–8, 383; préventive, 282; réforme, 362; comme science sociale, 266, 286; et le socialisme, 291–3; transnationale, 370; du travail, 339
médecine des preuves, 361–2, 363–4. *Voir aussi* essais contrôlés; evidence-based medicine
médecins: géographe/sociologue, 286–7; et l'insuline, 131–5; et la santé publique, 350; et le sida, 365–6, 368; et les statistiques, 344
media, 273, 364
medical arithmetic, 29–30, 35, 37, 67–74. *See also* statistics, medical
Medical Research Council (MRC), 309–27, 339; Patulin trial, 314, 322–3; pneumonia serum trial, 318–20; Statistical Research Unit (SRU), 339, 346; streptomycin trial, 312–13, 320, 321–2, 324, 326; Therapeutic Trials Committee, 314, 318–19; ultraviolet radiation trial, 314; whooping-cough vaccine trial, 320, 321
medical societies, 42
Medical Society of London, 42
médicaments: disponibilité, 368; évaluation, 362; information, 365–6; standardisation, 131–5. *Voir aussi* essais cliniques; essais contrôlés; therapeutics
medicine: alternative, 367–8, 383; communication in, 112–15; computers in, 388; in France, 222; government and, 101, 388, 394–400; history of, 37; journals of, 41, 42, 43; morality in, 53–6, 77–9, 130–1, 140–1; objectification of, 380; and politics, 55, 57–8; preventive, 43, 259; public versus private, 98, 206; scientific, 397–8; and social change, 101–2; as social science, 94, 286; students of, 208–10, 213; uncertainty in, 140–1, 396–7; and working class, 112–15. *See also* clinical medicine; médecine
Melamed, Myron, 180, 181
Mérieux, Charles, 348, 349
mesure: du sucre dans le sang, 133, 135; instruments de, 266–97; par le patient, 131, 134. *Voir aussi* measurement
métabolisme intermédiare (MI), 128–9
Metropolitan Life Insurance Company, 270, 271, 274, 275
microarrays. *See* DNA microarrays
microscopes, 175–83
midwives, 66, 208–10, 213, 221
Milbank Memorial Fund, 268, 271, 274, 275, 281, 284; administrators of, 277, 279, 288
Millar, John, 26, 37, 40, 41
Milmore, Benno K., 229–30

miscarriage, 71–4, 77
MIT Center for Genome Research, 188
Moheau, Jean-Baptiste, 67–70, 71, 74, 75, 77, 80
Mollaret, Henri, 348
Monro, Donald, 41
Montagu, Mary Wortley, 51–2
Montpellier (France), 80, 93, 97, 99–101
Montyon, Antoine Auget, Baron de, 67–70
morality: and experimentation, 158; in medicine, 53–6, 77–9, 130–1, 140–1; and mortality, 77–9; and quantification, 140; statistics and, 90–1
morbidity, 258, 339
Moreau, Dr, 212
Morgagni, Giovanni Battista, 43
morphology, 175–83, 189
mortalité: études de, 339; taux de, 274, 278; en termes monétaires, 274. *Voir aussi* mortality
mortality: from cancer, 227–8; in childbirth, 218, 221; differential, 258–63; inoculation and, 52, 81–2; occupational, 258–9; population density and, 261–3; in puerperal fever, 208–10; sanitation and, 262–3. *See also* bills of mortality; infant mortality; mortalité; mortality curves; statistics, mortality
mortality curves, 54, 255–6
Mosso, Angelo, 152
Mountin, J.W., 280
Mourgue, Jacques-Antoine, 67–70, 75–7
Mussy, François Guéneau de, 97

National Cancer Institute, 177, 180, 189–90, 339; Biostatistics Branch, 231; and cancer epidemiology, 227–9, 239–40; Cytology Automation Program, 179; Progress Review Group, 178
National Health Honor Roll, 274–5
National Health Service (NHS), 383
National Institute of Diabetes and Digestive and Kidney Diseases (NIDDK), 137
National Institutes of Health, 137, 339
National Pedagogical Institute (Poland), 150, 159
Nations Unies (ONU), 292
Newcastle Infirmary, 40
New Deal, 277, 279–80
New Haven health survey, 280–1, 283, 289, 290, 292
Newsholme, Arthur, 253, 263, 290
New York City, 272–3
New York state, 274
Niceforo, Alfredo, 276
Niemeyer, Felix, 114
Norfolk and Norwich Hospital, 30, 34–5
normalization, 109–10
normal versus pathological, 182, 184–6, 190, 193
nosography, 23, 32–7
nosology, 32–3, 38–9

objectivity: of body, 112–16; in diagnosis, 378, 380; government and, 118; of measurement, 113–15, 119–21; of medical opinion, 118, 377–8; and social change, 381, 382; and treatment, 378, 379
observation: documentation of, 23–4; improvement of, 27–9, 378; period of, 221; versus theory, 19–21, 24–7, 43, 213–14. *See also* empiricism
observatoires régionaux de la santé (ORS), 351
obstetrics, 34–5. *See also* fever, puerperal
OMS (Organisation mondiale de la santé). *See* World Health Organization (WHO)
oncogenes, 191
Organisation for Economic Co-operation and Development (OECD/OCDE), 292
Organisation mondiale du commerce (World Trade Organization), 360
organisations: non gouvernementales, 368–9; philanthropiques, 339–40. *Voir aussi les organisations particulières*
Orr, John Boyd, 282
Oswald, Wilhelm, 147

pain, 148–9, 151–2, 153
Palmer, Carroll E., 236–7, 240, 321
palsy, 34, 41
Papanicolaou, George, 176
Pap test, 176, 179–82
Parisot, Jacques, 283, 284–5, 288
Paris School, 212–13, 378. *See also* École clinique de Paris; Faculté de médicine (Paris)
Parry, Caleb, 313
patents, 371
pathologists, 183, 188–9, 191–2
pathology: biology and, 183, 185–6, 189,

193; of cancer, 173–94; versus normality, 182, 184–6, 190, 193; quantification and, 103–4, 140, 174, 176, 183, 193; tissue, 42, 192
pathophysiology, 43, 101
patients: and doctors, 94, 97–8, 113–15, 119; experiments involving, 133; feeding of, 114; as good or bad, 130, 140; point of view of, 114–15; versus populations, 386, 389; and research, 388; self-measurement by, 116, 119, 131, 133–5; and theory, 21. *See also specific medical conditions*
Paty, Michel, 51, 53
pauvreté, 286, 291
pays industrialisés, 336–7
Pearl, Raymond, 314
Pearson, Egon, 315
Pearson, Karl, 4, 10, 380–1, 398; on alternation, 310, 313–14, 320
pedagogy, 152. *See also* education
pedology, 145, 149, 156–60
Peirce, C.S., and J. Jastrow, 315, 316
pellagra, 236
Percival, Thomas, 41, 79–80, 81–2
Peruvian bark (cinchona), 31, 33, 40
peste bubonique, 269
Petty, William, 42
pharmaceutical industry, 381, 400. *See also* industrie pharmaceutique
photography, 153
physicians. *See* doctors; médecins
physics, 340, 397
physiologists, 131–5. *See also specific physiologists*; physiology
physiology, 398; and ergonomics, 152; experiments in, 397; and pedagogy, 152; and psychology, 153; as social science, 160–3
physique, 340
Pinel, Philippe, 35
Pinkel, Donald, 185
Pittaluga, Gustavo, 287
placebos, 29, 136, 314, 321
placenta praevia, 34–5
plague, 67, 269
pleurésie purulente, 205
pneumonia, 257, 318–20
Poisson, Siméon-Denis, 3, 91, 92, 95
Poland, 150–1, 159–60, 161
polio, 231, 233
politics, 55, 57–8. *See also* politique
politique: et sanitation, 271; de la santé publique, 338–9, 340; et le sida, 367–9; et statistiques de la santé, 279, 363. *Voir aussi* politics
populations: incidence of disease in, 257–8; individuals versus, 386, 389; rural, 271, 275, 280, 281, 286–7, 289
Positifs, 367
Posner, Stanislaw, 153
Price, Richard, 79
Principles of Medical Statistics (Hill), 312, 316, 320, 323–6, 327
Pringle, James, 40
probability, 385; calculus of, 58–9, 89, 91–2, 93–6, 342; of disease, 236; in nosography, 34; of recovery, 254; in selection, 234; and social questions, 53–5, 58–9; in statistics, 28, 310
propriété intellectuelle, 371
Prudential Insurance Company, 274, 281
PSA (prostate specific antigen), 178
psychiatry, 35, 37
psychology, 153, 159–60
public health, 395–6; in Britain, 251–63, 292, 343; in cities, 269–70; economics and, 282–3, 290; in Europe, 281–7, 288; and evidence-based medicine, 383; funding for, 273–4; government and, 346–7, 350–1; indices of, 271–3, 296; media and, 273; nutrition and, 282; and populations, 386; public and, 273–4; quantification in, 379; statistics and, 228–9, 397. *See also* public health conferences; U.S. Public Health Service
public health conferences: Alma-Ata (1978), 291; Bandoeng (1937), 283, 290, 291; européennes, 281, 283–4, 288; Mexico, 291; Moscow (1936), 283–4, 288
puerperal fever. *See* fever, puerperal
Pugh, Thomas, 239
pulse, 36–7
purging, 314

quantification: administrative, 6–7; in biology, 146, 182; as measurement, 174; and pathology, 103–4, 140, 174, 176, 183, 193; pathology and, 103–4, 140, 174, 176, 183, 193; of science, 397–8. *See also* quantification in medicine

quantification in medicine, 4, 43, 140; acceptance of, 379–80, 394–400; in Britain, 4, 22, 66–7; and commerce, 6; in diabetes, 128–31; in 18th century, 22–3; in France, 3–4, 67–70, 378–9; government and, 55–9, 101–2, 398, 400; models for, 380–1; morality and, 140; in 19th century, 377–80; and nosography, 32–7; in public health, 379; rejection of, 378–9; social effects of, 41–5, 146. *See also* medical arithmetic; objectivity; statistics
Quetelet, Adolphe, 396

Rabinbach, Anson, 146
Rajchman, Ludwik, 268, 276–7, 280, 282–4, 288, 291–2
randomization (in clinical trials): as concept, 314–15, 318; Hill on, 324–6; methods of, 324–5, 326–7; origins of, 315–18; reasons for, 309–12, 318–23; statisticians and, 316. *See also* allocation; controlled trials
Rankin, W.S., 271
rationalism, 19–21, 24–7, 43–4
Rayer, Pierre, 97
recherches, 336, 340, 362. *Voir aussi* épidémiologie
recovery curves, 255–6
Red Cross, 281
Reed, Lowell, 314
régime alimentaire, 128, 129–30, 136–7, 140. *Voir aussi* diet
Reide, Thomas, 26
research, 19–24; in Britain, 19–24, 42–3, 184–5; on cancer, 184–5, 232–4, 237–9, 336, 339, 340; case control in, 232–4; collaboration in, 317–18; on epidemiology, 336; on fatigue, 151–6; in France, 21, 99, 342; gender and, 161; in hospitals, 21, 23, 133, 232, 361; national differences in, 336–7; on pain, 148–9, 151–2; patient-centred, 388; strategic, 184–5. *See also* clinical trials; controlled trials; epidemiology; experiments
Réseau national de santé publique (RNSP), 351, 352
respiration, 36–7
rétinopathie, 138
Revue psychologique (ed. Joteyko), 149, 150, 153–4, 158
rheumatism (rhumatisme), 33–4, 206
Richet, Charles, 147, 151, 153, 161, 162
Ricord, Dr, 212
Rigby, Edward, 34–5
risk, 233–4, 272, 345
Risueño d'Amador, Benigno, 89, 91–6, 98–102, 378, 394, 397
Robbins, Lewis, 177
Robertson, Robert, 27, 40
Rochoux, J. André, 97
Rockefeller Foundation, 276, 284, 286, 290, 338, 339, 348
Rokintansky, Professor, 210
Romania, 286
Rosenberg, Charles, 98–9
Rousseau, Jean Jacques, 65–6
Rowley, William, 42
Royal College of Pathologists, 192
Royal College of Physicians, 42
Royal College of Surgeons, 42
Royal Infirmary (Glasgow), 320
Rubin, Donald, 316
Rumeau-Rouquette, Claude, 341, 344
Rusnock, Andrea, 6
Russell Sage Foundation, 270

Sackett, David, 383, 386
Sadowsky, Doris, 233
sages-femmes, 208–10, 213
saignée, 206. *Voir aussi* bloodletting
Salamon, Roger, 345–6
Sand, Ren, 285
sanitation, 262–3
sanométrie, 346
santé: de la collectivité, 292–3; identification, 128, 140; promotion, 337; rurale, 271, 275, 280, 281, 283–7; survols, 271, 276–90. *Voir aussi* health; santé publique
santé publique, 266–97; en Angleterre, 343; coûte, 267, 290; et l'épidémiologie, 335–6, 337, 344–8; aux États-Unis, 267, 269, 272, 346; formation, 346–7, 349; en France, 338–9, 348–52; indices numériques, 271–3; et les médecins, 350; normes, 267, 268–9, 289–90; politique de la, 338–9, 340; et la Société des Nations, 282–3; statistiques, 266–8. *Voir aussi* public health
Sauter, Guido, 189
Scadding, Guy, 318, 322, 323
scales, 115

scalpels, 98, 100
Scandinavia, 285, 337, 385
scarlet fever, 313
Schéma, 289, 291
Schneiderman, Marvin, 231
Schrek, Robert, 234
Schwartz, Daniel, 340–3, 346, 350; école de, 344, 345, 346, 350
science: debate in, 102; pure, 161–2, 163; quantification of, 397–8
screening, 176, 177–8, 182
scurvy, 27, 313
selection (for studies), 22–3, 232–4, 236, 385
séminaires Yves Biraud, 348, 349, 352
Semmelweis, Ignaz Philipp, 208–12, 220; presentation of statistical theory, 207–15; reaction to, 212–13, 214, 215–18, 223
septicémie, 223
Seven Years' War, 57
Shahar, Eyal, 385–6
Shattuck, Lemuel, 276
Shimkin, Michael B., 240
Short, Thomas, 40, 67, 74
Shyrock, Richard, 252
sick leave. *See* health insurance
sida, 347–8, 351, 359–71; associations, 363, 364–6, 367–8; causes, 371; controverses, 361; essais cliniques, 362–3, 364, 366; en France, 360; et les médecins, 365–6, 368; militants du, 360, 363, 364, 365–6, 371; mobilisation autour du, 361; et les organisations non gouvernementales, 368–9; et la politique, 367–9; statistiques, 279, 363; stigmatisation, 370–1
Sigerist, Henry, 291, 292
Silverman, William, 323
Simpson, James Young, 213, 214–15, 216, 218
smallpox, 34, 51, 254–5, 395. *See also* inoculation
smoking, 336. *See also* tobacco
Smyth, Carmichael, 42
Snow, John, 261
socialists, 102, 153–4
social science, 152, 163; medicine as, 94, 286; physiology as, 160–3
social status: and childbed mortality, 221; and clinical trials, 320; of doctors, 25, 41–2, 98, 385–6, 394; education and, 153–6, 160; and infant mortality, 79–80; measurement and, 117–21; and treatment, 115–16. *See also* workers
Société des Nations (SDN), 267–8, 276, 277, 281; enquêtes sur la santé, 281–90; et l'épidémiologie, 268, 276; et l'Est européen, 284–5, 286–7; Organisation d'hygiène, 268, 282–3, 291; et la santé publique, 282–3; et le système des indices, 284–5, 288–90, 291, 292
Société d'exploitation industrielle des tabacs et des allumettes (SEITA), 340
Société médicale d'accouchement, 222–3
Solvay, Ernest, 147, 152
Solvay Physiological Institute, 147, 157
Solvay Sociology Institute, 152, 157
Sorre, Maximilien, 287
specificity, 99, 237, 238–9, 379
spectrophotometer, 180, 181
Splawa-Neyman, J., 316
Stafford Hospital, 33
Stampar, Andrija, 281–2, 292
Stanford University, 189
statisticians, 316, 363
statistics: and clinical trials, 310, 327; development of, 252–3, 310, 380–1; and economic research, 278–80; as measuring device, 279; in 19th century, 256–7, 396; regularity in, 255–9. *See also specific types of statistics*; data; statistiques
statistics, medical, 43, 395–6; in aetiologic research, 226; age and, 29, 31; in Britain, 4, 19–24; doctors and, 344, 394; and epidemiology, 338, 345; in France, 89–104; geography and, 32, 75, 258, 259–61, 395; and individuals, 42–3, 55–9, 94; in insurance industry, 228; interpretation of, 220, 222–3, 235–6; and moral issues, 90–1; probability in, 28, 310; publication of, 21, 212; and public health, 228–9, 397; rejection of, 218, 221, 378–9, 394; and social issues, 41–2, 43, 90–1; and theory, 91–2, 94, 95; and therapeutics, 91–2, 94, 95; time and, 31–2; in United States, 266–97; value of, 12, 38–9; and variability, 94. *See also* medical arithmetic; quantification; statistics, mortality

statistics, mortality, 31, 39, 51–4, 59; diagnosis and, 257–8; Farr's analysis of, 258–63; insurance industry and, 399; and medical policy, 81–2; and public health policy, 228–9
statistics, vital, 40, 252–3, 256–7, 339; complexity of, 263; misreporting in, 257–8
statistiques: comparaisons, 267–8; contestation, 206–7; coopération internationale, 268, 276; crédibilité, 342; critique, 278, 279–80; du décès, 211, 218; enseignement, 343–4, 347; et l'épidémiologie, 336, 338, 345; inférentielles, 340, 343–4; et les médecins, 344; rejet, 215–23, 342; et la santé publique, 266–8; et le sida, 279, 363; tableaux, 266–8; théories, 207–15. *Voir aussi* statistics
status. *See* social status
Staudt, Louis M., 190
Stefanowska, Michalina, 146–9, 151, 152
Stephens, Joanna, 31
stethoscope, 98, 100
stillbirths, 71–4, 77
Stoker, Michael, 184
Stokes, William, 37
Stollberg, Gunnar, 116–17
Stouman, Knud, 280, 281, 285, 287, 289
streptococcal infections, 214, 223
streptomycin, 320, 321, 324
'Student,' 312, 316
studies, 232–5, 236, 238. *See also* clinical trials; controlled trials; experiments; research
Study Group on Smoking and Health, 239
sucre: dans le sang, 128, 133; dans l'urine, 128
surgeons, 25, 26–8, 41–2
surgery, 31, 214, 216
surveys. *See* studies
Sweden, 285
Sydenstricker, Edgar, 276, 277, 279, 280, 281, 293
syphilis, 339

tabac, 336, 340–1, 343
Tarnier, Stéphane, 220, 221, 222
Taylor, A.J.P., 284
Taylor, Frederick W., 155
Taylorism, 154–6, 267
technology, 188–9
telepathy, 315–16
temperature (body), 36–7, 109–22; measurement of, 110–12, 398; standardization of, 116–21. *See also* thermometers
10-City Cancer Morbidity Survey, 228–9
Tennessee Valley Authority, 287
Terray, Joseph Marie, 70
tests: laboratory, 380–1, 400; of perception, 315; psychological, 159, 161; qualitative, 184. *See also specific tests*
Theobald, G.W., 315
théories: étiologiques et prophylactiques, 215, 218; sous-détermination des, 216, 220–3; des statistiques, 207–15. *Voir aussi* theory
theory: about disease, 32, 236; versus observation, 19–21, 24–7, 43, 213–14; of statistical inference, 235–6; underdetermination of, 216, 220–3. *See also* théories
therapeutics, 38, 119; development of, 29–32, 34; evaluation of, 41, 98, 129, 317, 399–400; increases in, 381; objectification of, 378, 379; patients and, 21; research on, 20, 22–4, 29–32, 381; standardization of, 131–5; statistics and, 91–2, 94, 95. *See also specific conditions*; placebos; thérapeutique; treatments
thérapeutique, 129, 340. *Voir aussi* therapeutics; traitement
thermometers, 36–7, 109, 111–12, 117–20. *See also* temperature (body)
Thomson, Leonard, 131
Thorndike, E.L., and R.S. Woodworth, 315
tobacco, 226–40, 336, 340–1, 343
Tomcsik, J., 289
Toth, Ben, 319
trachéotomie, 205–6, 380
traitement: du croup, 205–6; du diabète, 130–1, 136–7, 138–9; moralisation du, 130–1; des tumeurs cancéreuses, 206. *Voir aussi* treatment
transparency, 42
Traube, Ludwig, 111
treatment: bloodletting as, 31, 33, 90, 92; of dropsy, 24; of fevers, 31–2, 40; social status and, 115–16; of tuberculosis, 314–15. *See also* surgery; traitement
Trousseau, A., 206

TRT-5, 366, 367
tubage, 205–6
tuberculosis (tuberculose), 34, 195, 230, 269, 274; studies of, 321, 339; treatments for, 314–15
typhus, 36

underdetermination: of medicine, 388; of theory, 216, 220–3
UNICEF, 291
Union of Soviet Socialist Republics (USSR) (URSS), 283–4
United Kingdom. *See* Britain
United Nations, 292
United States: AIDS in, 360, 364; and Europe, 288–9; health problems in, 269; health surveys in, 271, 276, 286; life insurance in, 399; Pap tests in, 182; public health initiatives in, 267, 269, 272–5, 346, 349; Social Security Act (1935), 277; statistical records in, 266–97. *See also specific cities, states, and government departments*; États-Unis
Université de France, 100
Université de Paris, 343
University of Edinburgh, 24, 28
University of Toronto, 133, 134, 135
urbanization. *See* cities
urine, 128, 135
U.S. Chamber of Commerce, 274–5
U.S. Health and Human Services Department, 348–9
U.S. Public Health Service (USPHS), 228–9, 276, 279, 280, 321, 339
U.S. Veterans Administration, 234
utilitarianism, 42, 95

vaccination, 59, 320, 321
Vaincre le sida (association), 363
Valleron, Jacques-Alain, 341
Vandenbroucke, Jan, 319, 320
Van Helmont, J.A., 314
Vatin, François, 146
Vienna Maternity Hospital, 208–9, 212–13
Villeneuve-Bargemont, Alban de, 102
Villermé, Louis-René, 102
Vincent, George E., 267
virus, 214–15
vitamins, 315, 339

Wagemann, Ernst, 278
Walker, W.F., 288
War on Cancer, 179
Waxweiler, Emile, 153, 157
Weindling, Paul, 281
Weisz, George, 102, 205–6
Westminster General Dispensary, 26, 40
wet-nurses, 65–6, 67, 80–1
White, Colin, 234
whooping cough, 320, 321
Wied, George, 181
Wieger, F., 212
Williams, Elizabeth, 99–100
Winch, W.H., 316
Winslow, Charles-Edward, 267, 271, 274–6, 279, 281, 283, 285, 292
Withering, William, 22–3, 28
workers: children as, 79–80; education for, 153, 154, 160; and health insurance, 120–1; industrialization and, 102; medicine and, 112–15; puerperal fever among, 221; theories about, 153–6
World Bank, 292
World Health Organization (WHO), 291, 292–3
Wright, Almroth, 380–1
Wunderlich, Carl August, 110–11, 113, 116
Wynder, Ernst L., 239, 343

Yerushalmy, Jacob, 235–7, 239
Yoshioka, Alan, 318, 321
Yule, G.U., 320